MEDICAL MANAGEMENT OF CANCER TREATMENT INDUCED EMESIS

MEDICAL MANAGEMENT OF CANCER TREATMENT INDUCED EMESIS

Edited by

MARIO A DICATO, MD
Department of Haematology-Oncology
Centre Hospitalier de Luxembourg
1210 Luxembourg
Luxembourg

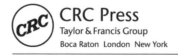

CRC Press
Taylor & Francis Group
Boca Raton London New York

CRC Press is an imprint of the
Taylor & Francis Group, an **informa** business

CRC Press
Taylor & Francis Group
6000 Broken Sound Parkway NW, Suite 300
Boca Raton, FL 33487-2742

© 1998 by Taylor & Francis Group, LLC
CRC Press is an imprint of Taylor & Francis Group, an Informa business

No claim to original U.S. Government works

Visit the Taylor & Francis Web site at
http://www.taylorandfrancis.com

and the CRC Press Web site at
http://www.crcpress.com

Contents

Preface

Supportive care, though long practised, has become a fast-developing field over the past decade, essentially because of the development of many new pharmaceutical agents such as antibiotics, cytokines, antiemetics and others. The pharmacological understanding of serotonin (5-hydroxytryptamine, 5-HT), the cloning of the serotonin receptors, and the clinical advent of new (5-HT$_3$) receptor antagonists have changed the clinician's attitude towards radiotherapy and chemotherapy-induced nausea and vomiting, which are ranked by patients as the most distressing side-effects of cytostatic treatment.

Once these 5-HT$_3$ receptor antagonists became part of clinical practice, numerous studies were undertaken, and the pivotal trials reviewed have identified the most appropriate dosages for the different cancer treatment schedules.

Many studies carried out over the past decade have lacked adequate end-points, and have had too small a patient cohort to draw any useful conclusions. A methodology for trials has therefore had to be established, and should be followed in future clinical trials.

Though major improvements have been made over the past few years in the treatment of acute emesis, in the case of nausea and delayed vomiting, the results have been far from satisfactory.

In addition to antiemetic treatment, other aspects have been addressed in this text, such as quality of life, the nurse's point of view, and side-effects of antiemetics. We have tried to bring together the state-of-the-art data in the various situations requiring antiemetic therapy, and I am very grateful to the outstanding contributors, all of whom are well known and established in this field.

Our thanks also go to the publishers, and especially to Alison Campbell, for their remarkable help and patience in the production of this book.

Mario A Dicato
Luxembourg

Contributors

David Cunningham, MD, FRCP
Head: GI & Lymphoma Units
The Royal Marsden Hospital
Downs Road
Sutton
Surrey SM2 5PT
UK

Albano Del Favero, MD
Department of Internal Medicine
and Oncological Sciences
University of Perugia
06122 Perugia
ITALY

Mario A Dicato, MD
Department of Hematology-Oncology
Centre Hospitalier de Luxembourg
L-1210 Luxembourg G.D.
LUXEMBOURG

Volker Diehl, MD
Klinik I für Innere Medizin
Medizinische Einrichtungen
University of Köln
Joseph-Stelzmann-Str. 9
D-50924 Köln
GERMANY

Andreas du Bois, MD
Frauenklinik
St. Vincentius Krankenhäuser Karlsruhe
76137 Karlsruhe
GERMANY

Caroline Duhem, MD
Department of Hematology-Oncology
Centre Hospitalier de Luxembourg
L-1210 Luxembourg G.D.
LUXEMBOURG

Petra Feyer, MD
Department of Radiotherapy
Medical School Charité Humboldt University
Schumannstrasse 20-21
D-10117 Berlin
GERMANY

Helen Gall, RN, RM
Department of Oncology
Academisch Ziekenhuis Vrije Universiteit
De Boelelaan 1117
1081 HV Amsterdam
THE NETHERLANDS

Richard J Gralla, MD
Ochsner Cancer Institute
1514 Jefferson Highway
New Orleans
LA 70121-2483
USA

Jørn Herrstedt, MD
Department of Medicine/Medical Oncology F
Hillerød Hospital
DK-3400 Hillerød
DENMARK

Stein Kaasa, MD, PhD
Palliative Medicine Unit
Department of Oncology and Radiotherapy
University Hospital
Trondheim
N-7006 Trondheim
NORWAY

Gary R Morrow, PhD, MS
University of Rochester
Cancer Center
601 Elmwood Avenue
Rochester
NY 14603-0704
USA

Robert J Naylor, PhD
Head, School of Pharmacy
University of Bradford
Bradford
West Yorkshire BD7 1DP
UK

Ian N Olver, MD, PhD
Clinical Director
Royal Adelaide Hospital Cancer Centre
North Terrace
Adelaide SA 5000
AUSTRALIA

Razvan A Popescu, MD, MRCP
The Royal Marsden Hospital
Downs Road
Sutton
Surrey SM2 5PT
UK

Fernand Ries
Department of Hematology-Oncology
Centre Hospitalier de Luxembourg
L-1210 Luxembourg G.D.
LUXEMBOURG

Fausto Roila, MD
Division of Medical Oncology
Policlinico Hospital
06122 Perugia
ITALY

Joseph A Roscoe, BS
University of Rochester
Cancer Center
601 Elmwood Avenue
Rochester
NY 14603-0704
USA

Michael Soukop, FRCP
Department of Medical Oncology
Glasgow Royal Infirmary
Glasgow G4 0SF
UK

Richard F Stevens, FRCP, FRCPath
Haematology/Oncology
Royal Manchester Children's Hospital
Hospital Road
Pendlebury
Manchester M27 4HA
UK

Anne L Swinbourne, MPsychol(Clin)
Department of Psychology A19
University of Sydney
NSW 2006
AUSTRALIA

Martin HN Tattersall, MD
Department of Cancer Medicine
The University of Sydney
NSW 2006
AUSTRALIA

Otto J Titlbach, MD
Department of Internal Medicine
Hospital Friedrichshain
Landsberger Allee 49
D-10429 Berlin
GERMANY

Maurizio Tonato, MD
Division of Medical Oncology
Policlinico Hospital
06122 Perugia
ITALY

Dimitris Voliotis, MD
Klinik I für Innere Medizin
Medizinische Einrichtungen
University of Köln
Joseph-Stelzmann-Str. 9
D-50924 Köln
GERMANY

1

The evolution of antiemetic treatment

Richard J Gralla

INTRODUCTION

The effective prevention of chemotherapy-induced emesis is a major achievement in cancer treatment. Among the research areas in oncology, developments in supportive care, including the prevention of emesis, have made possible many of the advances in the approach to the patient with cancer. Progress in antiemetic treatment has largely been made over the last 20 years; however, efforts in the 1960s served to underscore the areas of need. Methodology, identification of agents of potential activity, and increased knowledge of neuropharmacology have been helpful in achieving clinical benefits. The purpose of this chapter is to outline briefly the course of antiemetic progress.

EARLY APPROACHES AND EARLY STUDIES

The chemotherapy available in the 1950s and 1960s varied greatly in inducing emesis. Agents such as methotrexate, vinca alkaloids and 5-fluorouracil were in common usage, and only infrequently caused emesis. In contrast, nitrogen mustard and actinomycin D were legendary for their association with emesis. While there was clearly a need for improved control of emesis, chemotherapy was much less frequently given, and combination regimens containing the more emetogenic agents were just emerging in the practice of oncology (a term that itself was only newly applied to this field). Awareness of the problem was present, but appreciation of the magnitude was not great.

The physiology and neuropharmacology of emesis was studied during this period by Borison and his colleagues, among a few others. Their experimental studies and subsequent conclusions formed the framework that allowed an understanding of emesis and fostered logical approaches to clinical research.[1,2]

During this period, new medications with multiple pharmacological properties were introduced into practice. Among these landmark medications were the phenothiazines. In addition to their antipsychotic properties, an antiemetic effect had been noted. The marked impact of these agents on psychiatric care led to further pharmacologic research. It became apparent that phenothiazines interacted with dopamine receptors; some of their endocrine effects could also be explained by the blocking of these receptors. Coupling of this information with Borison's hypothesis that the area postrema in the medulla (containing the 'chemoreceptor trigger zone' or CTZ) was involved in emesis gave an enhanced insight for clinical approaches. Dopamine receptors, among many others, were found in the area postrema, and this further supported concepts for controlling emesis.

Clinical trials in the 1960s to prevent chemotherapy-induced emesis focused on agents that block dopamine receptors. While conflicting, and occasionally positive, results were reported, it was clear that none of the approaches were satisfactory.[3]

Several pharmacologic and methodologic problems are apparent in reviewing these earlier studies. From the pharmacologic viewpoint, questions arise such as: Why was the dose of the agent selected and what was the basis for the schedule of administration? Methodologically, it was common to combine in the same trial patients receiving different chemotherapy, patients with varying treatment exposures, and those with histories of differing clinical results with prior chemotherapy. Even the criteria establishing efficacy could be questioned. Thus, by the late 1970s, when agents that caused marked emesis (e.g. cisplatin) came into frequent clinical practice, no antiemetic of clear benefit had been identified.

Another avenue of clinical investigation was initiated in the 1970s. Anecdotal reports indicated that marijuana could have value as an antiemetic. Cannabinoids had been known to have a variety of clinical effects, and had been listed in many pharmacologic compendia for decades; modern studies also documented multiple side-effects, especially including autonomic effects. In addition to inhalant marijuana, the major psychoactive cannabinoid, delta-9-tetrahydrocannabinol (THC) had been purified and was available for clinical trials. Synthetic cannabinoid congeners, including nabilone and levonantradol, were developed to provide oral agents that were expected to preserve or improve upon the efficacy of THC, be easier to use than inhalant marijuana, avoid the social stigma of cannabinoids, and decrease the both-

ersome side-effects.[4]

The results of cannabinoid trials varied; however, the cannabinoids were frequently found to be superior to placebo, and equal to or superior to phenothiazines. The studies continued to be troubled by methodologic difficulties similar to those seen with phenothiazine trials. While some efficacy was seen, it appeared that with more emetogenic chemotherapy, the cannabinoids were less effective. This was seen with inhalant marijuana, THC and the synthetic agents.[5–7]

METOCLOPRAMIDE

By the late 1970s, it was clear that none of the commonly used agents, including the phenothiazines and the cannabinoids, were sufficiently potent to control the emesis observed in clinical practice. This caused many to call for increased investigations to help in controlling this problem, which was ranked as the leading concern of patients receiving chemotherapy.[8] A conference at the National Cancer Institute in 1980 outlined the approaches that were being undertaken. One of the leads pursued at the time was the use of metoclopramide; however, this investigation differed in that it was a formal phase I trial exploring unconventional doses of the agent.[9]

Early antiemetic trials with metoclopramide had alternately reported positive or modest results when the agent was given at traditional low doses.[10] The 10 mg or 20 mg doses generally used were based on the observed actions of the drugs in settings other than those related to antiemetic activity for cancer chemotherapy. The pharmacodynamics of metoclopramide indicated a variety of actions that occurred rapidly after administration. Its mode of action was debated. Older studies indicated actions mediated via cholinergic pathways, while others showed clear evidence of dopaminergic blockade.[11]

Prior to 1980, dose escalation studies with metoclopramide had not been reported. The study at Memorial–Sloan Kettering Cancer Center demonstrated that far higher doses of the agent were safe for general use, and could be given to patients with advanced cancer.[9] These initial studies showed that doses as high as 3 mg/kg every 2 hours intravenously (totalling up to 15 mg/kg over 8 hours) were well tolerated. Most importantly, the higher metoclopramide dose levels yielded marked antiemetic efficacy. Both intermittent bolus dosing and continuous-infusion phase I and II studies were conducted; no advantage was observed with the continuous infusions.[9]

The problem of inconsistent and unfocused methodology had held back progress in antiemetic studies. During the metoclopramide trials, a stricter methodology was employed. The primary endpoint was that of complete control of vomiting, measured by enumerating the number of vomiting episodes by direct observation. Separate evaluation of nausea, the duration of nausea and vomiting, and other related phenomena were also outlined.[12] Definitions of response were established, such as complete control of emesis and major control (two or fewer vomiting episodes). These categories were based on the prior observation that no patient receiving cisplatin had done this well with ineffective antiemetics. The emetic stimulus was standardized by testing patients receiving the same chemotherapy (initially with cisplatin in high doses, >100 mg/m^2, a dose that universally causes emesis). The confounding phenomenon of conditioned emesis due to prior poor experience was eliminated by evaluating only previously untreated patients. These and other criteria made the trials more difficult to conduct on a practical basis, but provided a framework for the accurate and reproducible evaluation of potential antiemetics.[9,12]

With the establishment of safety, and encouraging antiemetic results, and with a workable evaluation methodology, the next step was to conduct randomized trials. In that no agent was felt to be active, the first trial compared metoclopramide with placebo. This double-blind trial was followed by other random-assignment studies comparing metoclopramide in high intravenous doses (2 mg/kg every 2 hours, for 5 doses) with intramuscular prochlorperazine,

and then with oral delta-9-tetrahydrocannabinol.[6,12] Each of the comparisons showed marked benefit for treatment with the high-dose metoclopramide. In the three trials, the complete control rate of vomiting was 39%, and the major control rate was 64%.[6] The results of the placebo-controlled trial were soon reproduced.[13] Side-effects were fairly mild, with occasional dystonic reactions being the most prominent. Analysis of the first few hundred patients indicated a significant difference in dystonic reactions as determined by the patient's age. Those over age 30 had a 2% incidence of dystonic reactions, while younger patients had a nearly 20% rate.[14]

After the initial beneficial results with metoclopramide in cisplatin-induced emesis, a logical question that remained concerned whether this antiemetic would be active against the emesis induced by other chemotherapeutic drugs. A phase II study tested the same metoclopramide regimen in patients receiving dacarbazine, an agent that is chemically unrelated to cisplatin but induces nearly as much emesis as cisplatin when given in high doses. This trial indicated excellent efficacy for metoclopramide in the setting of dacarbazine-induced emesis as well.[15] The concept was then developed that if an antiemetic agent was effective against the apparently maximal stimulus of cisplatin, it would be at least as active with other chemotherapeutic drugs.

Further metoclopramide studies indicated that diphenhydramine may lower the dystonic reaction rate, but that it did not contribute to antiemetic efficacy.[16] These studies also indicated that when doses of metoclopramide of 3 mg/kg were given, only two doses were needed; thus the treatment period could be shortened from 8 to 2 hours, and antiemetic activity was preserved.

COMBINATION ANTIEMETICS

During the testing of metoclopramide, reports were starting to accumulate that corticosteroids could also be useful in controlling chemotherapy-induced emesis.[17] Formal trials confirmed the efficacy of these agents.[18] Although the mechanism of their action remained unclear, it appeared that corticosteroids likely exerted their activity via a mechanism different than that involved with metoclopramide. Additionally, the steroid-associated side-effects were not additive to those of metoclopramide.

Combination regimens with full doses of metoclopramide were reported as early as 1983, with a marked further improvement in antiemetic efficacy, with the majority of patients having complete control of cisplatin-induced emesis.[19,20] Testing demonstrated that multiple doses of dexamethasone, or treatments several hours prior to chemotherapy, were no more effective than a convenient single dose shortly before chemotherapy.[16] Although the optimal dose of dexamethasone, prednisone or methyprednisolone has not been defined, it appeared that 20 mg of dexamethasone was associated with maximal control of acute emesis.[16]

DEFINING REGIMENS AND RISK GROUPS

Studies in the late 1980s concentrated on simplifying antiemetic regimens, defining metoclopramide doses, examining different patient populations, and testing other agents when added to metoclopramide plus corticosteroid complications. It was demonstrated in trials that 3 mg/kg of metoclopramide given twice or 4 mg/kg given once yielded maximal efficacy when combined with dexamethasone.[21] Other agents did not appear to improve efficacy, but typically added side-effects. A possible exception was lorazepam, which added only a small improvement in complete control, but decreased chemotherapy-associated anxiety.[22]

An additional benefit of carefully conducted trials was the identification of groups of patients at higher risk of experiencing emesis with chemotherapy. Early studies demonstrated that the chemotherapy used (cisplatin as opposed to other agents, and those that do not cause emesis) was a prominent risk factor, as was prior poor control of emesis.[9] Subsequent analysis demonstrated that chronic, high alcohol exposure was associated with a greater likelihood of control of emesis.[23] Other trials have indicated that control is more difficult to achieve in women and in younger patients.[24,25]

The careful application of proper study methodology and identification of risk groups made future antiemetic trials more reliable and accurate.

THE NEXT STEP: SEROTONIN ANTAGONISTS

With established study methodology and a strong commitment in oncology to continue the improvement in supportive care, conditions were set for further advances in antiemetic control. The problem was that few new agents were available.

The clue leading to improvement was provided by metoclopramide. While it was clear that high doses of metoclopramide were more effective than traditional low doses,[12,26] it was not obvious why this was so. Metoclopramide has a fairly high affinity for dopamine receptors at lower doses, and marked improvement in efficacy would not have been predicted for higher doses if the dopamine mechanism was responsible for greater antiemetic control. In that it was accepted that metoclopramide is not a highly selective neurotransmitter blocking agent, it was reasonable to investigate other pathways as the possible explanation for the enhanced efficacy of higher-dose regimens.

Preclinical studies investigating serotonin (5-hydroxytryptamine, 5-HT) receptors provided an intersection with antiemetic clinical trials. Metoclopramide was found in several investigations to affect serotonin receptors. Later studies indicated that the newly defined type 3 (5-HT$_3$) receptor was the serotonin receptor particularly blocked by metoclopramide, and appeared an important receptor in chemotherapy-induced emesis.[27-30] Although metoclopramide blocked the 5-HT$_3$ receptor, it did not have great affinity for it; thus higher doses would be needed for improved blockade.

The theory was then developed that it should be possible to synthesize an agent with greater affinity for the 5-HT$_3$ receptor that would also be more selective. If this were possible then the efficacy of metoclopramide could be preserved or improved upon, while the side-effects associated with the dopamine pathway could be eliminated.

Trials with GR-C 507/75 or GR 38032F (later named ondansetron) rapidly demonstrated the efficacy and safety of a highly selective 5-HT$_3$ antagonist.[31,32] Dose-finding studies indicated a remarkable safety profile, but a lack of improved efficacy once adequate doses were given. This appeared to show that once the relevant receptors were saturated, maximal control was accomplished. Studies then followed with BRL43694A (granisetron), ICS 205-930 (tropisetron), RG 12915 and MDL 73147 (dolasetron), among others. These agents confirmed the efficacy, favorable side-effect profiles, and ease of use of the selective serotonin antagonists.

Clinical studies comparing the serotonin antagonists with metoclopramide showed a modest improvement in efficacy.[33-35] In general, the complete control rate was not improved significantly in many trials, but the complete-plus-major control rate (0–2 emetic episodes) was universally better with the newer agents. Importantly, the low side-effect profile of the new agents and the lack of schedule dependence made them easy to use and flexible for use in a variety of clinical settings and for nearly all patient populations. Later studies indicated that single doses of these agents were as effective as multiple administrations. This observation further added to the ease of use of these agents.

As in earlier studies, trials with combinations of antiemetics soon followed. It was found that the addition of corticosteroids improved the efficacy of serotonin antagonists.[25] This led to complete control in 70–80% of patients receiving cisplatin, and in 80–90% given moderately emetogenic chemotherapy.[25,36] Subsequent studies have concentrated on demonstrating the equivalence of the various serotonin antagonists,[37] and on the similarity of all oral antiemetic regimens with the intravenous route.[38,39]

CONTINUING PROBLEMS

Trials over the past several years have investigated a variety of additional emetic problems, including delayed emesis[40-42] and anticipatory emesis.[43] Improvements in both these areas have occurred. Nonetheless, as with the control of acute emesis, further improvement is desirable.

Research in controlling emesis in children receiving cancer chemotherapy, and for patients treated with radiation, has been conducted, but to a lesser extent than for the areas outlined above. The serotonin antagonists are particularly suited for use in pediatrics owing to their lack of dystonic side-effects (an age-related problem with dopamine-antagonist agents); however, formal dose-finding and comparison trials are lacking.

THE INFLUENCE OF PRIOR STUDIES ON FUTURE RESEARCH

It is clear that current therapy has logically built on prior trials. There is now a growing consensus that little further improvement is likely with altering schedules or doses of available agents. Studies over the last 20 years have demonstrated that a variety of neurotransmitter receptors are involved in the emesis occurring with anticancer treatment. Areas currently being investigated include the tachykinins, with several new agents that are substance P antagonists now entering clinical trials.

Elucidation of the more relevant pathways, development of new agents and the conduct of well-designed clinical studies have an excellent potential to provide further improvement in antiemetic control.

REFERENCES

1. Borison HL, Brand ED, Orkand RK, Emetic action of nitrogen mustard (mechlorethamine hydrochloride) in dogs and cats. *Am J Physiol* 1958; **192**: 410–16.
2. Borison HL, McCarthy LE, Neuropharmacology

of chemotherapy induced emesis. *Drugs* 1983; **25**: 8–17.

3. Moertel CG, Reitemeier RJ, Controlled clinical studies of orally administered antiemetic drugs. *Gastroenterology* 1969; **57**: 262–8.

4. Steele N, Gralla RJ, Braun DW et al, Double-blind comparison of the antiemetic effects of nabilone and prochlorperazine on chemotherapy-induced emesis. *Cancer Treat Rep* 1980; **64**: 219–24.

5. Levitt M, Faiman C, Hawks R et al, Randomized double blind comparison of delta-9-tetrahydrocannabinol (THC) and marijuana as chemotherapy antiemetics. *Proc Am Soc Clin Oncol* 1984; **3**: 91.

6. Gralla RJ, Tyson LB, Borden LA et al, Antiemetic therapy: a review of recent studies and a report of a random assignment trial comparing metoclopramide with delta-9-tetrahydrocannabinol. *Cancer Treat Rep* 1984; **68**: 163–72.

7. Chang AE, Shilling DJ, Stillman RC et al, A prospective evaluation of delta-9-tetrahydrocannabinol as an antiemetic in patients receiving adriamycin and cytoxan chemotherapy. *Cancer* 1981; **47**: 1746–51.

8. Coates A, Abraham S, Kaye SB et al, On the receiving end – patient perception of cancer chemotherapy. *Eur J Cancer Clin Oncol* 1983; **9**: 203–8.

9. Gralla RJ, Braun TJ, Squillante A et al, Metoclopramide: initial clinical studies of high dosage regimens in cisplatin-induced emesis. In: *The Treatment of Nausea and Vomiting Induced by Cancer Chemotherapy* (Poster D, ed.). New York: Masson, 1981: 167–76.

10. Kahn T, Elios EG, Mason GR, A single dose of metoclopramide in the control of vomiting from cisplatin. *Cancer Treat Rep* 1978; **62**: 1106–7.

11. Pinder RM, Brogden RN, Sawyer PR et al, Metoclopramide: a review of its pharmacological properties and clinical use. *Drugs* 1976; **12**: 81–131.

12. Gralla RJ, Itri LM, Pisko SE et al, Antiemetic efficacy of high-dose metoclopramide: Randomized trials with placebo and prochlorperazine in patients with chemotherapy-induced nausea and vomiting. *N Engl J Med* 1981; **305**: 905–9.

13. Homesley HD, Gayney JM, Jobsen VN et al, Double-blind placebo-controlled study of metoclopramide in cisplatin-induced emesis. *N Engl J Med* 1982; **307**: 250–1.

14. Kris MG, Tyson LB, Gralla RJ et al, Extrapyramidal reactions with high-dose meto-clopramide. *N Engl J Med* 1983; **309**: 433.

15. Tyson LB, Clark RA, Gralla RJ, High-dose meto-clopramide; control of dacarbazine-induced emesis in a preliminary trial. *Cancer Treat Rep* 1982; **66**: 2108.

16. Kris MG, Gralla RJ, Tyson LB et al, Improved control of cisplatin-induced emesis with high-dose metoclopramide and with combinations of metoclopramide, dexamethasone, and diphenhydramine. Results of consecutive trials in 255 patients. *Cancer* 1985; **55**: 527–34.

17. Lee BJ, Methylprednisolone as an antiemetic. *N Engl J Med* 1981; **304**: 486.

18. Aapro MS, Alberts DS, High-dose dexamethasone for prevention of cisplatin-induced vomiting. *Cancer Chemother Pharmacol* 1981; **7**: 11–14.

19. Tyson LB, Gralla RJ, Clark RA et al, Combination antiemetic trials with metoclopramide (MCP). *Proc Am Soc Clin Oncol* 1983; **2**: 91.

20. Allan SG, Cornbleet MA, Warrington PS et al, Dexamethasone and high dose metoclopramide: Efficacy in controlling cisplatin-induced nausea and vomiting. *Br Med J* 1984; **289**: 878–9.

21. Clark RA, Gralla RJ, Kris MG et al, Exploring very high doses of metoclopramide (4–6 mg/kg): preservation of efficacy and safety with only a single dose in a combination regimen. *Proc Am Soc Clin Oncol* 1989; **8**: 1286.

22. Kris MG, Gralla RJ, Clark RA et al, Antiemetic control and prevention of side effects of anti-cancer therapy with lorazepam or diphenhydramine when used in conjunction with metoclopramide plus dexamethasone. A double-blind, randomized trial. *Cancer* 1987; **69**: 1353–7.

23. D'Acquisto RW, Tyson LB, Gralla RI et al, The influence of a chronic high alcohol intake on chemotherapy-induced nausea and vomiting. *Proc Am Soc Clin Oncol* 1986; **5**: 257.

24. Dilly SG, Friedman C, Yocom K, Contribution of dexamethasone to antiemetic control with granisetron is greatest in patients at high risk of emesis. *Proc Am Soc Clin Oncol* 1994; **13**: 436.

25. Roila F, Tonato M, Cognetti F et al, Prevention of cisplatin-induced emesis: a double-blind multicenter randomized crossover study comparing ondansetron and ondansetron plus dexamethasone. *J Clin Oncol* 1991; **9**: 674–8.

26. Roila F, Tonato M, Basurto C et al, Protection from nausea and vomiting in cisplatin-treated patients: high dose metoclopramide combined with methylprednisolone versus metoclopramide combined with dexamethasone and diphenhydramine. A study of the Italian

Oncology Group for Clinical Research. *J Clin Oncol* 1989; **7**: 1693–700.

27. Fozard JR, Mobarok A, Blockade of neuronal tryptamine receptors by metoclopramide. *Eur J Pharmacol* 1978; **49**: 109–12.

28. Costall B, Domeney AM, Naylor RJ et al, 5-Hydroxytryptamine M-receptor antagonism to prevent cisplatin-induced emesis. *Neuropharmacology* 1986; **25**: 959–61.

29. Bradley P, 5-HT 3 receptors in the brain? *Nature* 1987, **330**: 696.

30. Bradley PB, Engel G, Feniuk W et al, Proposals for the classification and nomenclature of functional receptors for 5-hydroxytryptamine. *Neuropharmacology* 1986; **25**: 563–76.

31. Cunningham D, Pople A, Ford HT et al, Prevention of emesis in patients receiving cytotoxic drugs by GR 38032F, a selective 5HT-3 receptor antagonist. *Lancet* 1987; **i**: 1461–3.

32. Kris MG, Gralla RJ, Clark RA et al, Dose ranging evaluation of the serotonin antagonist GR-C 507/75 (GR38032F) when used as an antiemetic in patients receiving cancer chemotherapy. *J Clin Oncol* 1988; **6**: 659–62.

33. De Mulder PH, Seynaeue C, Vermorken JB et al, Ondansetron compared with high-dose metoclopramide in prophylaxis of acute and delayed cisplatin-induced nausea and vomiting. A multicenter, randomized double-blind crossover study. *Ann Intern Med* 1990; **113**: 834–40.

34. Hainsworth J, Harvey W, Pendergrass K, et al, A single-blind comparison of intravenous ondansetron with intravenous metoclopramide in the prevention of nausea and vomiting associated with high-dose cisplatin chemotherapy. *J Clin Oncol* 1991; **9**: 721–8.

35. Marty M, Pouillart P, Scholl S et al, Comparison of the 5-hydroxytryptamine 3 (serotonin) receptor antagonist ondansetron (GR38032F) with high-dose metoclopramide in the control of cisplatin-induced emesis. *N Engl J Med* 1990; **322**: 816–21.

36. The Italian Group for Antiemetic Trials, Dexamethasone, granisetron, or both for the prevention of nausea and vomiting during chemotherapy for cancer. *N Engl J Med* 1995; **332**: 1–5.

37. Riola F, DeAngelis V, Cognetti F et al, Ondansetron vs granisetron both combined with dexamethasone in the prevention of cisplatin-induced emesis. *Proc Am Soc Clin Oncol* 1995; **14**: 523.

38. Perez EA, Chawla SP, Kaywin PK et al, Efficacy and safety of oral granisetron versus IV ondansetron in prevention of moderately emetogenic chemotherapy-induced nausea and vomiting. *Proc Am Soc Clin Oncol* 1997; **16**: 43A.

39. Gralla RJ, Popovic W, Strupp J et al, Can an oral antiemetic regimen be as effective as intravenous treatment against cisplatin: results of a 1054 patient randomized study of oral granisetron versus IV ondansetron. *Proc Am Soc Clin Oncol* 1997; **16**: 52A.

50. Kris MG, Gralla RJ, Clark RA et al, Incidence, course, and severity of delayed nausea and vomiting following the administration of high-dose cisplatin. *J Clin Oncol* 1985; **3**: 1379–84.

41. Kris MG, Gralla RJ, Tyson LB et al, Controlling delayed vomiting: double-blind, randomized trial comparing placebo, dexamethasone alone, and metoclopramide plus dexamethasone in patients receiving cisplatin. *J Clin Oncol* 1989; **7**: 108–14.

42. The Italian Group for Antiemetic Research, Ondansetron versus metoclopramide, both combined with dexamethasone in the prevention of cisplatin-induced delayed emesis. *J Clin Oncol* 1997; **15**: 124–30.

43. Morrow GR, Morrell C, Behavioral treatment for the anticipatory nausea and vomiting induced by cancer chemotherapy. *N Engl J Med* 1982; **307**: 1476–80.

2

Methodology of trials for treating nausea and vomiting

Ian N Olver

INTRODUCTION

The design of trials for the control of chemotherapy-associated nausea and vomiting must take into account factors related to the emetic stimulus, the patient and the action of the antiemetic drugs.[1] Chemotherapy drugs are associated with varying patterns and severity of emesis.[2] Acute chemotherapy-induced emesis may be prolonged with cyclophosphamide or be followed by delayed emesis with cisplatin.[3,4] Severe post-chemotherapy emesis may result in anticipatory emesis over several chemotherapy cycles as a learned response.[5] Different study designs will be required to optimize antiemetic therapy, depending on the cytotoxic used. Early-phase studies should ensure that no adverse reactions are likely between the cytotoxic drugs and new antiemetics.

Clinical trials should search for new prognostic factors and further characterize known factors that will predict a patient's likelihood of emesis and that differ in the various phases of chemotherapy-induced emesis.[6] These factors must be balanced between the arms of randomized trials.

The introduction of the 5-HT$_3$ receptor antagonists has resulted in better control of acute post-chemotherapy emesis, although questions of optimal dosing and combinations of drugs remain.[7] There is a need for more research into the management of delayed emesis and a desire to determine its mechanism in preclinical studies.

Economic constraints have set new cost-effectiveness endpoints for antiemetic trial design.[8] For example, outpatient dosing schedules are highly desirable, and any toxicity that may decrease the productivity of a patient must be balanced against antiemetic efficacy in the overall evaluation of a drug.

Bioethical considerations not only focus on patient consent but also demand that a study be scientifically valid. Inert placebo control arms can be questionable, since no individual patient should be harmed by participation in a study, and randomized trial design can be problematic for patient autonomy.[9]

A schema for what parameters to measure should be developed. How the chosen endpoints are assessed and who assesses them can influence the result. Some standardization of approach is desirable to allow comparisons between studies.[6]

QUESTIONS TO BE ANSWERED PRECLINICALLY

The usefulness of animal models to guide the design of antiemetic clinical trials was evidenced by the discovery of the efficacy of high-dose metoclopramide for cisplatin-induced emesis in dogs.[10] Small laboratory animals such as rodents are unhelpful, because they do not vomit, although indirect measures have been proposed.[11] The ferret has become the most widely used model of acute post-chemotherapy emesis.[12]

Discovering the mechanisms of nausea and emesis in animals has been useful in the development of the 5-HT$_3$ receptor antagonists. Cisplatin-induced acute emesis in the ferret could be completely inhibited by 5-HT$_3$ antagonists.[13] Anticipatory emesis, however, cannot be studied in this model, and delayed emesis after cisplatin did not occur. Also, in animals complete control of emesis was achieved, which cannot be achieved in man – suggesting the possibility of other mechanisms of emesis operating in man that still need to be characterized.

Information about a drug's selectivity and affinity for a receptor gained from preclinical studies may allow more rational design of antiemetic dosing and scheduling. For example, the early studies of 5-HT$_3$ receptor antagonists employed widely differing dosing schedules to maintain plasma concentrations to saturate receptors, yet no clear dose–response relationship was observed.[13] Since the plasma kinetics did not provide sufficient information to guide dosing, preclinical studies of the binding of the drugs to their receptors may provide vital information to guide study design.

A delayed-emesis model has been developed in ferrets, but further preclinical work is required to elucidate the mechanism of this form of emesis, which does not respond as well to 5-HT$_3$ receptor antagonists and seems best controlled by steroid combinations.[12]

Preclinical models would be ideal for testing a number of the possible antiemetic drug combinations prior to selecting the most promising for clinical trials. Information on interactions between antiemetics and cytotoxics would be best derived preclinically. Whereas it could be postulated that steroids may have adverse effects, some interactions may be favourable, such as those reported for the antiemetic benzquinamide, which inhibits p-glycoprotein-mediated drug efflux and potentiates anticancer agent cytotoxicity in multidrug-resistant cells.[14,15]

EARLY-PHASE ANTIEMETIC TRIALS

Phase I trials of antiemetics seek to establish the optimal safe dose and schedule for later studies of efficacy. These trials should incorporate pharmacokinetics, but the plasma concentrations of the drugs may not parallel their activity. Rather, affinity for receptors may be the important factor. The 5-HT$_3$ receptor antagonist tropisetron has a plasma half-life of 8 hours, yet is active on a daily dosing schedule.[16]

There are some methodological differences in the endpoints of such studies of supportive-care drugs compared with cytotoxics. First, the identification of a maximum tolerated dose should be replaced by the definition of a minimum effective dose, perhaps using similar trial designs as employed in identifying the most effective dose of biologic agents, which also differs from a maximum tolerated dose.[17] This minimum effective dose would ensure that the toxicity of the antiemetic was minimized. This dosage may vary according to the emetic stimulus. Phase I studies may need to be duplicated in different patient populations, depending on whether highly emetogenic cytotoxic drugs such as cisplatin are used or the chemotherapy is moderately emetogenic. Different schedules may be required for drugs with a rapid onset of emesis, such as nitrogen mustard, as compared with the later and prolonged emesis of cyclophosphamide.[2,18] Newer antiemetics have been subject to formal phase I studies. In the past, phase I studies have established the safety of higher doses of antiemetics such as metoclopramide or prochlorperazine.[19,20] These have proven more effective against chemotherapy-induced emesis than the lower doses previously used to control emesis of other aetiologies. The optimum dose and indeed the optimum steroid to use as an antiemetic are still not well characterized.[21]

Separate phase I studies will explore different routes of administration. Oral, sublingual or per rectal routes will be favoured for ease of outpatient administration. Pharmacokinetic studies are required to determine whether different formulations will deliver bioequivalent doses.

Early-phase studies are also required to test combinations of antiemetics. It is now recognized that the combination of a serotonin antagonist and dexamethasone is the most effective antiemetic therapy for cisplatin and chemotherapy of moderate emetic potential.[22] Newer combinations will explore serotonin and dopamine antagonists.[23] These studies will determine whether there are not only any adverse interactions between classes of antiemetics but also interactions between antiemetics and cytotoxics. Potential interactions between 5-HT$_3$ receptor antagonists and cytotoxics have been questioned.[24]

PROGNOSTIC FACTORS FOR EMESIS

Before considering phase III study design issues, it is important to explore the variables that will determine the likelihood of a patient developing acute post-chemotherapy emesis, prolonged emesis or anticipatory emesis, since these will need to be considered in evaluating an antiemetic (Table 2.1).

Table 2.1 Prognostic factors for nausea and vomiting

Acute	Delayed	Anticipatory
Highly emetogenic chemotherapy	Dose of cisplatin	Acute post-chemotherapy emesis
Prior exposure to chemotherapy	Severity of post-chemotherapy emesis	Young age
	Female gender	Motion sickness
Young age		
		'Weakness' post-chemotherapy
Prior alcohol intake		'Sweating' post-chemotherapy
Setting of the chemotherapy (inpatient vs outpatient)		'Warmth' post-chemotherapy
		Anxiety
Motion sickness		Setting of chemotherapy (environment of outpatients)
Sickness with pregnancy		
Type of cancer		
Weight		
Performance status		
Psychosocial		

Acute post-chemotherapy emesis

We have discussed the necessity of identifying the optimum dose, schedule and route of administration of an antiemetic in early-phase studies, since these will influence the drug's efficacy. Patients receiving chemotherapy are a heterogeneous population, and variable characteristics of the patient will determine the propensity to vomit. The nausea and vomiting associated with different chemotherapeutic agents varies greatly in its severity and duration. The most important prognostic factors have been reported as the chemotherapy and the antiemetics used. Inconsistencies reported for prognostic factors have been related to the inability to separate treatment from patient and environmental characteristics.[25]

The emetic stimulus

Antineoplastic drugs can be categorized according to the severity of the emesis that they produce (Table 2.2). Such groupings usually refer to bolus standard dosing. Nitrosoureas given in high doses with either bone marrow or peripheral blood stem cell support can cause more severe emesis than at conventional doses. With cisplatin, the bolus dose is likely to be the most significant predictor of emesis, but continuous infusions of the drug are associated with only mild emesis.[25] The efficacy of steroids and 5-HT$_3$ receptor antagonists varies according to the type of chemotherapy used; particularly whether it is a cisplatin or non-cisplatin regimen.[25]

The different patterns of acute emesis, such as the late onset after cyclophosphamide, will impact on the perceived intensity of the emetic response.[2] Much of the data on the severity of emesis rely on empirical observation rather than direct comparisons.[26]

The timing of the chemotherapy administration has been reported as altering the likelihood of emesis in relation to circadian rhythms.[27] In an analysis by Pater et al[25] of four large trials this factor was significant on a unifactorial analysis in patients receiving cisplatin regimens, but did not retain significance in a multifactorial analysis.

Combinations of cytotoxic drugs may result

Table 2.2 Emetogenic potential bolus cytotoxic agents at conventional doses

Most severe	Intermediate	Least severe
Cisplatin	Anthracyclines	Methotrexate
Dacarbazine	Cyclophosphamide	5-Fluorouracil
Nitrogen mustard	Cytosine arabinoside	Bleomycin
Streptozotocin	Carboplatin	Vinca alkaloids
Actinomycin D	Nitrosoureas	Chlorambucil
	Mitomycin C	Epipodophyllotoxins
	Procarbazine	Busulphan
		Melphalan
		Hydroxyurea
		6-Thioguanine
		Taxanes
		Gemcitabine

in additive emetic potential. The antiemetic regimen will need to account for the severity and pattern of emesis of the combination.

Prior exposure to chemotherapy that has caused severe emesis will make patients more refractory to antiemetics in subsequent courses.[27] This may be a learned response, much like anticipatory emesis, so that patients have the expectation of vomiting with subsequent exposure to cytotoxic drugs.[28] Pretreatment expectations have been postulated to influence post-treatment outcomes.[29]

Age

Patients' ages are a factor predicting their likelihood of emesis after cytotoxic chemotherapy. This factor has been reported as more consistently associated with outcome with non-cisplatin chemotherapy regimens.[25] Younger patients do not respond as well to antiemetics such as metoclopramide or tropisetron as older patients.[30-32] Tetrahydrocannibinol, however, had its greatest efficacy in younger patients.[33] Younger patients are more likely to experience extrapyramidal reactions from metoclopramide and prochlorperazine, and yet tolerate the dysphoric reaction caused by tetrahydrocannabinol more easily.[34-36]

Sex

Female gender is associated with more difficulty in controlling post-chemotherapy-induced emesis, particularly that associated with cisplatin.[31,37] The reason for this is unclear. We have postulated a hormonal aetiology and investigated oestradiol levels in women receiving tropisetron for cisplatin-induced emesis. There was a trend towards better response rates in women with oestradiol levels less than 40 pmol/l, although this did not reach statistical significance.[32] Certainly emesis during pregnancy has been recognized as a prognostic factor for acute post-chemotherapy emesis, suggesting an association between hormonal factors and the propensity to vomit.[38] Hormonal factors impact on post-anaesthetic vomiting, where nausea and vomiting is more likely in young women undergoing laparoscopy if this is performed during menstruation.[39] A possible difference in the distribution of neuroreceptor sites or drug-binding characteristics between men and women has been postulated.[40]

Prior alcohol intake

Patients with a chronic alcohol intake of more than 100 g/day were found to experience less nausea and vomiting following cisplatin chemotherapy, with a complete protection rate increasing from 52 to 93%.[41] This was confirmed in a retrospective study.[42] Acute alcohol administration intravenously does not show an antiemetic effect, suggesting that decreasing the sensitivity of the chemoreceptor trigger zone is a long-term effect.[43] In a prospective analysis of alcohol intake during an antiemetic study of tropisetron for cisplatin-induced emesis, it was shown that both an alcohol intake spanning more than 20 years and binge drinking over the previous year were linked with a higher complete response rate than in patients who drank less alcohol, but, surprisingly, a similar response rate was seen in non-drinkers. The frequency of consumption or the amount consumed at each session if less than the 100 g defined as bingeing were unrelated to antiemetic efficacy.[32]

Setting of the chemotherapy

The setting in which the chemotherapy is given can influence the incidence of nausea and vomiting.[25,44] In a large multicentre randomized study for patients receiving cisplatin, complete protection from nausea was obtained in 77.6% of inpatients and 48.4% of outpatients.[31] Inpatients may be more tolerant of side-effects because of a greater feeling of security. This is an inconsistent prognostic factor. In an analysis of 582 patients on four clinical trials, those receiving non-cisplatin chemotherapy and 5-HT$_3$ receptor antagonists had less nausea when treated as inpatients but more nausea if they were treated with ineffective antiemetics when they were inpatients as opposed to outpatients.[25]

Motion sickness

Patients who report susceptibility to motion sickness have more post-chemotherapy nausea and vomiting.[45] Some patients are more constitutionally vulnerable to gastrointestinal disturbance, and will have more post-chemotherapy emesis.[46] Scopolamine has been successfully added to a treatment regimen for cisplatin-induced emesis, suggesting a vestibular component to this emesis, which this antiemetic, useful for motion sickness, controls.[47]

Other prognostic factors

Other reported prognostic factors for acute post-chemotherapy emesis have included the type of cancer, weight and performance status, although the impact of these factors has been variably described.[30,31,48,49]

Psychosocial factors such as stress, depression and social support require further investigation to determine their impact on emesis.

Delayed emesis

The prognostic factors for the delayed emesis seen after cisplatin differ from those for acute emesis.

Dose of cisplatin

The incidence and severity of delayed emesis is influenced by the dose of cisplatin administered. Comparing studies with placebo controls, the reported incidence of delayed emesis is higher for patients having $120 \, mg/m^2$ cisplatin than less than $100 \, mg/m^2$.[4,50,51]

Complete control of emesis in the first 24 hours is associated with a lower likelihood of a patient developing delayed emesis.[4,51] Roila et al[51] showed that prior experience of acute vomiting was associated with worse delayed emesis. Female gender also predicted a greater likelihood of developing delayed emesis, although Roila et al[51] found no effect of age, prior exposure to chemotherapy, other cytotoxics administered with cisplatin, or performance status, unlike with acute post-chemotherapy emesis.

Anticipatory emesis

Anticipatory nausea and vomiting occurs prior to a second or subsequent course of chemother-

apy, and displays elements of a conditioned response.[28] Factors predicting its occurrence have been described.

Post-treatment emesis

Anticipatory emesis only occurs if post-treatment side-effects have occurred. The frequency increases linearly with the number of chemotherapy cycles, and the more severe the post-treatment side-effects, the more likely is the development of anticipatory emesis.[28]

Patient characteristics

Morrow[52] reported that patients with four or more of eight characteristics had developed anticipatory nausea and vomiting by their fourth cycle of chemotherapy. These were age less than 50, nausea and/or vomiting after the first chemotherapy, post-treatment nausea or vomiting described as 'moderate', 'severe' or 'intolerable', susceptibility to motion sickness, feelings of generalized weakness following treatment, sweating following treatment, or feeling warm or hot all over after treatment.[52]

Other factors

Anxiety has been investigated as having a role in the development of anticipatory emesis. It may not be a direct cause but rather a mediating factor and predictor of patients at risk.[53] The setting of the chemotherapy may be important for anticipatory emesis in that patients in a large room within sight of others were more likely to develop anticipatory systems than those who were treated individually.[48]

RANDOMIZED TRIAL DESIGN

A recommended design for phase III antiemetic studies is a prospective, randomized, double-blind parallel-subjects design stratifying for established prognostic factors.[1]

Prospective trial

The above discussion of prognostic factors highlights why historical controls are problematic for antiemetic studies. These are unlikely to be matched when comparing an old with a new antiemetic. Sallan et al[54] demonstrated the unpredictability of historical controls when they reported that a significant number of historical non-responders responded to the same therapy when it was the control arm of a randomized trial. If a study is conducted over multiple courses, a patient's physical condition could change over time. These confounding factors are addressed by a prospective trial where the conditions can be specified in advance and are identical and in the same time frame for the treatment groups being compared.

Randomization

Randomly allocating patients to the treatment arms of a clinical trial attempts to ensure that any unknown prognostic factors are equally distributed between the new treatment and standard treatment arms of the study according to a known random distribution so that their effects can be allowed for in tests of statistical significance.[55] This helps to ensure that significant differences between the two arms are due to true treatment effects. Randomly allocating patients also avoids any selection bias.

Stratification

Stratification ensures that the prognostic variables that we have discussed previously and that are known will be equally distributed between the treatment arms before measuring the treatment-related variables. Stratification can be planned prior to randomization or at the time of analysis, when interactions can be identified where the treatment effect varies for a subset. The problem with stratifying the analysis is that there may not be sufficient numbers in any one identified subset to give a clinically meaningful result. Pretreatment stratification ensures that the population size to allow for different subsets can be planned in advance.

The factors that may require stratification are discussed above, but some may be taken in account not by stratification but by limiting the patient population. For example, the eligibility criteria for many studies are restricted to patients receiving cisplatin who are chemotherapy-naive. Patients may also be excluded if they have another potential source of emesis such as metabolic causes, tumour compression of the gastrointestinal tract or cerebral metastases, or if they are receiving medication, such as corticosteroids for other conditions, that may also have an antiemetic effect. Any limitation in the patient population means that the results apply only to patients with the same characteristics as those eligible for the trial, and the results should not be extrapolated to a wider patient population. We have seen that there are differences, for example between the outcome of inpatients receiving 5-HT$_3$ receptor antagonists, depending upon whether they were receiving cisplatin- or non-cisplatin-containing chemotherapy.[25]

Double blinding

A double-blind study design, where neither patients nor investigators know which arm of the study has been randomly assigned, serves to eliminate any effects due to expectation or suggestion by the investigator or the patient. Patients may be influenced by the information about side-effects on a consent form.[56] Blinding is particularly important in an antiemetic trial where subjective endpoints such as nausea are being assessed. It can be very difficult to achieve in practice if one of the antiemetics has easily recognizable side-effects, such as was demonstrated by Seipp et al[57] in trials of tetrahydrocannabinol. However, as long as the assessor is blinded, even if the nurse administering the treatment is not, a satisfactory result may be obtained. Blinding may not be as vital with objective measures such as number of vomits.

Placebo control

The control arm of a randomized study testing a new agent should be the best treatment available at the time. A placebo control should only be used if no active treatment is available or where the incidence of vomiting is low, the patient can be rescued if they vomit, and perhaps the effects of vomiting need to be balanced against the possible toxicity of the antiemetic. It would be unethical, however, to use an inert placebo control when investigating high-dose cisplatin-induced emesis, where every patient would be expected to vomit and some active prophylactic antiemetic therapy is available. Randomized trials can be problematic for patients who often desire, even if non-rationally, to choose one arm or the other. This is more likely when the arms are very different, such as between a treatment and no treatment. The control arm of a study may not even be a single antiemetic. For cisplatin-induced emesis the combination of a 5-HT$_3$ receptor antagonist and dexamethasone would be considered the current best available treatment.[58]

Parallel-subjects design

The two most common trial designs for antiemetic studies are the parallel-subjects design and the crossover design. In the parallel-subjects design patients are randomized to receive either the study drug or the control for one or more courses and the two groups of patients are compared. In a simple two-period crossover study each patient receives both the study drug and the control in successive courses in random order. By avoiding inter-patient variability and evaluating each patient over both treatments, the crossover design is more powerful and requires fewer patients.

Although it is intuitively more appealing to have patients act as their own controls by directly comparing the two treatments and indicating a preference, particularly because many of the endpoints are subjective, there are problems with evaluating this approach. The crossover design can be difficult to analyse if there is a difference in the conditions and response in each period, there is an effect that carries over from one period to the next, or many patients (>5%) are lost between the first

period and the second. If one could assume that these effects were negligible then the crossover design would be appropriate but these effects can occur in antiemetic studies. The development of anticipatory nausea and vomiting can carry over between one treatment and the next. The patients' physical condition may change between treatments, depending on the response of the cancer to the treatment. A difference in treatment efficacy may appear greater for the second period with subjective self-evaluated endpoints in patients who had ineffective control in the first period, as opposed to a new patient receiving treatment for the first time.[1] Although these period effects could be allowed for in the analysis, the sample size calculated on the assumption of no period effects may be too small to reliably compare treatments. Modifications to the two-period crossover design have been proposed, but either no longer use patients as their own controls or require more than two periods, which increases the chance of the further loss of patients between periods.[59,60]

Another problem with the parallel-subjects design is a bioethical dilemma. If a patient has no nausea and vomiting in the first period and no toxicity from the antiemetic, is it ethically sound to cross them over to another treatment that at best could only be as good?

Although a greater number of patients are required for the parallel-subjects design, it is easier to analyse and interpret, and comparisons between studies are simpler to make. There can be no loss of patients between periods, since the initial assessment is made on the first course. More importantly, the parallel-subjects design allows the evaluation of an antiemetic over multiple cycles, which parallels the clinical situation.

Sample size

The sample size of an antiemetic study must be determined in advance to have the statistical power to detect the smallest difference that would be regarded as clinically important. Randomized studies that are too small may not

Table 2.3 Required patient numbers for a parallel-subjects study

Differences in CR[a] rate to be detected (%)[b]:	10	15	20	25
Total patients required[c]	796	330	196	132

[a] CR = complete response.
[b] Assuming that CR rate on control arm is 25%.
[c] Total number of patients needed to have an 80% power to detect the relevant differences using a two-tailed test of significant at significance level $\alpha = 0.05$: assumes that approximately equal numbers of patients will be randomized to each arm.

detect a difference between two arms, but this may be an indeterminate result rather than a negative result. This can be determined if confidence intervals rather than p values are reported. The numbers required for a study can be estimated from the results of prior trials. For example, if the complete response rate on the control arm is 25% and one wished to detect a 25% difference for a new drug then to have an 80% power to detect that difference using a 2-tailed test of significance at significance level $\alpha = 0.05$, 132 patients would need to be randomized, assuming a one-to-one randomization. If the detection of smaller differences is desirable, larger numbers are required (Table 2.3).

Interim analyses

The target sample size should be specified at the outset of a trial so that the trial is not stopped early with a spuriously positive result because of multiple interim analyses. The timing of interim analyses should be preplanned. It is important to note that the probability of finding a significant difference by chance in repeated analyses of the same normally distributed data is greater than the significance level used for each analysis.[61] For example, the probability of statistically significant ($p = 0.05$)

results where none actually exist by chance alone can exceed 20% if interim analyses are performed every six months in a four-year study.[62] Termination of a trial before the target sample size would require a much more extreme p value than $p = 0.05$.

Design of trials of delayed emesis

The investigation of delayed emesis requires a separate trial methodology rather than just continuing acute post-chemotherapy trials for a few days longer. The inferior response of delayed emesis to 5-HT$_3$ receptor antagonists and a second vomiting peak at 18 hours after the acute peak at 4 hours suggests a different aetiology from acute post-chemotherapy emesis.[63]

A trial in delayed emesis should consider the prognostic factors. Since the incidence of delayed emesis is related to the cisplatin doses, the best patient population to study would be those being treated with cisplatin at a dose of 100 mg/m^2 and above.[4,51] The control of acute emesis impacts on the incidence of delayed emesis, but ethically the patient should be receiving the optimal drug combination for acute emesis. This currently would be a 5-HT$_3$ receptor antagonist and dexamethasone. This should be the same for all patients to avoid differences in delayed emesis being due to the treatment of acute emesis in the first 24 hours. Finally if female gender is a prognostic factor, as has been suggested, then stratification for this in a randomized trial should be considered.[51]

The timing of the randomization proposed for studies of delayed emesis has varied from prior to chemotherapy to at the time of delayed emesis.[26,50] I would favour the first. A patient population at high risk of delayed emesis would be randomly assigned to antiemetics designed to prevent the occurrence of delayed emesis. This avoids patient drop-out on the basis of their acute emesis experience. The time at which the antiemetic regimen for acute emesis should be commenced is also controversial, since some investigators have detected a vomiting peak at 18 hours and therefore would advocate starting at 16 hours, while others start delayed emesis prophylaxis at 24 hours.[26,63] Since this is prophylactic treatment, I would advocate commencing at the earlier time until more data is available.

The design of an antiemetic regimen for delayed emesis will need to take into account the outpatient setting of delayed emesis when deciding scheduling and the route of administration. Parameters to be measured will have to be recorded over several days, and then the method of reporting response, either over the whole period, the worst day, or day by day can be determined.

Methodology of studies of anticipatory nausea and vomiting

Anticipatory vomiting has decreased in frequency as post-chemotherapy acute emesis has been better controlled. Anticipatory nausea is less severe, but its frequency should be the same because the frequency of post-chemotherapy nausea is unchanged.[28] The patient population to be studied will be those having severe post-treatment side-effects and displaying the prognostic characteristics discussed above. The likelihood that a patient will become eligible for study will increase with the number of treatment cycles. Further observations may serve to identify other prognostic factors that will predict which patients to treat.

Prospective randomized studies of treatments for anticipatory emesis have been conducted to test relaxation-based behavioural treatments rather than pharmacological treatments, and represent the appropriate study design.[5] It may be helpful if the patients had received the same emetic stimulus and antiemetic therapy for acute emesis to ensure that the severity of anticipatory emesis was the same in each treatment group. From the above discussion, such studies should also be controlled for the degree of patient anxiety in each arm.[53] However, the ideal management of anticipatory emesis is to eliminate post-treatment emesis, without which the learned response does not develop.

Multiple-day chemotherapy

It may be inappropriate to extrapolate the results of the antiemetic control of acute emesis for single doses of a cytotoxic to when the drug is administered in smaller doses over multiple days, as occurs in some regimens with cisplatin for testicular cancer. Firstly, the extrapyramidal toxicities of metoclopramide may be more severe.[64] Secondly, with cisplatin, acute emesis may overlap with delayed emesis. In non-randomized studies, the efficacy of single agent, ondansetron, decreased from 78% on day 1 to 57% on day 5.[65] If the problem is overlapping types of emesis, this may be improved by adding a corticosteroid, since this is the most effective treatment for delayed emesis and improves the response rate in acute emesis in combination with 5-HT$_3$ receptor antagonists. The addition of steroids in multiple-day regimens has been shown to increase efficacy.[66] The design issues relevant to both delayed and acute emesis apply to studies of antiemetics for multiple-day therapy.

Analysis of trials over multiple cycles

One reason for choosing the parallel-subjects design for randomized trials of antiemetics is that this allows the study to parallel the clinical situation of multiple courses of chemotherapy. However, it cannot be assumed that the results obtained with the initial cycle of chemotherapy will be maintained. In a review of granisetron, efficacy was maintained except in a subgroup of patients receiving high-dose cisplatin.[67]

There are methodological issues that need to be considered so that the data from trials over multiple chemotherapy cycles can be interpreted. First, the number of patients will decrease over the duration of the study. This must be anticipated so that there are sufficient numbers at the end of the study to make meaningful comparisons between the two arms. It is also important that the prognostic factors remain balanced. Not only must the chemotherapy dose remain as intense in the two arms of a randomized study, but also patient withdrawals must be monitored to ensure that there is no imbalance between factors such as age, gender and prior alcohol intake. The development of delayed emesis and anticipatory emesis may all confound the assessment of the ability of an antiemetic regimen to control acute emesis over multiple chemotherapy cycles.[6]

Soukop[68] reported the control of nausea and vomiting over six scheduled courses of cyclophosphamide-based chemotherapy, randomly comparing dexamethasone combined with either ondansetron or metoclopramide and showed the superiority of the former. He applied a Markov-chain statistical model to the data to determine the prognostic value of the complete control of emesis in one cycle on the subsequent cycle. This is an important consideration in evaluating multiple cycles. The hypothesis upon which the model is based is that the response in a given treatment course depends not only on the efficacy of the antiemetic treatment but also on the response obtained in the previous course. A change in the numbers of complete responders will depend on the likelihood of achieving a complete response in the first course and the probabilities that the response will remain either complete or incomplete between two successive treatments. Applying it to the trial allowed comparison of the efficacy of the two regimens over the six courses. The 5-HT$_3$ regimen was the most effective over repeated cycles. It would be predicted, however, that using this regimen to rescue failures on the other arm of the study would not yield the same efficacy as it would if the superior regimen had been used from the beginning. More studies are needed to determine strategies for rescuing patients from failure of regimens containing 5-HT$_3$ receptor antagonists.

EVALUATION OF ANTIEMETIC EFFICACY

There are no widely accepted standards for measuring and reporting the efficacy of antiemetics. I favour at least reporting raw data, since response categories can vary between studies. The assessment of an antiemetic should reflect its ability to control acute, delayed and anticipatory nausea and vomiting, the toxicities of the antiemetic, and an assessment by the patients of their overall rating of the antiemetic, balancing efficacy with toxicity (Table 2.4).

Scales of measurement

Many scales have been used to score the parameters in antiemetic studies.[69] The most common is the simple numerical scale with up to 10

Table 2.4 Assessment of antiemetics

Vomiting
     Anticipatory, acute post-treatment and delayed
     Number of episodes (includes retching)
     Duration

Nausea
     Anticipatory, acute post treatment and delayed
     Severity: four-point scale (none, mild, moderate, severe)
     Duration

Toxicities
     Severity: four-point scale
     Duration
     (specify whether specific or spontaneous reporting)

Cost effectiveness
Global quality of life   Pre- and post-treatment

Overall tolerance
     Four-point scale (very poor to very good)
     Record reason for choice

points. Having a large number of points does not necessarily increase the accuracy of the patients' assessment of a subjective sensation, since they may only be able to discriminate between broad categories. Making up an aggregate score from multiple variables only adds to the complexity of the assessment.

Visual analogue scales for subjective sensations such as nausea have been validated and found reliable.[3] Such scales provide continuous variables for statistical analysis, but this does not mean that the patient will score any more accurately – in particular, they need to be instructed in the use of the scales.

I prefer simple numerical scales scoring none, mild, moderate and severe for subjective sensations. An even number of points avoids the problem of over-selection of a neutral middle category, although this has been found to come from both extremes of the scale, balancing the result.[70]

Reporting results

The most unequivocal result is complete control of vomiting or nausea. These are probably better reported separately, since they are separate parts of the emetic response and one does not necessarily parallel the other. Lesser responses are probably best reported as number of emetic episodes or the severity of nausea on a simple numerical scale. Response categories, particularly a major response (two or fewer vomits) have become common, but are not universal, and if reported should be so in addition to the raw data on which the response category was assigned.

Simple numerical scales can also be used for reporting the toxicities of an antiemetic. It is important to record whether the patient was specifically asked about the occurrence of a side-effect or whether it was spontaneously reported, since the former will usually yield the higher incidence.

A study report should include the planned accrual target. Ineligibility criteria and patient exclusions are important to define the patient population to which the study applies.

Patient and observer assessments

Assessments of emesis can be recorded by both patients and observers, since both provide useful perspectives on the trials. Objective assessments such as the number of vomiting episodes may best be recorded by an observer. Subjective sensations can only be reported by a patient who also records outpatient data.

In an analysis of patient and observer assessments over three consecutive antiemetic studies, we found that differences between the two can occur.[71] In a parallel-subjects study there was no significant difference between patients' and nurses' assessment of the number of vomiting episodes, but the duration of vomiting, the severity and duration of nausea and the side-effects of the antiemetics were given higher scores by the nurses. In two crossover studies the patients recorded more vomiting episodes, while the nurses recorded that the patients had more severe anxiety and sedation than the patients reported. This resulted in the patients detecting a difference between the side-effects of the treatments that was not apparent to the nurses. Many of the differences reflected differences in the timing and frequency of data collection that has been previously reported.[3] Nurses collected data regularly during their shifts, but patients completed their reports at 24 hours. Any more-frequent observations by the patient may have intruded upon their treatment experience. There is no external standard against which the accuracy of the patients and nurses can be tested. However, in general the correlations between the two are good. The potential advantage of having two data sets is that side-effects such as sedation may compromise the accuracy of the patients' reports.

Vomiting

There are three parameters of vomiting that could be recorded. The most commonly recorded is the number of vomiting episodes as part of asessing the severity of emesis. Usually this includes retching, since this involves the same response to an emetic stimulus without the expulsion of gastric contents. The duration of emesis should include anticipatory emesis pretreatment, acute post-chemotherapy emesis and delayed emesis. The volume of emesis is not a particularly useful measure unless correlated with a patient's intake.

Nausea

Nausea, being a subjective sensation, has to be assessed by the patient, since the correlation of objective criteria such as pulse and blood pressure with the experience of nausea is poor. The main parameters of nausea are severity and duration. Del Favero et al[72] studied scales of nausea, but could find no advantages to using analogue rather than simple numerical scales. They found that the maximal intensity of nausea is the most valid way to quantify this parameter.

It has been demonstrated that in antiemetic studies protection from vomiting can be a confounding factor in protection from nausea, and if there is a correlation between the probabilities of vomiting and nausea then a multifactorial analysis may be required to establish the ability of an antiemetic to protect from nausea.[73]

Cost effectiveness

Large phase III trials of antiemetics will require the assessment of new endpoints. One is the prospective evaluation of the cost benefit of the antiemetic. There are considerable methodological difficulties in evaluating this endpoint.[74] Direct drug costs are easy to obtain, and medical, nursing and bed costs are only slightly more difficult to obtain. It is the indirect costs that are difficult to assess. Patients with poorly controlled post-treatment emesis are unproductive, and if this side-effect compromises their anticancer treatment then there will be a permanent loss of productivity. How can that be accurately and reproducibly assessed? Routes and schedules of administration would also figure in a study looking at cost benefit, since outpatient regimens would be more desirable. Many

studies are tackling the problem of demonstrating whether the 'setrons' are cost-effective.[75]

Quality of life

Another measure that could be incorporated as an endpoint into large antiemetic trials is an assessment of global quality of life. The scoring instrument used is important, and a scale that scores each domain and symptom separately may be the most useful.[76] Indeed, not only does a global quality-of-life score ascertain the impact of nausea and vomiting on health-related quality of life, although post-chemotherapy other factors exist, but the pretreatment scores have been found to be predictive of the likelihood of developing post-treatment nausea and vomiting.[76]

Overall assessment

In a parallel-subjects study design, the patient should be asked to make a global assessment of the success of their antiemetic regimen. This will balance the efficacy and toxicity of the antiemetic, and these assessments can be compared between the two arms. Some of the toxicities may be beneficial. Sedation can enhance antiemetic efficacy for some patients.[70] A simple numerical scale could be used to quantify this global satisfaction.

CONCLUSIONS

Antiemetic studies provide many methodological challenges. Three distinct types of nausea and vomiting must be considered, and a number of prognostic factors influencing emesis must be allowed for to ensure that the antiemetic treatment effect is what is being measured. New endpoints such as cost benefit and quality of life can be incorporated into the large prospective randomized double-blind parallel-subject design studies advocated for comparing the efficacy of new agents with established treatments once they have shown promise in early-phase studies.

REFERENCES

1. Olver IN, Simon RM, Aisner J, Antiemetic studies: a methodological discussion. *Cancer Treat Rep* 1986; **70**: 555–63.
2. Martin M, The severity and pattern of emesis following different cytotoxic agents. *Oncology* 1996; **53**(Suppl 1): 26–31.
3. Fetting JH, Grochow LB, Folstein MR et al, The course of nausea and vomiting after high-dose cyclophosphamide. *Cancer Treat Rep* 1982; **66**: 1487–93.
4. Kris MG, Gralla RJ, Clark RA et al, Incidence, course and severity of delayed nausea and vomiting following the administration of high-dose cisplatin. *J Clin Oncol* 1985; **3**: 1379–84.
5. Morrow GR, Lindke J, Black PM, Anticipatory nausea development in cancer patients: replication and extension of a learning model. *Br J Psychol* 1991; **82**: 61–72.
6. Olver IN, Antiemetic study methodology: recommendations for future studies. *Oncology* 1996; **53**(Suppl 1): 96–101.
7. Hesketh PJ, Treatment of chemotherapy-induced emesis in the 1990's: impact of the 5-HT$_3$ receptor antagonists. *Supportive Care Cancer* 1994; **2**: 286–92.
8. O'Brien BJ, Rusthoven J, Rocchi A et al, Impact of chemotherapy-associated nausea and vomiting on patients' functional status and on costs: survey of five Canadian centres. *Can Med Assoc J* 1993; **149**: 296–302.
9. Beauchamp TL, Childress JF, *Principles of Biomedical Ethics*. New York: Oxford University Press, 1989: 349–53.
10. Gylys JA, Doran KM, Buyniski JP, Antagonism of cisplatin induced emesis in the dog. *Res Commun Chem Pathol Pharmacol* 1979; **23**: 61–8.
11. Olver IN Roos IAG, Thomas K, Hillcoat BL, Development of a murine gastric distension model for testing the emetic potential of new drugs and efficacy of antiemetics. *Chem Biol Interactions* 1989; **69**: 353–7.
12. Naylor RJ, Rudd JA, Mechanisms of chemotherapy/radiotherapy-induced emesis in animal models. *Oncology* 1996; **5**(Suppl 1): 8–17.
13. Costall B, Domeney AM, Naylor RA, Tattersall FD, 5-Hydroxytryptamine M-receptor antagonism to prevent cisplatin-induced emesis. *Neuropharmacology* 1986; **25**: 959–61.
14. Haid M, Steroid antiemesis may be harmful. *N Engl J Med* 1981; **304**: 1237.
15. Mazzanti R, Croop JM, Gatmaitan Z et al, Benzquinamide inhibits p-glycoprotein mediated drug efflux and potentiates anticancer agent cytotoxicity in multidrug resistant cells. *Oncol Res* 1992; **4**: 359–65.
16. Olver IN, Assessing the comparative clinical value of tropisetron. *Aust NZ J Med* 1995; **25**: 523–7.
17. Simon R, Design and conduct of clinical trials. In: *Cancer Principles and Practice of Oncology* (De Vita VT Jr, Hellman S, Rosenberg SA, eds). Philadelphia: Lippincott, 1993: 420–1.
18. Borison HL, McCarthy LE, Neuropharmacology of chemotherapy induced emesis. *Drugs* 1983; **25**: 8–17.
19. Gralla RJ, Itri LM, Pisko SE et al, Antiemetic efficacy of high dose metoclopramide: randomised trials of placebo and prochlorperazine in patients with chemotherapy-induced nausea and vomiting. *N Engl J Med* 1981; **305**: 905–9.
20. Olver IN, Webster LK, Bishop JF et al, A dose finding study of prochlorperazine as an antiemetic for cancer chemotherapy. *Eur J Cancer Clin Oncol* 1989; **25**: 1457–61.
21. Cersasimo RJ, Karp DD, Adrenal corticosteroids as antiemetics during cancer chemotherapy. *Pharmacotherapy* 1986; **6**: 118–27.
22. Roila F, Tonato M, Ballatori E, Del Favero A, Comparative studies of various antiemetic regimens. *Support Care Cancer* 1996; **4**: 270–80.
23. Herrstedt J, Sigsgaard T, Boesgaard M et al, Ondansetron plus metopimazine compared with ondansetron alone in patients receiving moderately emetogenic chemotherapy. *N Engl J Med* 1993; **328**: 1076–80.
24. Aamdal S, Can ondansetron hydrochloride (Zofran) enhance the nephrotoxic potential of other drugs? (letter). *Ann Oncol* 1992; **3**: 774.
25. Pater L, Slamet L, Zee B et al, Inconsistency of prognostic factors for post-chemotherapy nausea and vomiting. *Support Care Cancer* 1994; **2**: 161–6.
26. Tonato M, Roila F, Del Favero A, Ballatori E, Methodology of trials with antiemetics. *Support Care Cancer* 1996; **4**: 281–6.
27. Hrushesky WJM, Roemeling R, Chemotherapy-induced vomiting: circadian drug timing as a source of predictable within-patient variability. *Cancer Treat Rep* 1986; **70**: 1347–8.
28. Morrow GR, Rosenthal SN, Models, mechanisms and management of anticipatory nausea and emesis. *Oncology* 1996; **53**(Suppl 1): 4–7.
29. Cassileth BR, Lusk EJ, Bodenheimer BJ et al,

Chemotherapeutic toxicity – the relationship between patients' pretreatment expectations and post-treatment results. *Am J Clin Oncol* 1985; **8**: 419–25.

30. Pollera CF, Giarnelli D, Prognostic factors influencing cisplatin-induced emesis. Definition and validation of a predictive logistic model. *Cancer* 1989; **64**: 1117–22.

31. Roila F, Tonato M, Basurto C et al, Protection from nausea and vomiting in cisplatin-treated patients: high dose metoclopramide combined with methylprednisolone vs metoclopramide combined with dexamethasone and diphenhydramine: a study of the Italian Oncology Group for Clinical Research. *J Clin Oncol* 1989; **7**: 1693–700.

32. Olver IN, Craft PS, Glingan PR et al, An open multicentre study of tropisetron for cisplatin-induced nausea and vomiting. *Med J Aust* 1996; **164**: 337–40.

33. Sallan SE, Zinberg NE, Frei E III, Antiemetic effect of delta-9 tetrahydrocannabinol in patients receiving cancer chemotherapy. *N Engl J Med* 1975; **293**: 795–7.

34. Goslin RH, Garnick MB, Metoclopramide as an antiemetic in patients receiving cisplatin. In: *The Treatment of Nausea and Vomiting Induced by Cancer Chemotherapy* (Poster DS, Penta JS, Bruno S, eds). New York: Masson, 1981: 159–65.

35. Kris MG, Tyson LB, Gralla RJ et al, Extrapyramidal reactions with high-dose metoclopramide. *New Engl J Med* 1983; **309**: 433–8.

36. Fritak S, Moertel CG, O'Fallon J, Delta-tetrahydrocannabinol as an antiemetic in patients treated with cancer chemotherapy: a double comparison with prochlorperazine and a placebo. *Ann Intern Med* 1979; **91**: 825–30.

37. De Mulder HM, Seynaeve C, Vermorken JB et al, Ondansetron compared with high-dose metoclopramide in prophylaxis of acute and delayed cisplatin-induced nausea and vomiting. A multicenter, randomized, double-blind, crossover study. *Ann Intern Med* 1990; **113**: 834–40.

38. Tonato M, Roila F, Del Favero A, Methodology of antiemetic trials: a review. *Ann Oncol* 1991; **2**: 107–14.

39. Forrest JB, Beattie WS, Goldsmith CH, Risk factors for nausea and vomiting after general anaesthesia. *Can J Anaesth* 1990; **37**: Part II, 590.

40. Roila F, Tonato M, Del Favero A, Prognostic factors of chemotherapy-induced emesis. In: *Antiemetic Therapy: Current Status and Future Prospects* (Diaz Rubio E, Martin M, eds). Madrid:

Creaciones Elba, 1992: 97–104.

41. D'Acquisto RW, Tyson LB, Gralla RJ et al, The influence of a chronic high alcohol intake on chemotherapy-induced nausea and vomiting. *Proc Am Soc Clin Oncol* 1986; **5**: 257.

42. Sullivan JR, Leyden MJ, Bell R, Decreased cisplatin-induced nausea and vomiting with chronic alcohol ingestion. *N Engl J Med* 1983; **309**: 796.

43. Speiss JL, Adelstein DJ, Hines JD, Evaluation of ethanol as an antiemetic in patients receiving cisplatin. *Clin Ther* 1987; **5**: 1994–7.

44. Carey MP, Burish TG, Brenner DE, Delta-9-tetrahydrocannabinol in cancer chemotherapy: research problems and issues. *Ann Intern Med* 1983; **99**: 106–14.

45. Morrow GR, The effect of susceptibility to motion sickness on the side effects of cancer chemotherapy. *Cancer* 1985; **55**: 2766–70.

46. Jacobsen PB, Andrykowski MA, Redd WH et al, Non pharmacologic factors in the development of post-treatment nausea with adjuvant chemotherapy for breast cancer. *Cancer* 1986; **61**: 379–85.

47. Meyer BR, O'Mara V, Reidenberg MM, A controlled clinical trial of the addition of transdermal scopolamine to a standard metoclopramide and dexamethasone antiemetic regimen. *J Clin Oncol* 1987; **5**: 1994–7.

48. Cohen RE, Blanchard EB, Ruckdeschel JC et al, Prevalence and correlates of post-treatment and anticipatory nausea and vomiting in cancer chemotherapy. *J Psychosom Res* 1986; **30**: 643–54.

49. Parikh PM, Charak BS, Banavali SD et al, A prospective, randomized double-blind trial comparing metoclopramide alone with metoclopramide plus dexamethasone in preventing emesis induced by high-dose cisplatin. *Cancer* 1988; **62**: 2263–6.

50. Hesketh P, Management of cisplatin-induced delayed emesis. *Oncology* 1996; **53**: 73–7.

51. Roila F, Boschetti E, Tonato M et al, Predictive factors of delayed emesis in cisplatin treated patients and antiemetic activity and tolerability of metoclopramide and dexamethasone. *Am J Clin Oncol* 1991; **14**: 238–42.

52. Morrow GR, Clinical characteristics associated with the development of anticipatory nausea and vomiting in cancer patients undergoing chemotherapy treatment. *J Clin Oncol* 1984; **2**: 1170–8.

53. Cull A. Psychological effects of anti-cancer ther-

apy. In: *Emesis in Anti-Cancer Therapy: Mechanisms and Treatment* (Andrews PLR, Sanger GJ, eds). London: Chapman & Hall Medical, 1993: 211–28.

54. Sallan SE, Cronin C, Zelen M et al, Antiemetics inpatients receiving chemotherapy for cancer: a randomized comparison of delta-9-tetrahydrocannabinol and prochloperazine. *N Engl J Med* 1980; 302: 135–8.

55. Wendel HA, Randomisation in clinical trials. *Science* 1978; 199: 368.

56. Olver IN, Buchanan L, Laidlaw C, Poulton G, The adequacy of consent forms for informing patients entering oncological clinical trials. *Ann Oncol* 1995; 6: 867–70.

57. Seipp CA, Chang AE, Shilling DJ et al, In search of an effective antiemetic: a nursing staff participates in marijuana research. *Cancer Nurs* 1980; 3: 271–6.

58. Tonato M, Roila F, Del Favero A, Ballatori E, Antiemetics in cancer chemotherapy: historical perspective and current state of the art. *Support Care Cancer* 1994; 2: 150–60.

59. Ebbut AF, Three-period crossover designs for two treatments. *Biometrics* 1984; 40: 69–79.

60. Laska E, Meisner M, Kushner HB, Optimal crossover designs in the presence of carryover effects. *Biometrics* 1983; 39: 1087–91.

61. Morrow GR, Black PM, Dudgeon DJ, Advances in data assessment. Application to the aetiology of nausea reported during chemotherapy, concerns about significance testing, and opportunities in clinical trials. *Cancer* 1991; 67: 780–7.

62. Fleming TR, Green SJ, Harrington DP, Considerations for monitoring and evaluating treatment effects in clinical trials. *Controlled Clinical Trials* 1984; 5: 55–66.

63. Kris MG, Pisters KMW, Hinkley L, Delayed emesis following anticancer chemotherapy. *Support Care Cancer* 1994; 2: 297–300.

64. Kris MG, Tyson LB, Gralla RJ et al, Extrapyramidal reactions with high-dose metoclopramide (letter). *N Engl J Med* 1983; 309: 433–4.

65. Hainsworth JD, The use of ondansetron in patients receiving multiple-day cisplatin regimens. *Semin Oncol* 1992; 19(Suppl 10): 48–52.

66. Bremer K (on behalf of the Granisetron Study Group), A single-blind study of the efficacy and safety of intravenous granisetron compared with alizapride plus dexamethasone in the prophylaxis and control of emesis in patients receiving 5-day cytostatic therapy. *Eur J Cancer* 1992; 28: 1018–22.

67. Blijham GH (on behalf of the Granisetron Study Group), Does granisetron remain effective over multiple cycles? *Eur J Cancer* 1992; 28A(Suppl 1): S17–21.

68. Soukop M, Management of cyclophosphamide-induced emesis over repeated courses. *Oncology* 1996; 53(Suppl 1): 39–45.

69. Morrow GR, The assessment of nausea and vomiting. Past problems, current issues and suggestions for future research. *Cancer* 1974; 53(Suppl): 2267–78.

70. Presser S, Schuman H, The measurement of a middle position in attitude surveys. *Public Opinion Q* 1980; 44: 70–85.

71. Olver IN, Matthews JP, Bishop JF, Smith RA, The roles of patient and observer assessments in antiemetic trials. *Eur J Cancer* 1994; 30A: 1223–7.

72. Del Favero A, Roila F, Basurto C et al, Assessment of nausea. *Eur J Clin Pharmacol* 1991; 38: 115–20.

73. Italian Group for Antiemetic Research, On the relationship between nausea and vomiting in patients undergoing chemotherapy. *Support Care Cancer* 1994; 2: 171–6.

74. Plosker GL, Milne RJ, Ondansetron. A pharmacoeconomic and quality-of-life evaluation of its antiemetic activity in patients receiving cancer chemotherapy. *Pharmacoeconomics* 1992; 2: 285–304.

75. Aapro MS, Costs and benefits of antiemetic therapy. *Support Care Cancer* 1994; 2: 304–6.

76. Osoba D, Zee B, Warr D et al, Quality of life studies in chemotherapy-induced emesis. *Oncology* 1996; 53(Suppl 1): 92–5.

3

Pharmacology of serotonin and its receptors

Robert J Naylor

INTRODUCTION

Page and colleagues[1] were the first to isolate and chemically characterize a vasoconstrictor substance released from platelets in clotting blood. It was called serotonin, which was then realized to be the same substance as enteramine, an indole previously shown to occur in high concentration in the gastrointestinal mucosa, platelets and the central nervous system (CNS),[2] where it was hypothesized to exert a neurotransmitter role.[3] Subsequently, serotonin or 5-HT (3-(β-aminoethyl)-5-hydroxyindole) was shown to be widely distributed in animals and plants. 5-HT is synthesized from the essential amino acid tryptophan, which is taken up into neurones by an active uptake process, subject to tryptophan hydroxylase forming L-5-hydroxytryptophan, which is then decarboxylated by aromatic L-amino acid decarboxylase to 5-hydroxytryptamine. It is metabolized mainly by monoamine amine oxidase enzymes and aldehyde dehydrogenase to 5-hydroxyindoleacetic acid (5-HIAA).[4]

Five decades of pharmacological analysis has revealed an effector role for 5-HT in[5]

- contracting many cardiovascular preparations;
- contracting or relaxing gastrointestinal smooth muscle and modifying secretion within the gastrointestinal tract;
- modifying hormonal release at hypothalamic and peripheral sites;
- modifying the function of the immune system;
- exerting a trophic role in cell development;
- within the CNS to influence temperature, feeding, sleep, memory, mood, sexual and motor behaviour.

This provides for an extraordinary breadth of activities for a single neurotransmitter substance, and pharmacological studies have provided a wealth of opportunities for the creation of new therapies for human illness. Thus, selective 5-HT receptor ligands now afford the most successful treatment of migraine, 5-HT reuptake inhibitors provide the most successful treatment for depression, agents with mixed dopamine and 5-HT receptor blocking actions provide the most effective treatment for chronic schizophrenia, and 5-HT$_3$ receptor antagonists have revolutionized the treatment of sickness in the cancer patient. From the enormous breadth of research on 5-HT, the present chapter focuses on emesis.

Over the last ten years, there has been a renaissance of research in nausea and emesis; this has been due to the pharmacological demonstration of the antiemetic profile of ondansetron and other 5-HT$_3$ receptor antagonists in animal models and in cancer patients receiving chemotherapy and radiation treatment. Such research has revealed the potential role of other 5-HT receptors in emesis, and the present chapter will focus mainly on the pharmacology of 5-HT and the different 5-HT receptor types and the drugs available to modify 5-HT function, relevant to an understanding of the peripheral and central mechanisms involved in the induction and antagonism of nausea and vomiting (Figure 3.1).

MULTIPLE 5-HT RECEPTORS

Pharmacological and therapeutic interest in 5-HT receptor ligands is focused on the different 5-HT receptors and their location; a single receptor type would negate any attempt to selectively manipulate a particular function. It would appear that 5-HT receptors have been present from the earliest beginnings of life. A primordial 5-HT receptor was present some 800 million years ago, and its subsequent evolution has endowed numerous species with multiple 5-HT receptor subtypes.[7] Classical pharmacology, using the rank order of agonist potencies and selective 5-HT receptor antagonists, in functional and other assays, established the beginnings of a 5-HT receptor classification. Thus Gaddum and Picarelli[8] proposed the existence of two 5-HT receptor subtypes, which they termed M and D, in the guinea pig ileum: the former (which are blocked by morphine) are located on parasympathetic nerve endings to control the release of acetylcholine, the latter (which are blocked by dibenzline) are located on smooth muscle, and activation of either causes muscle contraction. A second major advance came with the development of radioligand binding assays, Peroutka and Snyder

providing the first clear evidence of two distinctive recognition sites for 5-HT in the rat brain.[9] Using [^{3}H]spiperone and [^{3}H]5-HT, recognition sites, described as 5-HT$_1$, were shown to have a high affinity for [^{3}H]5-HT, whereas 5-HT$_2$ recognition sites have a low affinity for [^{3}H]5-HT and a high affinity for [^{3}H]spiperone. Such binding assays, whilst providing no direct evidence of a function role for the recognition site, have been of considerable importance in characterizing receptors and establishing their location. The third major advance came with the development of molecular biology, which established the actual structure of receptors, and the homology of receptor proteins.[7,9] Based on data from the functional and other assays, and receptor structure, the classification scheme of Hoyer et al[10] is widely accepted (Table 3.1).

5-HT$_1$ receptors

All members of the 5-HT$_1$ receptor family are negatively coupled to adenyl cyclase. The ability of 5-HT and 5-HT receptor agonists to inhibit 5-HT release was initially shown using rat brain synaptosomes and cortical slices. Subsequent studies showed that the presynaptic autoreceptors regulating the release of 5-HT are located throughout the brain.[11] However, there are interesting species differences in the 5-HT$_1$ receptors that mediate the inhibitory response: 5-HT$_{1B}$ receptors are involved in the mouse and rat whereas 5-HT$_{1D}$ mediate the response in guinea pig and man. Also, heteroreceptors located on the 5-HT nerve terminals, e.g. prostaglandin and α_2-adrenoceptors, can also inhibit 5-HT release.[12] Furthermore, 5-HT heteroreceptors located on cholinergic and glutaminergic nerves can moderate transmitter release.[11] 5-HT$_{1A}$ receptors are also located on postsynaptic structures in the forebrain and on 5-HT-containing cells in the raphé nuclei in the midbrain. In the raphé nuclei the 5-HT$_{1A}$ receptor functions as a somatodendritic autoreceptor to switch off the release of 5-HT in the forebrain. The use of selective 5-HT$_{1A}$ receptor agonists and antagonists has facilitated investigations of the role of 5-HT$_{1A}$ receptors, but there remain cautions in an interpretation of drug

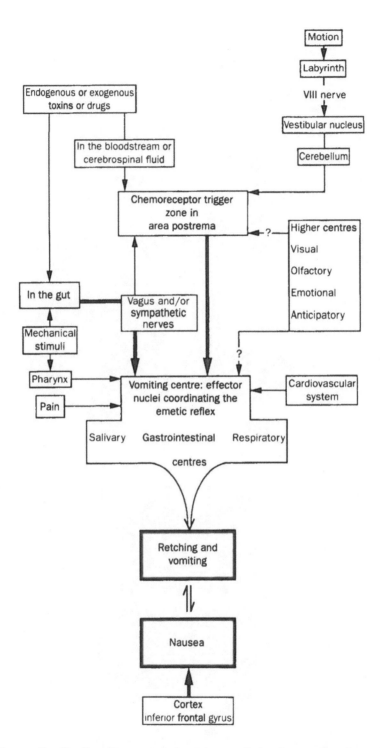

Figure 3.1 The major emetic stimuli, pathways and structures mediating the emetic reflex and nausea. With the exception of the vagus input to the chemoreceptor trigger zone and nucleus tractus solitarius, where 5-HT$_3$ receptors are present on the vagus nerve endings, the chemical nature of the neurotransmitter systems and sites of antiemetic drug action are not known.

Table 3.1 Classification of 5-HT receptors after Hoyer et al.[10] The signal transduction mechanisms of the seven major 5-HT receptor subtypes and examples of their location and function are given. Selective agonists and antagonists are available for only a restricted number of 5-HT receptor subtypes

Receptor subtype	Signal transduction	Localization	Function	Selective agonists[a]	Selective antagonists[a]
5-HT$_{1A}$	Inhibition of adenyl cyclase	Raphé N, forebrain structures	Autoreceptor	8-OH-DPAT	WAY100135
5-HT$_{1B}$ (5-HT$_{1D\beta}$)		Subiculum, substantia nigra	Autoreceptor	?	?
5-HT$_{1D}$ (5-HT$_{1D\beta}$)		Cranial blood vessels	Vasoconstrictor	Sumatriptan	?
5-HT$_{1E}$		Cortex, striatum	?	?	?
5-HT$_{1F}$ (5-HT$_{1E\beta}$)		Brain, periphery	?	?	?
5-HT$_{2A}$ (D receptor)	Activation of phospholipase C	Brain, smooth muscle, platelets	Platelet aggregation		Ketanserin, ICI170809
5-HT$_{2B}$		Stomach fundus, brain	Contraction	DOI	Ritanserin, SB204741
5-HT$_{2C}$		Choroid plexus	?		SB200646A
5-HT$_3$	Ligand-operated ion channel	Brain, peripheral nerves	Neuronal excitation	2-methyl-5-HT	Ondansetron, tropisetron, granisetron
5-HT$_4$	Activation of adenylyl cyclase	Brain, gastrointestinal tract, adrenal medulla, hippocampus	Neuronal excitation	?	GR113808, SB204070
5-HT$_{5A}$	Unknown	?			
5-HT$_{5B}$				?	?
5-HT$_6$	Activation of adenylyl cyclase	Striatum	?	?	?
5-HT$_7$	Activation of adenylyl cyclase	Hypothalamus, intestine	?	?	?

[a] ICI170809 = 2-(2-dimethylamino-2-methylpropylthio)-3-phenylquinoline; SB204741 = N-(1-methyl-5-indolyl)-N'-(3-methyl-5-isothiazolyl)urea; SB200646A = N-(1-methyl-5-indolyl)-N'-(3-pyridyl)urea; WAY100135 = (S)-N-t-butyl-3-[4-(2-methoxyphenyl)piperazine-1-yl]-2-phenylpropanamide; GR113808 = 1-[2-(methylsulphonylamino)ethyl]-4-piperidinyl-1-methyl-1H-indole-3-carboxylate maleate; SB204070 = 8-amino-7-chloro-(N-butyl-4-piperidyl)methylbenzo-1,4-dioxan-5-carboxylate hydrochloride.

induced effects. Thus the 5-HT$_{1A}$ receptor ligand MDL73005EF acts as an antagonist at the 5-HT$_{1A}$ receptors mediating hyperpolarization in the hippocampus and ACTH release, a partial agonist at postsynaptic 5-HT$_{1A}$ receptors mediating forepaw treading, and a full agonist on spontaneously firing dorsal raphé neurones and those mediating an inhibition of 5-HT release in the hippocampus.[13] Variations in receptor reserve and 5-HT tone between different brain systems may contribute to such differences. With the exception of WAY100135, which is a selective 5-HT$_{1A}$ receptor antagonist, there are no selective ligands for the 5-HT$_1$ receptor subtypes.

5-HT$_2$ receptors

5-HT$_2$ receptors are linked to phospholipase C, with the generation of second messengers inositol phosphate (which releases intracellular stores of calcium) and diacylglycerol (which activates protein kinase C). The 5-HT$_{2A}$ receptor is found throughout the brain and in platelets, 5-HT$_{2B}$ receptors were originally described in the stomach to mediate contraction responses, and 5-HT$_{2C}$ receptors achieve a high density in the choroid plexus.[10] α-Methyl-5-HT and 1-(2,5-dimethoxy-4-iodophenyl)isopropylamine (DOI) are relatively selective 5-HT$_2$ receptor agonists; ritanserin and ICI170809 are essentially non-selective 5-HT$_{2A}$ receptor antagonists, whereas ketanserin retains selectivity for the 5-HT$_{2A}$ receptors, SB200646A has both 5-HT$_{2B}$ and 5-HT$_{2C}$ receptor selectivity, and SB204741 possesses high affinity for 5-HT$_{2B}$ receptors but not 5-HT$_{2A}$ or 5-HT$_{2C}$ receptors.[14]

5-HT$_3$ receptors

The 5-HT$_3$ receptor is the only monoamine neurotransmitter receptor that functions as a ligand-operated ion channel. It corresponds to Gaddum and Picarelli's M-receptor, and has only been located on neurones, in central and peripheral autonomic, sensory and enteric systems. The highest densities of 5-HT$_3$ receptors in the brain are located in the area postrema, nucleus tractus solitarius and dorsal vagal motor nucleus.[15] They mediate a rapid depolarizing response, associated with an increase in membrane conductance following the opening of cation-selective channels; the influx of sodium and potassium contribute importantly to the response.[16] The response to 5-HT is usually described as a cooperative effect, where the occupation of one receptor subunit enhances the binding of other agonist molecules. The 5-HT$_3$ receptor has probably evolved to mediate rapid synaptic events. However, it should be noted that in all 5-HT$_3$ systems examined, repeated challenge to 5-HT is met by desensitization and a rapid decline in the amplitude of depolarization. Zinc, cadmium and copper ions also inhibit the 5-HT$_3$ receptor-mediated response.

There are a number of reasonably selective 5-HT$_3$ receptor agonists whose profiles have been established in many preparations and species, namely 2-methyl-5-HT, 1-phenylbiguanide and m-chlorophenylbiguanide.[17,18] There are species differences: 1-phenylbiguanide has no action on peripheral nerves in the guinea pig, but has full or partial agonist action in the rat and mouse.[18]

There are also highly selective 5-HT$_3$ receptor antagonists: MDL72222 was the first,[19] followed by tropisetron,[20] ondansetron[21] and granisetron.[22] With the possible exception of ondansetron, the other antagonists have competitive/insurmountable antagonisms.[16,21,23]

It is widely accepted that there are major species variations in the properties of 5-HT$_3$ receptors. The affinity values for 5-HT$_3$ receptor antagonists in the guinea pig are much lower than in the rat or rabbit, but there is no evidence of tissue dependence.[16] The determination of antagonist potencies against 5-HT-induced depolarization responses or 5-HT-evoked inward membrane currents recorded under voltage clamp conditions also support their lower potency in guinea pig tissue. The differences detected with (+)tubocurarine were particularly notable, being low in the guinea pig and particularly high in the mouse.[16] The latter may reflect an interspecies variant of the 5-HT$_3$ receptor.

A splice variant of 5-HT$_3$ R-A termed 5-HT$_3$ R-As has been cloned from NIE-IIS neuroblastoma cells and NG108-15 hybridoma cells.[24,25] The cloning and characterization of species homologues of the 5-HT$_3$ R-A is a most useful technique in identifying interspecies receptor heterogeneity. Thus Hope and colleagues[24] and Belelli and colleagues[25] have recently reported that an EDNA encoding a 5-HT$_3$ receptor subunit isolated from a human amygdala CDNA library was cloned into a eukaryotic expression vector transfected into HEK293 cells; RNA transcripts of the human CDNA were also injected into xenogenous oocytes.[25] The inward current response to 5-HT was antagonized potently by ondansetron at picomolar concentrations, but only by micromolar concentrations of (+)tubocurarine, showing major differences with those obtained in the murine 5-HT$_3$ R-A receptor.[26] The use of agents such as (+)tubocurarine in conjunction with site-directed mutagenesis may facilitate an understanding of the amino acid residues essential to ligand binding sites. In turn, this may elucidate differences between 5-HT$_3$ receptors in the human and other species. This has important implications in the preclinical studies used to predict drug effects in man.

5-HT$_4$ receptors

5-HT$_4$ receptors were first discovered in fetal mice colliculi neurons, their activation stimulating adenylyl cyclase and causing a decrease in K$^+$ conductance and a slow depolarizing response.[27] Subsequently, they were found in other brain areas and to enhance peristalsis and contraction responses in the gut, cause relaxation of the oesophagus, increase heart rate and cause the release of steroids from the adrenal medulla.[28] 5-Methoxytryptamine is a relatively selective 5-HT$_4$ receptor agonist, benzamide derivatives (e.g. cisapride, zacopride and metoclopramide) also have agonist/partial agonist/antagonist potential, whilst GR113808 and SB204070 are highly selective 5-HT$_4$ receptor antagonists.[29-31] Two-splice variants of the 5-HT$_4$ receptor have recently been determined.[32]

5-HT$_5$, 5-HT$_6$ and 5-HT$_7$ receptors

These three new receptor families have recently been cloned, and their functions are being determined.[32]

THE NEUROTRANSMITTER AND NEUROMODULATORY ROLES OF 5-HT

The neurotransmitter role of 5-HT is self-explanatory. It involves the neuronal release of 5-HT into the synapse to stimulate pre- and/or postsynaptic 5-HT receptors, to respectively moderate its own release or the firing of other cells (see Figure 3.2). Yet, within the CNS, there remain additional actions of 5-HT to modulate neuronal activity independent of or additional to the classical neurotransmitter role. Sizer and colleagues[33] have defined a neuromodulatory response to 5-HT as one that should influence the response to an excitatory amino acid without having any detectable effect on the passive electrical properties of the neurone. In their review of the literature and from their own studies, Sizer and colleagues[33] found that iontophoretically applied 5-HT can profoundly alter the response of rat cortical and other brain neurones to iontophoretically applied glutamate, quisqualate, aspartate or N-methyl-D-aspartic acid. The effect of 5-HT in either reducing or enhancing the effect of the excitatory amino acids appeared to depend on the brain area investigated; the effects are blocked by cinanserin, ketanserin or methysergide, and in some experiments were mimicked by 5-carboxamidotryptamine.[33] The importance of these studies is that the effects of 5-HT may appear profound or absent, dependent on the degree of excitatory amino acid challenge.

PHARMACOLOGICAL MANIPULATIONS OF 5-HT FUNCTION

There are two possibilities.

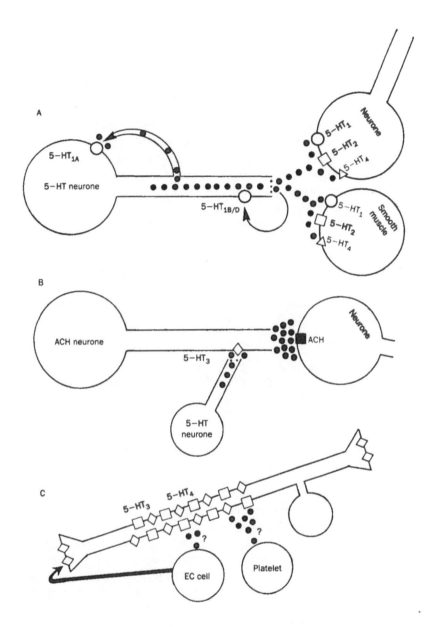

Figure 3.2 Diagrammatic representation of the possibilities of control by 5-HT of the functioning of the 5-HT and other neurones via 5-HT receptor subtypes.

(A) 5-HT synthesized in the 5-HT neurone is transported (a) via the collateral fibre to exert an autoinhibitory role on 5-HT$_{1A}$ somatodendritic receptors to switch off the release of 5-HT, and (b) is released at the synapse where it may (i) stimulate presynaptic inhibitory 5-HT$_{1B/D}$ (species-dependent) receptors to attenuate the synaptic release of 5-HT or (ii) stimulate postsynaptic 5-HT$_1$, 5-HT$_2$ and 5-HT$_4$ receptors to moderate neuronal cell firing or relax or contract smooth muscle cells.

(B) 5-HT is released to stimulate 5-HT$_3$ receptors, causing rapid depolarization of neuronal terminals and the release of neurotransmitters from within the cholinergic or other neurones.

(C) Speculatively, 5-HT released from a non-neuronal source, e.g. enterochromaffin cells (EC) or platelets, and diffusing through tissues or via the bloodstream, may stimulate 5-HT$_3$ or 5-HT$_4$ receptors located on the vagus nerve, causing a rapid or slow depolarizing response respectively.

Non-specific manipulations of 5-HT function

Early experiments in animals that attempted to increase or decrease 5-HT function in the brain or periphery inevitably caused a generalized effect throughout the system. Thus the systemic administration of 5-hydroxytryptophan to increase the synthesis or release of 5-HT would increase activity in all serotonergic neurones.[34] Attempts to reduce the metabolism of 5-HT using monoamine oxidase inhibitors also cause a generalized and dramatic increase in 5-HT throughout the brain, and also noradrenaline and dopamine in other monoamine-containing neurones, since these also are normally metabolized by oxidase enzymes.

Attempts to reduce 5-HT function have focused on electrolytic or neurotoxic lesions of the central 5-HT systems, or the peripheral administration of the tryptophan hydroxylase inhibitor p-chlorophenylalanine.[35] The latter agent causes an effective reduction in brain levels of 5-HT; peripheral toxicity precludes its routine use in man. Fenfluramine provides a further pharmacological tool to disrupt 5-HT release from neurones, and can be used in both animals and man.[36] The use of 5-HT reuptake inhibitors such as fluoxetine or citalopram provides a further means to influence 5-HT function. Inhibition of neuronal reuptake would act to increase the synaptic concentration of 5-HT to theoretically enhance postsynaptic-mediated events. However, there is little evidence in animals or man to support this hypothesis. It is probably more likely that the acute effect of a 5-HT reuptake inhibitor in enhancing synaptic concentrations of 5-HT actually facilitates stimulation of presynaptic 5-HT autoreceptors to reduce any further 5-HT release.[37] A longer-term effect may be to downregulate the autoreceptors.[38]

Specific manipulations of 5-HT function

Specific manipulations of 5-HT function are limited to the manipulation of a specific 5-HT receptor subtype. Thus the 5-HT receptor antagonists such as WAY100135, ritanserin,

ondansetron and GRI 13808 selectively block the 5-HT_{1A}, 5-HT_2, 5-HT_3 or 5-HT_4 receptor-mediated events respectively. But all the effects mediated by any one of the individual receptor subtypes are indiscriminately blocked by the selective antagonist.

It should also be noted that, in terms of manipulating 5-HT function, there is considerable evidence for a functional heterogeneity between different 5-HT systems, some with opposing actions and some with facilitatory actions.[39,40] This can greatly complicate an understanding of the role of 5-HT.

PHYSIOLOGY OF NAUSEA AND VOMITING

Nausea is a highly subjective and unpleasant sensation that precludes other mental and physical activity; it is usually relieved by an emetic episode. However, the presence of chronic nausea is to severely reduce the quality of life. It is usually accompanied by a vasomotor disturbance causing pallor and sweating and a relaxation of the lower part of the oesophagus and abdominal muscles, the latter tending to increase tension on the gastric and oesophagal muscles. A contraction of the upper small intestine is closely followed by contraction of the pyloric sphincter and the pyloric portion of the stomach. Such changes empty the contents of the upper jejunum, duodenum and pyloric portion of the stomach into the fundus and body of the stomach: the stomach, cardiac sphincter, oesophagus and oesophageal sphincter are all relaxed. The system is thus prepared for retching and vomiting which is reflex in origin and serves to remove the contents of the upper gastrointestinal tract.

The emetic reflex involves a series of highly coordinated changes in gastrointestinal motility and respiratory movements. Emesis, which is initiated by a deep and sharp inspiration, is immediately followed by reflex closure of the glottis and a raising of the soft palate, to prevent the passage of vomitus into the lungs and nasal cavity. The abdominal muscles then contract in the rhythmic manner of 'retching' movements, which compress the stomach between the contracted diaphragm and abdominal organs. The inevitable increase in intragastric pressure causes evacuation of the stomach contents through the relaxed oesophagus.

STIMULI GIVING RISE TO NAUSEA AND VOMITING

Stimuli may be single or, more frequently, multifactorial.

Gastrointestinal irritation

The stimulation of mechanoreceptors caused by distension or obstruction in the gut, or chemoreceptors responsive to bacterial endotoxins, alcohol or a wide range of therapeutic agents, e.g. non-steroidal anti-inflammatory agents and antibiotics, can induce nausea and emesis.

Motion sickness

The sickness caused by movement may contribute importantly to nausea and vomiting in medical practice. An essential function of the vestibular system is to develop compensatory eye movements that will stabilize the retinal image of visual target in the presence of head movement. This reflex is inappropriate, and generates sensory conflict where the visual world shares the same motion as that of the head; nausea and vomiting follow.

Pregnancy sickness

Nausea has been shown to occur in the majority of pregnant women during the first trimester; the 'morning sickness' (which can actually occur at any time) then sharply declines. The continued vomiting of hyperemesis gravidarum is rare. The cause of nausea and vomiting is likely to involve

- altered gastric function, e.g. delayed gastric emptying;

- changes in intra-abdominal pressure;
- changes in metabolism;
- alterations in hormonal function;
- psychogenic influences.

Intracranial pathology

A sudden bout of vomiting associated with severe headache may be a consequence of raised intracranial pressure. This may be due to a direct influence on the central structures coordinating the vomiting reflex, with additional inputs from nociceptors present in the vascular smooth muscle.

Metabolic disorders

A wide variety of metabolic disorders may induce nausea and vomiting, e.g. hypoglycaemia or uraemia following kidney damage.

Psychogenic nausea and retching or vomiting

Chronic 'psychogenic vomiting' (or usually retching) and anorexia nervosa and bulimia have a well-established psychopathology where retching/vomiting is a symptom of psychiatric illness. Also, certain sights, smells or feelings can trigger revulsion or fear that can cause immediate nausea and vomiting. Further, anticipatory nausea and vomiting has occurred in up to 30% of cancer patients, and is a learned response, the patients having associated their emetic treatment with the hospital and its personnel, which can trigger emesis on sight. A raised level of anxiety also predisposes to nausea and emesis.

Pain

The severe discomfort of somatic or cardiac pain or that caused by distension of the bile or urethral ducts can induce nausea and vomiting.

Drug- and radiation-induced emesis

The major classes of drugs where nausea and vomiting are a predictable consequence of their administration are as follows.

- Cancer chemotherapy and radiation: many cytotoxic treatments, when administered to the cancer patient, cause the most severe nausea and vomiting of any treatment, dependent on the drug regimen and doses used. Nausea and vomiting induced by radiation are also related to the dose used and to the area and extent of the body that is irradiated.
- Drugs with dopamine agonist properties that are used in the treatment of Parkinson's disease all have the potential to induce nausea and vomiting.
- Morphine and related opioid analgesics have complex actions influencing nausea and vomiting. The acute administration of such agents to opioid naive patients frequently induces nausea and sometimes vomiting, although tolerance develops rapidly to such effects. Indeed, the first treatment is usually shown to antagonize the emetic effects to a second opioid injection or indeed other emetogens.
- Cardiac glycosides such as digoxin induce abdominal pains, nausea and vomiting. Drugs enhancing 5-hydroxytryptamine (5-HT) function, e.g. 5-hydroxytryptophan, have been reported to induce nausea, which may relate to increased 5-HT activity in both central and gut tissues.
- Miscellaneous agents: heavy-metal components, such as copper sulphate, when administered orally, have an irritant action in the gut, triggering the emetic reflex via vagal and splanchnic nerves. The ipecacuanha alkaloids also stimulate peripheral and central mechanisms.

Post-operative nausea and vomiting (PONV)

This provides one of the best examples of the multifactorial nature of nausea and vomiting, which may be triggered by the following factors:

- inhalation agents, intravenous anaesthetics and spinal anaesthesia are potentially emetogenic;
- the nature of the surgery, e.g. gynaecological and paediatric strabismus surgery have a high incidence of nausea and vomiting;
- pain resulting from surgery or disease;
- hypoxia, hypotension and carbon dioxide retention;
- clumsy movement of the patient causing labyrinthine disturbance;
- the nature of any pre- or postoperative drug treatments, e.g. opioid analgesics;
- psychogenic factors such as anxiety.

CENTRAL AND PERIPHERAL SYSTEMS MEDIATING NAUSEA AND EMESIS

A key structure is the 'chemoreceptor trigger zone' (CTZ), which is located within the area postrema, a circumventricular organ located at the caudal end of the fourth ventricle. This structure lacks an effective blood–brain barrier, and will detect emetic agents in both the systemic circulation and the cerebrospinal fluid. Lesion of the CTZ abolishes the emetic response to many emetogens. The area postrema has afferent and efferent connections with underlying structures, the subnucleus gelatinosus and nucleus tractus solitarius.[41] These brain regions are also important structures in the emetic reflex, receiving (with the area postrema) vagal afferent fibres from the gastrointestinal tract, a major source of emetic stimuli, on which are located 5-HT$_3$ receptors within the emetic circuit.[42]

A second major 'structure' is the 'vomiting centre', an area located in the brainstem medullary structures, which is described as a collection of effector nuclei rather than a discrete brain area.[43,44] It receives major inputs from the CTZ, and a vagal and sympathetic input from the gut, the cardiovascular system and a number of limbic brain nuclei, e.g. the olfactory tubercle, amygdala, hypothalamus and ventral thalamic nucleus. Electrical stimulation of all these structures can induce emesis. The latter nuclei may be involved respectively in olfactory, emotional/anticipatory, hormonal, and stress- and pain-induced vomiting.

Finally, the brain regions that produce the sensation of nausea have been difficult to assess; nausea is a subjective human experience, and animal models are not available. However, recently non-invasive magnetic source imaging in man has revealed that neuronal activation occurs in the cortex in the inferior frontal gyrus in volunteers made nauseous with ipecacuanha or vestibular stimulation. This brain area may be important in the perception or sensation of nausea.[45]

ROLE OF 5-HT IN NAUSEA AND EMESIS

There is considerable evidence that an enhanced 5-HT function can facilitate nausea and vomiting. Thus 5-hydroxytryptophan can induce nausea and vomiting in man, and one of the most significant side-effects of treatment with 5-HT reuptake inhibitors is gastrointestinal irritation and nausea.[46] However, these clinical data provide no evidence as to whether a stimulation of all 5-HT receptors or a subtype is required to induce the effect. Such evidence comes from the use of more selective 5-HT receptor agonists and antagonists in animal models of emesis.

Agonist action at the $5-HT_{1A}$ receptor may encompass a 'broad spectrum' antiemetic profile. Thus the $5-HT_{1A}$ receptor agonist 8-hydroxy-2-(di-*n*-propylamino)tetralin (8-OH-DPAT) was first shown to reduce motion-, cisplatin- and xylazine-induced emesis in the cat[47] and subsequently motion- and cisplatin-induced emesis in *Suncus murinus*[48] and copper sulphate-, morphine- and apomorphine-induced emesis in the ferret.[49,50] Other $5-HT_{1A}$ receptor agonists, e.g. buspirone, flesinoxan and gepirone, have a similar antiemetic spectrum in the ferret[50] and other species.[51] However, 8-OH-DPAT as a prototypical $5-HT_{1A}$ receptor agonist has known actions in animals to induce sedation and repetitive motor behav-

iour.[52] In addition, 8-OH-DPAT can actually induce emesis in the cat and ferret,[50,53] and exacerbates cisplatin-induced emesis in the ferret,[50] which limits its clinical relevance as an antiemetic agent.

However, lesopitron, a selective and specific $5-HT_{1A}$ receptor agonist that lacks the sedative potential or the motor effects of 8-OH-DPAT[54,55] and antagonizes motion-, copper sulphate- and cisplatin-induced emesis in *Suncus murinus* and the ferret (Naylor, unpublished data) may provide a further therapeutic opportunity.

There is little evidence for a $5-HT_2$ receptor involvement in emesis. However, the administration of the $5-HT_1/5-HT_2$ agonist *d*-lysergic acid diethylamide in the dog prevented emesis induced by apomorphine and other chemical emetogens,[56] and the more selective $5-HT_{2A/2C}$ receptor agonist DOI was shown to dose-dependently antagonize both motion- and cisplatin-induced emesis in *Suncus murinus*.[57] The antiemetic effects of DOI were attenuated by the selective $5-HT_2$ receptor antagonist ketanserin, although such actions were compromised by the ability of ketanserin alone to prevent cisplatin-induced emesis in *Suncus murinus*.[58]

Agonist action at the $5-HT_3$ receptor can induce emesis. Thus in the ferret, cat or *Suncus murinus*, the oral (in particular) or intraperitoneal injection of the selective $5-HT_3$ receptor agonists 2-methyl-5-HT, 1-phenylbiguanide or chlorophenylbiguanide induced emesis that was antagonized by granisetron or other selective $5-HT_3$ receptor antagonists.[59-62] Indeed, it is the use of the $5-HT_3$ receptor antagonists that has unequivocally established a role for 5-HT in emesis, revolutionized the treatment of emesis in man and caused a renaissance of emesis research. Highly selective $5-HT_3$ receptor antagonists such as ondansetron, tropisetron and granisetron inhibit emesis induced by cancer chemotherapy and radiation in the ferret,[63,64] dog,[65] cat,[66] *Suncus murinus*[67] and cancer patient.[68] The antagonism is selective, the $5-HT_3$ receptor antagonists failing to reduce motion sickness or the effects of other emetogenic agents such as apomorphine or copper sulphate in animal models.

SITES OF ACTION OF 5-HT RECEPTOR AGONISTS AND ANTAGONISTS TO INDUCE OR ANTAGONIZE EMESIS

Preclinical studies have investigated the possibility of a central or peripheral site of action for drugs to induce or antagonize emesis.

Central role for 5-HT receptors in mediating emesis

A central site of action for emetogenic agents initially came from brain-lesion studies, showing, for example that lesion of the area postrema in cat and dog could prevent cisplatin emesis.[69,70] and that emesis induced by cisplatin injected into the cerebroventricular system of cats and ferrets, albeit at a reduced intensity, could be antagonized by the 5-HT$_3$ receptor antagonist zacopride.[71,72] The most detailed study was afforded by Higgins et al,[73] who demonstrated an antagonism of (peripherally administered) cisplatin-induced emesis by the direct central injection into the vicinity of the area postrema of the 5-HT$_3$ receptor antagonists ondansetron, MDL72222 and GR65630.

It was therefore an unexpected finding that intracerebroventricular injection of 5-hydroxytryptophan, 5-HT or 2-methyl-5-HT into the cat or ferret failed to induce a convincing or consistent emetic response[73,74] (Naylor, unpublished data). However, a number of hypotheses could be advanced to explain this unexpected failure. First, 5-HT may have stimulated 5-HT$_{1A}$ receptors to attenuate 5-HT release and therefore reduce emesis, whilst an agonist action at the 5-HT$_3$ receptors would act to induce emesis. These mutually antagonistic effects would cause a null response. Secondly, the response to the selective 5-HT$_3$ receptor agonist 2-methyl-5-HT may have caused a rapid densitization of the 5-HT$_3$ receptor precluding a persistent depolarizing response.

Further attempts to elucidate a central site of antiemetic action came from the use of agents with reduced ability to penetrate the blood–brain barrier, but with inconclusive results. Thus a quaternary 5-HT$_3$ receptor antagonist LY191617, with limited access to structures within the blood–brain barrier, fails to prevent cisplatin-induced emesis in the dog,[75] suggesting that the antiemetic site of action of 5-HT$_3$ receptor antagonists in this species lies within the brain. However, in the ferret, quaternarized ICS 205-930 is able to prevent emesis.[76] This suggests that a site of action outside the blood–brain barrier is more important in this species, and may indicate true species differences. However, it should also be considered that the area postrema has an incomplete blood–brain barrier.

A peripheral role for 5-HT receptors to mediate emesis

Studies have been restricted to the 5-HT$_3$ receptor, which is present on afferent vagal fibres and in the gastrointestinal tract at the mucosal–submucosal junction.[77] The intragastric administration of 2-methyl-5-HT, 1-phenylbiguanide or chlorophenyl biguanide provoked a more intense emesis in the ferret than that induced by intraperitoneal injection, and this was abolished by a combined vagotomy plus greater splanchnic nerve section.[62] Similar data have been obtained in the cat.[60] This strongly suggests that emesis induced by 5-HT$_3$ receptor stimulation is mediated via the abdominal visceral innervation. However, Ravenscroft et al[62] performed a further experiment based on the observation that 5-HT administered intravenously rarely causes emesis, whilst clearly evoking cardiovascular changes. They injected phenylbiguanide intravenously upon an established emetic response: the vomiting was blocked. This antiemetic potential was attributed to the activation of cardiopulmonary vagal afferents that can modulate somatic reflexes. It should also be noted that lesion studies in animals indicate that the vagus and splanchnic nerves are important in mediating chemotherapy-induced emesis.[78]

From all the above evidence, it is reasonable to conclude that emesis induced by 5-HT agonist challenge may reflect both central and peripheral effects. The important question is how this pharmacological data relates to a role for endogeneous 5-HT.

ROLE OF ENDOGENOUS 5-HT IN THE EMETIC RESPONSE

The hypothesis that endogenous 5-HT, as distinct from erogenous 5-HT agonist challenge, has a role in a drug-induced emetic response is indicated first by the ability of p-chlorophenyl-alanine to inhibit 5-HT synthesis and prevent cisplatin-induced emesis in the ferret, pigeon and *Suncus murinus*.[79] Secondly, and at least as importantly, there is the proven class action of all 5-HT$_3$ receptor antagonists in inhibiting chemotherapy- and radiation-induced emesis in man.[79] These two observations have led to the concept that an agent such as cisplatin can cause an inappropriate increase in 5-HT function at 5-HT$_3$ receptors involved in the modulation of the emetic reflex.

There is also further evidence in humans that cisplatin chemotherapy increases urine and plasma levels of 5-hydroxyindoleacetic acid (5-HIAA), the main metabolite of 5-HT, and the increases appeared to correlate well with the incidence of nausea and vomiting.[80,81] In addition, in animal models, cisplatin has been reported to raise 5-HT/5-HIAA levels in the plasma,[82] although others have failed to find such changes in the ferret.[83].

The rise in both 5-HT and 5-HIAA in the plasma and urine of different species has been hypothesized to originate from the enterochromaffin cells of the gastrointestinal tract. Thus these cells found in the mucosa contain approximately 90% of the total body 5-HT content,[84] and cisplatin causes mucosal damage[85,86] and alters 5-HT levels in the mucosa of animals.[86,87] It remains an interesting observation that cyclophosphamide is a potent emetogen, yet fails to induce changes in 5-HT release and that the carcinoid syndrome rarely encompasses emesis.[88]

Under normal circumstances, it seems unlikely that 5-HT released from peripheral stores in the enterochromaffin cells could reach the AP to contribute to the emetic response.

This would be prevented by the active uptake by platelets and rapid degradation by monoamine oxidases in the epithelial linings of many organs.[89] Also, such increases would presumably manifest as cardiovascular problems, and such effects have not been observed. Therefore if 5-HT is released then its effects are probably mediated locally within the close vicinity of 5-HT$_3$ receptors located on afferent vagal nerve fibres.

MECHANISM OF 5-HT RELEASE FROM ENTEROCHROMAFFIN CELLS (EC)

The mechanism by which cytotoxic drugs, radiation or indeed other forms of gastrointestinal irritation or assault cause a release of 5-HT from EC cells is unknown. From studies on the guinea pig isolated intestine (although the guinea pig is a non-vomiting species), it has been suggested that a cisplatin-induced release of 5-HT from guinea pig EC cells is mediated by a cascade of events that involves stimulation of neuronal 5-HT$_3$ receptors.[90] However, this seems unlikely, since the concentrations of ondansetron and tropisetron that were required to block cisplatin-induced 5-HT release are not consistent with the antagonism of 5-HT$_3$ receptors. Further, clinically effective doses of ondansetron do not affect cisplatin-induced 5-HT release in man.[81] It has also been suggested that a subtype of the 5-HT$_3$ receptor (the existence of which has not been established) and 5-HT$_4$ receptors are located on EC cells and are involved in an autoregulatory feedback mechanism by which the amount of 5-HT released from EC cells is modulated. Inhibition of release is achieved via 5-HT$_4$ receptors and facilitation of release is mediated via atypical 5-HT$_3$ receptors.[91] However, the 5-HT$_4$ receptor antagonist GR125487, which would be expected to remove any inhibitory feedback mechanism, does not increase emesis following cisplatin, copper sulphate or zacopride, and does not influence the efficacy of ondansetron or granisetron following cisplatin in the ferret. These results indicate strongly that 5-HT$_4$ receptors are not involved in the emetic response

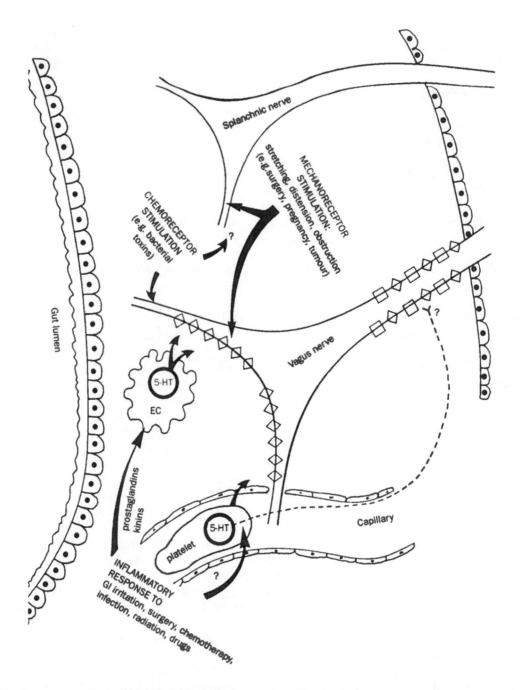

Figure 3.3 Peripheral stimuli that may activate the emetic reflex within the gut. An inflammatory response to infection, surgery and particularly chemotherapy and radiation is envisaged to activate the enterochromaffin cell (EC), causing the release of 5-HT, which may stimulate 5-HT$_3$ receptors (◇) located on the afferent vagus nerve terminals, triggering vagus firing and initiating the emetic reflex. An inflammatory response may influence the capillary blood flow and platelets to again release 5-HT, which could influence the 5-HT$_3$ receptors on the afferent vagus nerve terminals or possibly the 5-HT$_4$ (□) receptors located on the vagus axons. Chemoreceptor and mechanoreceptor stimuli due to toxins, surgery, pregnancy and other causes mediate their effects via the vagus nerve to trigger emesis; the splanchnic nerves may also play a role.

induced by cisplatin, copper sulphate or zacopride in the ferret.[92] Furthermore, it was suggested that atypical 5-HT$_3$ receptors on EC cells are more sensitive to blockade by gransetron and tropisetron compared with ondansetron.[91] Whilst further work is needed to substantiate this claim, it is unlikely to be clinically relevant, since there is no difference in the antiemetic efficacy of ondansetron and granisetron in the clinic.[93]

BREADTH OF ANTIEMETIC ACTION OF 5-HT$_3$ RECEPTOR ANTAGONISTS

The 5-HT$_3$ receptor antagonists are established as the single most effective therapy in the cancer patient for the treatment of acute (first-day) emesis and, when combined with dexamethasone, for the treatment of delayed emesis (after the first day).[94] Also, it has been demonstrated that ondansetron is clinically the preferred treatment to reduce postoperative nausea and vomiting, with a notable absence of significant side-effects.[95,96] The latter finding is particularly important and indicates an ability of a 5-HT$_3$ receptor antagonist to reduce emesis in the presence of a multifactorial aetiology. This may involve the potential of ondansetron to reduce nausea and vomiting induced by morphine.[97] There is also preliminary evidence that ondansetron can relieve the nausea and vomiting induced by antibiotics,[98] 5-HT re-uptake inhibitors,[99] hyperemesis gravidarum,[100] uraemia,[101] neurological trauma[102] and baclofen.[103] Examples of the ability of such stimuli to trigger nausea and vomiting are shown in Figure 3.3.

Further studies on the sites and mechanisms of interaction between the 5-HT$_3$ receptor antagonist and the various emetogenic challenges may broaden understanding of the role of 5-HT in the emetic reflex, the potential of other 5-HT receptor ligands to reduce emesis, and how to secure an optimal therapeutic control of nausea and vomiting in man. It remains clear that such control may be exerted at both peripheral and central sites of action.

REFERENCES

1. Page IH, The discovery of serotonin. *Perspect Biol Med* 1976; **20**: 1–8.

2. Erspamer V, *5-Hydroxytryptamine and Related Indoleaklylamines. Handbuch der Experimentellen Pharmakologie* Vol 19. Berlin: Springer-Verlag, 1966.

3. Brodie BB, Shore PA, A concept for the role of serotonin and norepinephrine as chemical mediators in the brain. *Ann NY Acad Sci* 1957; **66**: 631–42.

4. Sanders-Bush E, Mayor SE, 5-Hydroxytryptamine (serotonin) receptor agonists and antagonists. In: *Goodman and Gilman's Pharmacological Basis of Therapeutics*, 19th edn (Hardman JS, Limbird LE, Molinoff PB, eds). New York: McGraw-Hill, 1996: 2249–63.

5. Vanhoutte PM, Saxena PR, Paoletti R et al, *Serotonin from Cell Biology to Pharmacology and Therapeutics*. Dordrecht: Kluwer, 1993.

6. Fozard JR, Saxena PR, *Serotonin: Molecular Biology, Receptors and Functional Effects*. Basel: Birkhäuser, 1991.

7. Peroutka SJ, Howell TA, The molecular evolution of G protein-coupled receptors: focus on 5-hydroxytryptamine receptors. *Neuropharmacology* 1994; **33**: 319–24.

8. Gaddum JH, Picarelli ZP, Two kinds of tryptamine receptors. *Br J Pharmacol* 1957; **12**: 323–8.

9. Boess FG, Martin IL, Molecular biology of 5-HT receptors. *Neuropathology* 1994; **33**: 275–317.

10. Hoyer D, Clarke DE, Fozard JR et al, VII International Union of Pharmacology classification of receptors for 5-hydroxytryptamine. *Pharmacol Rel* 1994; **46**: 157–203.

11. Gothert M, Presynaptic effects of 5-HT. In: *Aspects of Synaptic Transmission LTP, Galatnin, Opioids, Autonomic and 5-HT* (Stone TW, Taylor M, Francis L, eds). London: Taylor & Francis, 1991: 314–29.

12. Gothert M, Schlickler E, Regulation of serotonin release in the central nervous system by presynaptic heteroreceptors. In: *Presynaptic Regulation of Neurotransmitter Release* (Feigenbaum JL, ed.). Tel Aviv: Freund Publishing House, 1990: 321–56.

13. Boyce MJ, Hinze K, Haegle D et al, MDL73005EF, a novel 5-HT1A receptor ligand and pentative anxiolytic. In: *Serotonin: Molecular Biology, Receptors and Functional Effects* (Fozard JR, Saxena PR, eds). Basel: Birkhäuser, 1991: 471–82.

14. Baxter G, Kennett G, Blaney F et al, 5-HT₂ receptor subtypes: a family reunited? *Trends Pharmacol Sci* 1995; 16: 105–10.

15. Reynolds DJM, Where do 5-HT3 receptor antagonists act as anti-emetics? In: *Serotonin and the Scientific Basis of Anti-Emetic Therapy* (Reynolds DJM, Andrews PLR, Davis DJ, eds). Oxford: Oxford Clinical Communications, 1995: 111–23.

16. Peters JA, Lambert JJ, Malone RM, Electrophysiological studies of 5-HT₃ receptors. In: *5-Hydroxytryptamine-3 Receptor Antagonists* (King FD, Jones BJ, Sanger GJ, eds). Boca Raton: CRC Press, 1994: 115–53.

17. Wallis DI, Nash H, Relative activities of substances related to 5-hydroxytryptamine as depolarising agents of superior cervical ganglion cells. *Eur J Pharmacol* 1981; 70: 381–92.

18. Kilpatrick GJ, Butler A, Burridge J et al, 1-(*m*-chlorophenyl)-biguanide, a potent high affinity 5-HT₃ receptor agonist. *Eur J Pharmacol* 1990; 2: 193–7.

19. Fozard JR, MDL72222: a potent and highly selective antagonist at neuronal 5-hydroxytryptamine receptors. *Naunyn Schmiedeberg's Arch Pharmacol* 1984; 326: 36–44.

20. Richardson BP, Engel G, Donatsch M et al, Identification of serotonin M-receptor subtypes and their specific blockade by a new class of drugs. *Nature* 1985; 316: 126–31.

21. Butler A, Hill JM, Ireland SJ et al, Pharmacological properties of GR38032F, a novel antagonist at 5-HT₃ receptors. *Br J Pharmacol* 1988; 94: 397–412.

22. Plosker GL, Goa KL, Granisetron – a review of its pharmacological properties and therapeutic use as an antiemetic. *Drugs* 1991; 42: 805–24.

23. Newberry NR, Cheshire SH, Gilbert MJ, Evidence that the 5-HT₃ receptors of the rat, mouse and guinea pig cervical ganglion may be different. *Br J Pharmacol* 1991; 102: 615–20.

24. Hope AG, Brown AM, Peters JA et al, Characterisation of a cloned human 5-HT₃ receptor subunit stably expressed in HEK293 cells. *Br J Pharmacol* 1995; 116: 82P.

25. Belelli D, Balcarek JM, Hope AG et al, Cloning and functional expression of a human 5-hydroxytryptamine type 3AS receptor (5-HT₃R-As) subunit. *Mol Pharmacol* 1995; 48: 1054–62.

26. Gill CH, Peters JA, Lambert JJ, An electrophysiological investigation of the properties of a murine recombitant 5-HT₃ receptor for stably expressed in HEK293 cells. *Br J Pharmacol* 1995; 114: 1211–21.

27. Dumuis A, Bouhelal R, Sabben D et al, A non-classical 5-hydroxytryptamine receptor positively coupled with adenylate cyclase in the central nervous system. *Mol Pharmacol* 1988; 34: 880–7.

28. Ford APDW, Clarke DE, The 5-HT₄ receptors. *Med Res Rev* 1993; 13: 633–50.

29. Gale JD, Grossman CJ, Whitehead JWF et al, GRI 13808, a novel selective antagonist with high affinity at the 5-HT₄ receptor. *Br J Pharmacol* 1994; 111: 332–8.

30. Wardle KA, Ellis ES, King FD, SB204070: a highly potent and selective 5-HT₄ receptor antagonist. *Br J Pharmacol* 1993; 110: 96P.

31. Eglen RM, Wong EIU, Dumuis A et al, Central 5-HT₄ receptors. *Trends Pharmacol Sci* 1995; 16: 391–7.

32. Lucas JJ, Hen R, New players in the 5-HT receptor field: genes and knockouts. *Trends Pharmacol Sci* 1995; 16: 246–52.

33. Sizer AR, Long SK, Robert MHT, A modulatory function of 5-hydroxytryptamine in the central nervous system. In: *Serotonin, CNS Receptors and Brain Function* (Bradley PB, Handley SC, Cooper SJ et al, eds). Oxford: Pergamon Press, 1992: 135–46.

34. Cheng CHK, Costall B, Kelly ME et al, Actions of 5-hydroxytryptophan to inhibit and disinhibit mouse behaviour in the light/dark test. *Eur J Pharmacol* 1994; 255: 39–49.

35. Koe BK, Wiseman A, *p*-chlorophenylalanine – a specific depletor of brain serotonin. *J Pharmacol Exp Ther* 1966; 154: 499–506.

36. Costall B, Naylor RJ, Tattersal FD, The actions of fenfluramine and interaction with 5-HT₃ receptor antagonists to inhibit emesis in the ferret. *J Pharm Pharmacol* 1990; 42: 94–101.

37. Langer SZ, Moret C, Citalopram antagonises the stimulation by lysergic acid diethylamide of presynaptic inhibitory autoreceptors in the rat hypothalamus. *J Pharmacol Exp Ther* 1982; 222: 220–6.

38. Maura G, Raiteri M, Functional evidence that chronic drugs induce adaptive changes of central autoreceptors regulating serotonin release. *Eur J Pharmacol* 1984; 97: 309–13.

39. Hjorth S, Functional differences between ascending 5-HT systems. In: *Serotonin, CNS Receptors and Brain Function* (Bradley PB, Handley SC, Cooper SJ et al, eds). Oxford: Pergamon Press, 1992: 203–18.

40. Costall B, Naylor RJ, The pharmacology of the 5-HT$_4$ receptor. *Int Clin Psychopharmacol* 1993; **2**: 11–18.

41. Leslie RA, Comparative aspects of the area postrema: fine structural considerations help determine its function. *Cell Mol Neurobiol* 1986; **6**: 95–120.

42. Leslie RA, Reynolds DJM, Andrews PLR et al, Evidence for presynaptic 5-hydroxytryptamine 3 recognition sites on vagal afferent terminals in the brainstem of the ferret. *Neurosci* 1990; **38**: 667–73.

43. Davis CJ, Harding RK, Leslie RA, Andrews PLR, The organisation of vomiting as a protective reflex. In: *Nausea and Vomiting: Mechanisms and Treatment* (Davis CJ, Lake-Bakaar GV, Grahame-Smith DG, eds). Berlin: Springer-Verlag, 1986: 65–75.

44. Miller AD, Bianchi AL, Bishop BP, *Neural Control of the Respiratory Muscles*. Boca Raton: CRC Press, 1996.

45. Miller AD, Rowley HA, Roberts TPL et al, Human cortical activity during vestibular and drug induced nausea detected using MSI. *Ann NY Acad Sci* 1996; **781**: 670–2.

46. Boyer WF, Feighner JP, *Selective Serotonin Reuptake Inhibitors*. Chichester: Wiley, 1991.

47. Lucot JB, Crampton GH, 8-OH-DPAT suppresses vomiting in the cat elicited by motion, cisplatin or xylazine. *Pharmacol Biochem Behav* 1989; **33**: 627–31.

48. Okada F, Torri Y, Saito H, Matsukl N, Antiemetic effects of serotonergic 5-HT$_{1A}$ receptor agonists in *Suncus murinus*. *Jap J Pharmacol* 1994; **64**: 109–14.

49. Bunce KT, Naylor RJ, Rudd JA, Effect of 8-OH-DPAT on drug induced emesis in the ferret. *Br J Pharmacol* 1992; **106**: 101P.

50. Rudd JA, Naylor RJ, Modulation of emesis by 5-HTIA receptors. *Pathophysiology* 1994; **1**: 267–8.

51. Lucot BJ, 5-HT$_{1A}$ receptor agonists as antiemetics. In: *Serotonin and the Scientific Basis of Anti-Emetic Therapy* (Reynolds DJM, Andrews PLR, Davis CJ, eds). Oxford: Oxford Clinical Communications, 1995: 222–7.

52. Pranzatelli MR, Pluchino RS, The relation of central 5-HTIA and 5-HT$_2$ receptors: low dose agonist-induced selective tolerance in the rat. *Pharmacol Biochem Behav* 1991; **39**: 407–13.

53. Lucot JB, Prevention of motion sickness by 5-HTIA agonists in cats. In: *Mechanisms and Control of Emesis* (Bianchi AL, Grélot L, Miller AD et al, eds). Paris: Colloque Inserm/John Libbey Eurotext, 1992: 195–9.

54. Costall B, Domeney AM, Farré AJ et al, Profile of action of a novel 5-hydroxytryptamine$_{1A}$ receptor ligand E-4424 to inhibit aversive behaviour in the mouse, rat and marmoset. *J Pharmacol Exp Ther* 1992; **262**: 90–8.

55. Haj-Dahmane S, Jolas T, Laporte AM et al, Interactions of lesopitron with central 5-HT$_{1A}$ receptors: in vitro and in vivo studies in the rat. *Eur J Pharmacol* 1994; **255**: 185–96.

56. Dhawan BN, Gupta GP, Antiemetic activity of *d*-lysergic acid diethylamide. *J Pharmacol Exp Ther* 1961; **131**: 137–9.

57. Okada F, Saito H, Matsuki N, Blockade of motion- and cisplatin-induced emesis by a 5-HT$_2$ receptor agonist in *Suncus murinus*. *Br J Pharmacol* 1995; **114**: 931–4.

58. Torri Y, Saito H, Matsuki N, Selective blockade of cytotoxic drug-induced emesis by 5-HT$_3$ receptor antagonism in *Suncus murinus*. *Jap J Pharmacol* 1991; **55**: 107–13.

59. Matsuki N, Torri Y, Ueno S, Saito H, *Suncus murinus* as an experimental model for emesis and motion sickness. In: *Mechanisms and Control of Emesis* (Bianchi AL, Grélot L, Miller AD et al, eds). Paris: Colloque Inserm/John Libbey Eurotext, 1992: 323–9.

60. Miller AD, Nonaka S, Mechanisms of vomiting induced by serotonin-3 receptor agonists in the cat – effect of vagotomy, splanchnicectomy or area postrema lesion. *J Pharmacol Exp Ther* 1992; **260**: 509–17.

61. Sancilio LF, Pinkus LM, Jackson CB et al, Studies on the emetic and antiemetic properties of zacopride and its enantiomers. *Eur J Pharmacol* 1991; **192**: 349–53.

62. Ravenscroft M, Wells U, Bhandari P et al, Agonist evidence for the involvement of 5-HT(3) receptors in emesis in the ferret. In: *Mechanism and Control of Emesis* (Bianchi AL, Grélot L, Miller AD et al, eds). Paris: Colloque Inserm/John Libbey Eurotext, 1992: 251–2.

63. Costall B, Domeney AM, Naylor RJ, Tattersall FD, 5-hydroxytryptamine M-receptor antagonism to prevent cisplatin-induced emesis. *Neuropharmacology* 1986; **25**: 959–61.

64. Miner WD, Sanger GJ, Inhibition of cisplatin-

induced vomiting by selective 5-hydroxytrypt-amine M-receptor antagonism. *Br J Pharmacol* 1986; 88: 497–9.

65. Smith WL, Jackson CB, Proakis AG et al, Zacopride: a unique and potent inhibitor of cancer chemotherapy induced emesis in dogs. *Proc Am Soc Clin Oncol* 1986; 5: 260.

66. Lucot JB, Blockade of 5-hydroxytryptamine₃ receptors prevents cisplatin-induced but not xylazine-induced emesis in the cat. *Pharmacol Biochem Behav* 1989; 32: 207–10.

67. Torri Y, Saito H, Matsuki N, Selective blockade of cytotoxic drug-induced emesis by 5-HT₃ receptor antagonists in *Suncus murinus*. *Jap J Pharmacol* 1991; 55: 107–13.

68. Butcher ME, Global experience with ondansetron and future potential. *Oncology* 1993; 50: 191–7.

69. Bhandari P, Gupta YK, Seth SD et al, Cisplatin-induced emesis: effect of chemoreceptor trigger zone ablation in dogs. *Asia Pacific J Pharmacol* 1989; 4: 209–11.

70. McCarthy LE, Borison HL, Cisplatin-induced vomiting eliminated by ablation of the area postrema in cats. *Cancer Treatment Rep* 1984; 68: 410–14.

71. Smith WL, Callahan EM, Alphin RS, The emetic activity of centrally administered cis-platin in cats and its antagonism by zacopride. *J Pharm Pharmacol* 1988; 40: 142.

72. Tattersall FD, 5-Hydroxytryptamine control of emesis and gastrointestinal activity. PhD thesis, University of Bradford, 1988.

73. Higgins GA, Kilpatrick GJ, Bunce KT et al, 5-HT₃ receptor antagonists injected into the area postrema inhibit cisplatin-induced emesis in the ferret. *Br J Pharmacol* 1989; 97: 247–55.

74. Feldberg W, Sherwood SL, Injections of drugs into the lateral ventricle of the cat. *J Physiol* 1954; 123: 148–67.

75. Robertson DW, Cohen ML, Krushinski JH, LY191617, a 5-HT₃ receptor antagonist which does not cross the blood brain barrier. In: *Proc 2nd IUPHAR Meeting on Serotonin, Basel, July 1990*, 149.

76. Buchheit KH, Buschner HH, Gamse R, The antiemetic profile of the 5-HT₃ receptor antago-nist ICS205-930 and its quaternary derivative. In: *Proc 2nd IUPHAR Meeting on Serotonin, Basel, July 1990*, 148.

77. Kilpatrick GJ, Bunce KT, Tyers MB, 5-HT₃ receptors. *Med Res Rev* 1990; 10: 441–75.

78. Andrews PLR, Davis CJ, Maskell L, The abdominal visceral innervation and the emetic reflex: pathways, pharmacology and plasticity. *Can J Physiol Pharmacol* 1990; 68: 325–45.

79. Naylor RJ, Rudd JA, Emesis and antiemesis. In: *Cancer Surveys, Vol 21: Palliative Medicine: Problem Areas in Pain and Symptom Management* (Hanks GW, Sidebottom E, eds). New York: Cold Spring Harbour Laboratory Press, 1994: 117–35.

80. Cubeddu LX, Hoffman IS, Fuenmayor NT et al, Changes in serotonin metabolism in cancer patients: its relationship to nausea and vomit-ing induced by chemotherapeutic agents. *Br J Cancer* 1992; 66: 198–203.

81. Cubeddu LX, Hoffman IS, Fuenmayor NT et al, Efficacy of ondansetron (GR38032F) and the role of serotonin in cisplatin-induced nausea and vomiting. *N Eng J Med* 1990; 322: 810–16.

82. Endo T, Minami M, Monma Y et al, Vagotomy and ondansetron (5-HT₃ antagonist) inhibited the increase of serotonin concentration induced by cytotoxic drugs in the area postrema of fer-rets. *Biogenic Amines* 1992; 9: 163–75.

83. Rudd JA, Bunce KT, Cheng CHK et al, The effect of cisplatin on plasma 5-HT and 5-HIAA levels during emesis in the ferret. *Br J Pharmacol* 1992; 105: 274P.

84. Racké K, Schwörer H, Regulation of serotonin release from the intestinal mucosa. *Pharmacol Res* 1991; 23: 13–25.

85. Allan SG, Smyth JF, Small intestinal mucosal toxicity with platinum analogues and dexa-methasone. *Br J Cancer* 1986; 53: 355–60.

86. Stables R, Andrews PLR, Bailey HF et al, Antiemetic properties of the 5-HT₃ receptor antagonist, GR38032F. *Cancer Treatment Rev* 1987; 14: 333–6.

87. Milano S, Simon C, Grélot L, In vitro release and tissue levels of ileal serotonin after cis-platin-induced emesis in the cat. *Clin Auton Res* 1991; 1: 275–80.

88. Andrews PLR, 5-HT3 receptor antagonists and antiemesis. In: *5-Hydroxytryptamine-3 Receptor Antagonists* (King FD, Jones BJ, Sanger GJ, eds). Boca Raton: CRC Press, 1994: 255–317.

89. Gillis CN, Peripheral metabolism of serotonin. In: *Serotonin and the Cardiovascular System* (Vanhoutte PM, ed.). New York: Raven Press, 1985: 27–36.

90. Showörer H, Racké K, Kilbinger H, Cisplatin increases the release of 5-hydroxytryptamine (5-HT) from the isolated perfused small intes-tine of the guinea pig: involvement of 5-HT₃

receptors. *Naunyn Schmiedebergs Arch Pharmacol* 1991; **344**: 143–9.

91. Gebauer A, Merger M, Kilbinger H, Modulation of 5-HT$_3$ and 5-HT$_4$ receptors of the release of 5-hydroxytryptamine from the guinea-pig small intestine. *Naunyn Schmiedeberg's Arch Pharmacol* 1993; **347**: 137–40.

92. Twissel DJ, Bountra C, Dale TJ et al, 5-HT$_4$ receptors are not involved in emesis in the ferret. *Br J Pharmacol* 1994; **113**: 22P.

93. Ruff, P, Paska W, Goedhals et al, Ondansetron compared with granisetron in the prophylaxis of cisplatin-induced acute emesis: a multicentre double-blind, randomised, parallel group study. *Oncology* 1994; **51**: 113–18.

94. Naylor RJ, Rudd JA, Mechanisms of chemotherapy/radiotherapy-induced emesis in animal models. *Oncology* 1996; **53**: 8–17.

95. McKenzie R, Kovac A, O'Connor T et al, Comparison of ondansetron versus placebo to prevent post operative nausea and vomiting in women undergoing ambulatory gynecological surgery. *Anesthesiology* 1993; **78**: 21–8.

96. Larijani GE, Gratz L, Afshar M et al, Treatment of post operative nausea and vomiting with ondansetron – a randomised, double blind comparison with placebo. *Anaesthesia Analgesia* 1991; **73**: 246–9.

97. Koch KL, Bingaman S, Effects of ondansetron on morphine-induced nausea, vasopressin and gastric myoelectrical activity in healthy humans. *Gastroenterology* 1993; **104**: A535.

98. Gompels M, McWilliams S, O'Hare M et al, Ondansetron usage in HIV positive patients – a pilot study on the control of nausea and vomiting in patients on high dose co-trimoxazole for *Pneumocytis carinii* pneumonia. *Int J STD AIDS* 1993; **4**: 293–6.

99. Bailey J, Potokar J, Nutt D, Can the GI disturbance produced by SSRIs be attenuated by a 5-HT$_3$ antagonist? *Neuropsychopharmacology* 1994; **10**: 220.

100. Sullivan CA, Johnson CA, Roach H et al, A pilot study of intravenous ondansetron for hyperemesis gravidarum. *Am J Obstet Gynecol* 1996; **174**: 1565–8.

101. Andrews PA, Quan V, Ogg CS, Ondansetron for the symptomatic relief in terminal uraemia. *Nephrol Dial Transplant* 1995; **10**: 140.

102. Kleinerman KD, Deppe SA, Sargent AI, Use of ondansetron for control of projectile vomiting in patients with neurosurgical trauma: two case reports. *Ann Pharmacother* 1993; **27**: 566–8.

103. Broggi U, Dones I, Servello D et al, A possible pharmacological treatment of baclofen overdosage. *Ital J Neurol Sci* 1996; **17**: 179–80.

4

Clinical aspects and prognostic factors of nausea and vomiting after chemotherapy

Dimitris L Voliotis, Volker Diehl

INTRODUCTION

The number of patients treated with several chemotherapeutic regimens has increased continuously over the past few years. It must be recognized that a large proportion of antineoplastic therapies can have only a palliative intent. Furthermore, the curative potential of other chemotherapeutic regimens used today (e.g. some high-dose regimens with stem cell support or autologous bone marrow transplantation) is currently under investigation, and cannot yet be exactly determined. A rational decision for the use of any cancer chemotherapy therefore always has to carefully weigh benefits (i.e. antitumor effects) against costs (i.e. side-effects).

Most chemotherapeutic regimens bring about at least one and frequently several side-effects in addition to the numerous symptoms caused by the malignant disease itself.

The undesirable effects of cytostatic therapy have consequences for the treatment results: compliance with therapy decreases when patients experience difficulty with side-effects of treatment. A bad patient compliance can result in therapy delay or even refusal of further treatment, with negative effects on treatment outcome.

Cancer chemotherapy can be associated with a considerable number of unpleasant or even sometimes life-threatening side-effects: for example bone marrow depression and immunological dysfunction resulting in infections or bleeding complications, organ failure, mucous membrane damage, hair loss, pain, central nervous symptoms, etc. Nevertheless, it seems that these problems are not the most important ones in patients' own perception of therapy-induced adverse effects.

In fact, nausea and vomiting are the two most distressing symptoms experienced by cancer patients undergoing chemotherapy. Nausea and vomiting after chemotherapy can sometimes be so intense that patients decide to withdraw from further treatment, even if they definitely know that this can reduce their chances of cure or survival.

Besides this, nausea and vomiting can have a multitude of consequences for the patient. Possible results are anorexia, impaired alimentation status, serious metabolic complications (metabolic alkalosis, dehydration and electrolyte disturbances), gastric or esophageal trauma, and deterioration of physical and mental status, as well as psychological and family problems.

Nausea is a very characteristic unpleasant sensation experienced in the pharyngeal and/or the gastric area that can (but not necessarily) result in vomiting. Vomiting itself is a physiologic process of forceful emptying of the contents of the stomach or small bowel through the oral cavity. Although nausea can result in vomiting, some studies indicate that these two phenomena are different entities with distinct components. For patients, the feeling of nausea seems to be even more disturbing than vomiting.

The severity and clinical presentation of chemotherapy-induced emesis depend on several factors. The emetogenic potential of an antineoplastic therapy varies with the particular drug used (see Table 4.1), ranging from cisplatin, which results in severe emesis in almost all patients, to vinca alkaloids and hormone preparations, with only minimal (if any) inducible emesis. In addition, the emetic activity and pattern of the drugs used depends distinctly on the dosage and administration schedule: lower doses of cisplatin (about 20 mg/m^2) induce less nausea and vomiting than high-dose regimens (50 mg/m^2 or above), bolus application is more emetogenic than continuous application, and combination therapy can induce more side-effects than monotherapy. Besides this, individual patient characteristics must be taken into account: age, gender, alcohol consumption, susceptibility to motion-sickness, psychosocial situation, and several other factors (see below).

In the last few years there have been considerable advances in the treatment of chemotherapy-induced emesis, especially with the use of antagonists to 5-hydroxytryptamine type 3 (5-HT$_3$) receptors. Despite this, nausea and vomiting after cytostatic therapy are still of major clinical relevance, especially for a subgroup of patients and with some of the drugs used.

CLINICAL PRESENTATION OF CHEMOTHERAPY-INDUCED EMESIS

A multitude of somatic problems can induce nausea and vomiting in cancer patients. The

Table 4.1 Emetogenic potential of selected single-agent chemotherapeutic drugs depending on dosage

High
Cisplatin >50 mg/m^2
Cyclophosphamide >1500 mg/m^2
Carmustine
Nitrogen mustard
Dactinomycin
Streptazocin
Dacarbazine

Moderately high
Carboplatin
Cisplatin <50 mg/m^2
Cyclophosphamide 750–1500 mg/m^2
Ara-C >1000 mg/m^2
Doxorubicin and daunorubicin >60 mg/m^2
Methotrexate >1000 mg/m^2
Procarbazine
Lomustine

Moderate
Cyclophosphamide <750 mg/m^2 and cyclophosphamide oral
Doxorubicin and daunorubicin 20–60 mg/m^2
Ifosfamide
Idarubicin
Mitoxantrone
Methotrexate 250–1000 mg/m^2

Low
Methotrexate <250 mg/m^2
Taxols
Etoposide
5-Fluorouracil
Gemcitabine
Mitomycin
Vincristine
Vinblastine
Asparaginase
Azacytidine
Thiotepa
6-Mercaptopurine
Thioguanine
Bleomycin
Hydroxyurea
Busulfan

course of the malignant disease itself can lead to emesis by several complications, for instance by metastasis to the central nervous system, by gastrointestinal obstruction or by inducing metabolic and electrolyte imbalances. Concurrent medication such as opioids, which are used frequently in cancer patients, can induce nausea and vomiting. Furthermore, infections or uremia related to renal insufficiency can also contribute to the development of emesis in cancer patients. Even some primarily unrelated factors such as gastroenteritis or gastrointestinal ulcers as well as several psychological components can cause symptoms. After exclusion of such causes, emesis related directly to the application of antineoplastic therapy is to be viewed as being caused by these drugs and is called chemotherapy-induced emesis.[1–3]

Nausea and vomiting after cytostatic therapy are commonly divided into three categories: acute chemotherapy-induced emesis, delayed emesis and anticipatory emesis. It is important to distinguish between these entities, because their causes and treatments can differ significantly.[2–6]

Acute chemotherapy-induced nausea and vomiting

The incidence of nausea and vomiting after chemotherapy is affected by the kind of chemotherapeutic agent given and also by its dose and the route of administration. If combination chemotherapy is given, each drug has to be taken into consideration individually. The agents that are most often associated with emesis also induce the greatest severity of symptoms (see Table 4.1), with differences occurring from patient to patient and among different treatment courses in the same patient.

Acute nausea and vomiting occur within a variable time period from the moment of drug administration to the occurrence of symptoms, but, by definition, always within the first 24 hours. When the term 'acute emesis' is used, it usually means the occurrence of nausea and vomiting within the first 1 or 2 hours after the application of cytostatic drugs in a patient who

has not received any previous chemotherapy.[7–10]

There are two important exceptions: with the chemotherapeutic agents carboplatin and (high-dose) cyclophosphamide, the onset of acute emesis can occur even 10–20 hours after administration. This late onset should not be confused with delayed emesis, which is caused by different underlying mechanisms and occurs at the earliest 24 hours after chemotherapy (see Figure 4.1).[7–10]

In contrast, the pattern of emesis induced by cisplatin is quite different. In general, nausea and vomiting are best studied in patients given cisplatin, since this is regarded as the most emetogenic chemotherapeutic agent. It causes nausea and vomiting in virtually 100% of patients. Cisplatin-induced emesis follows a biphasic course: after application, there is an intense phase of emesis, which is completed within the first 12 hours, and is followed by a second phase, which culminates after 48–72 hours and is called 'delayed emesis'.[7–13]

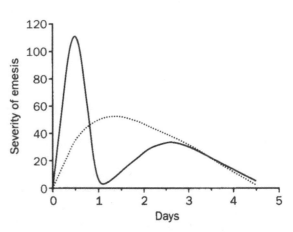

Figure 4.1 Different patterns of nausea and vomiting after cisplatin (biphasic: acute, delayed emesis) and carboplatin/cyclophosphamide (monophasic: late onset). Cisplatin, ———; carboplatin/ cyclophosphamide, ·········.

Delayed emesis

The importance of delayed emesis has increased as the control of acute chemotherapy-induced emesis has improved in the past years. With combination treatments consisting of 5-HT$_3$ antagonists, dexamethasone and other antiemetics such as metoclopramide, a high proportion of patients receiving high emetogenic drugs do not experience substantial acute nausea and vomiting after chemotherapy. However, those patients treated successfully for acute emesis can still develop symptoms at a later time point. Delayed nausea and vomiting are defined to occur after the acute phase, that is, more than 24 hours after chemotherapy is given, and can sometimes persist for several days. The underlying mechanisms and the course of delayed emesis are not yet completely understood. Delayed emesis is associated with a high percentage of morbidity, and treatment options for this side-effect are few and difficult to manage effectively. Between 20% and 85% of patients subject to cisplatin-based chemotherapy present this form of emesis. The wide range may probably be related to several prognostic factors associated with this phenomenon. The problem is again best described in patients receiving cisplatin in high doses (>100 mg/m^2 per dose). The clinical problem of delayed emesis seems to differ from acute emesis with regard to the underlying etiologic mechanisms: it is not simply the postponement of acute emesis to a later time period. Although delayed emesis is less severe, it still causes considerable discomfort to patients as well as difficulties with nutrition and peroral hydration. Even when the control of emesis during the acute phase is successful, delayed emesis can occur in the patients treated. Most patients who are given high-dose cisplatin experience delayed emesis to some degree, usually after 48–72 hours post chemotherapy, with the intensity of nausea decreasing within the next 1–3 days. Patients with poor control of acute emesis are more likely to develop delayed emesis after cisplatin. Although delayed emesis was initially described in patients receiving cisplatin at dosages above 100 mg/m^2, it has also been reported in patients receiving lower doses of cisplatin or some other cytotoxic drugs, especially cyclophosphamide, doxorubicin and ifosfamide when given at high doses or repeated on several days. Even though treatment of delayed emesis is difficult, appropriate therapy can significantly diminish patients' complaints.[11-17]

Anticipatory nausea and vomiting

This problem is defined as nausea or vomiting beginning before the administration of chemotherapy, approximately within a 24-hour period. Patients experience these symptoms when going to the hospital, on seeing nurses preparing an injection or with the sight of the attendant physician. These emetic symptoms, which are not directly produced by chemotherapeutic drugs, can also occur outside the hospital, when patients perceive certain tastes, smells or images that they associate with the chemotherapy. Several characteristics of anticipatory nausea and vomiting suggest that it represents a respondent learning model. The sight of the physician or the nurse, or the perception of certain smells (e.g. a disinfectant alcohol swab) or tastes acts here as a neutral or conditioned stimulus, while the unconditioned stimulus (the chemotherapy itself) induces an unconditioned response, namely nausea and vomiting. After several repeats of chemotherapy, which then act as a learning process, the conditioned stimulus can lead to a conditioned response, which in this case is anticipatory nausea and vomiting.[11-17]

Anticipatory nausea and vomiting does not seem to develop unless treatment-induced emesis has appeared at least once, and it is typically presented in patients with poor control of emesis (acute or delayed) with previous chemotherapy. There seems to be a clear relationship between the severity of post-chemotherapy side-effects and the development of anticipatory symptoms. The frequency of anticipatory nausea and vomiting increases with the number of chemotherapy cycles given. After several cycles (usually four to five), an estimated 25% of all patients are likely to develop this form of emesis. Anticipatory nausea and vomiting is important not only for the discomfort it can cause by itself to the patients, but also because of its influence on post-treatment side-effects, since patients with anticipatory nausea and vomiting are again more susceptible to post-treatment nausea and vomiting. Also, there is convincing evidence that the grade of anticipatory nausea and vomiting experienced by a given patient is strongly influenced by that patient's anxiety level.[11–17,24]

The treatment of anticipatory nausea and vomiting is difficult. Once it has occurred, it cannot be treated with antiemetics. The best treatment methods are based on behavioral approaches, and include relaxation-based approaches as well as systematic desensitization together with anxiolytic medication.[14–19,24]

CLINICAL RISK FACTORS ASSOCIATED WITH THE DEVELOPMENT OF NAUSEA AND VOMITING WITH CHEMOTHERAPY

There are several variables that may influence the occurrence of nausea and vomiting with chemotherapy. In the following, prognostic characteristics that are associated with anticipatory nausea and vomiting as well as with post-chemotherapy nausea and vomiting are discussed separately. In Table 4.2, the most important clinical risk factors that are important for the development of chemotherapy-induced emesis are briefly summarized. The most important prognostic factors are discussed below.

Prognostic factors associated with the development of post-chemotherapy nausea and vomiting

Post-chemotherapy nausea and vomiting appears after a variable time period when chemotherapy is given. Its intensity depends mainly on the emetogenicity of the cytostatics or the drug combination used and on several individual patient characteristics, which may differ substantially from one patient to another

Table 4.2 Factors influencing the development of nausea and vomiting with chemotherapy

Patient-associated factors
  Experience of emesis during previous chemotherapy
  Degree of emesis after last chemotherapy
  Lengthy treatment infusions
  Feeling of warmth or heat after chemotherapy
  Sweating after chemotherapy
  Psychogenic factors and perception (anxiety, conditioning mechanisms, psychosocial distress, decreased coping ability, greater absorption)
  Gender (female)
  Age (<50 years)
  History of alcohol consumption
  Susceptibility to motion sickness
  Physical function
  Quality of life
  Fatigue
  Anorexia
  Pain
  Diarrhea
  Experience of generalized weakness after chemotherapy
  Alimentation, smells

Chemotherapy-associated factors
  Agent
  Dose
  Schedule
  Route

and must be taken into account when conducting the appropriate antiemetic regimen.

Type of cytostatic drugs and chemotherapy combinations

This seems to be the most important factor. First, the importance of the individual emetogenic potential of each cytostatic drug together with the dose intensity has already been mentioned (see Table 4.1). Cytostatic drugs can be divided into different categories according to their individual emetogenic potential and the dosage used. This may allow the development of risk-adapted strategies to treat emesis after chemotherapy. Second, the combination of two or more cytotoxic drugs within a chemotherapeutic schedule potentates the side-effects, producing a synergistic effect on the emetogenic potential. This synergistic effect also has to be taken into consideration when designing a chemotherapeutic schedule. Third, the same drug combination can cause different intensities of emesis, depending on the way the drugs are given. The same drug when given as a bolus injection or short infusion causes more severe emesis than as a continuous infusion, because the peak levels of drug concentration in vivo are higher with short-time application. Furthermore, there is evidence that a drug combination administered as an adjuvant therapy has a higher emetogenic potential than the same combination administered non-adjuvantly. The reason for this is not known. Fourth, another factor influencing the emetogenicity of a chemotherapy combination can involve the setting where the treatment is performed: chemotherapy given on an outpatient basis may be better tolerated than in hospitalized patients. Fifth, there is increasing probability of an agent or a combination treatment causing emesis after several repeated cycles of therapy.[20-25]

Patient characteristics

If patients have *previous experience with poorly controlled emesis*, they are more likely to develop nausea and vomiting after chemotherapy in response to a new treatment. Here it is not only the occurrence of emesis in the past that is important but also the degree of the side-effects experienced. If, during previous chemotherapy, the emetic control was sufficient, the percentage of patients who do not experience emesis in subsequent chemotherapy courses is larger than in patients with insufficient previous antiemetic treatment. In fact, with regard to treatment with cisplatin, the protection

obtained in previous cycles is the most important prognostic factor.

Sex is probably also one of the most important individual prognostic factors in predicting emesis: female gender predisposes, irrespective of the antiemetic treatment, the chemotherapy regimen or the cancer site, for an increased probability of developing nausea and vomiting after chemotherapy. Women vomit and experience nausea more frequently and with greater intensity than men when receiving cytostatic drugs as cisplatin, cyclophosphamide and high-dose Ara-C. The reasons for this phenomenon are not known. Although hormonal regulations with central nervous effects are supposed to be involved, there is still uncertainty about the underlying mechanisms.

Age appears to be another important prognostic factor that influences nausea and vomiting after chemotherapy. Younger patients (i.e. <50 years) experience more severe nausea and vomiting after chemotherapy than older patients (>65 years). The reasons are altogether unknown, although there is some evidence for a difference in tolerance to several antiemetic regimens with age.

Alcohol intake is another factor that can influence the level of chemotherapy-induced emesis. Studies have indicated that a history of chronic heavy alcohol abuse (more than 100 g/day) may be associated with better control of chemotherapy-induced emesis. It has been assumed that chronic alcohol exposure results in a decreased sensitivity of the chemoreceptor trigger zone, but knowledge of this area is still incomplete.

Another factor involved in the appearance of emesis after chemotherapy is the experience of *motion sickness*. It has been found that patients susceptible to motion sickness report both a greater frequency of nausea following chemotherapy and a greater severity and longer duration of each episode of post-treatment emesis. In general, patients susceptible to motion sickness experience much more common side-effects after chemotherapy than those who are not. Susceptibility to motion sickness appears to be another determinant of patients experiencing side-effects with cytostatic therapy. A possible explanation is in the assumption that the multiple neuronal afferent pathways involved in the nausea and vomiting response to chemotherapy are, at least in part, similar to the pathophysiologic processes that cause nausea and vomiting in motion sickness.[20-28]

The patient-to-patient differences concerning frequency, duration and intensity of post-treatment nausea and vomiting must also to be taken into consideration, since it is known, for instance, that bleomycin causes nausea in about 15% of patients in the USA but in about 50% of patients in Japan.[28-30]

Surely the wide variability of post-treatment nausea and vomiting cannot be explained by biological factors alone. Furthermore there are several other problems contributing to the development of nausea and vomiting after chemotherapy. The most important are psychogenic factors: anxiety, expectations, negative experiences with previous chemotherapy, decreased coping ability and classical conditioning mechanisms. All of these factors usually result in an increased incidence of nausea and vomiting after application of chemotherapy. The exact mechanisms by which these factors influence chemotherapy-induced emesis are poorly understood.[15,18,24,31]

In summary, the characteristics of patients form a large group of factors that can, each by itself or in combination, modulate the occurrence of nausea and vomiting after chemotherapy.

Factors associated with the development of anticipatory nausea and vomiting

Anticipatory nausea and vomiting occur prior to treatment as a classically conditioned response to specific stimuli associated with chemotherapeutic treatment. For instance, a cytostatic agent acts as an unconditioned stimulus that may be paired with a smell inside the clinic or the sight of a nurse preparing an infusion, which represent the neutral or conditioned stimulus at the time of chemotherapy administration. Then, the patient experiences nausea and vomiting after chemotherapy as an unconditioned response. In the future, after

several pairings or repeated applications of chemotherapy, the smell for instance of a disinfectant alone or the sight of the nurse or the physician becomes the conditioned stimulus, which then again leads to nausea and vomiting as a conditioned response. There is some evidence that the neutral triggering stimuli in anticipatory nausea and vomiting may be predominantly smells, tastes and thinking of the treatment. Approximately 25–30% of patients undergoing anticancer chemotherapy may develop anticipatory nausea and vomiting by the time of their third or fourth treatment cycle. The time of onset varies among patients, usually occurring up to 24 hours before chemotherapy.[24,26,28,42]

Anticipatory nausea and vomiting represent a major clinical problem in the management of chemotherapy-induced side-effects. As the treatment of post-chemotherapy nausea and vomiting has improved substantially over the past years, the problem of anticipatory nausea and vomiting has become more and more important, because it is refractory to standard pharmacological antiemetic treatment.

Factors associated with the development of anticipatory nausea and vomiting have been extensively studied, and are summarized here separately from the factors influencing post-treatment emesis, although there are some overlaps within the several features involved in post-chemotherapy as well as anticipatory symptoms.[24,26,28,35-42]

Anxiety

Independently of the chemotherapeutic regimen used, patients show a wide variability in developing nausea and vomiting before and after treatment. One factor that is supposed to be important in this issue is anxiety. Anxiety is especially suggested to be relevant to the development of anticipatory nausea and vomiting. Many patients experience adverse reactions to their treatment, and as a result of a conditioning mechanism then develop anxiety and anticipatory nausea and vomiting before the application of chemotherapy. Again the development of anticipatory symptoms is related to post-treatment emesis, since anxiety seems to increase when post-chemotherapy induced emesis is suddenly augmented. Besides that, anxiety may be just one more factor involved in the stressful perception of chemotherapy, and may therefore lead to anticipatory symptoms, since it is known that anxious patients are more susceptible to environmental stimuli and can therefore more easily develop classical conditioning responses to chemotherapeutic treatment.

In summary, there is considerable evidence that anxiety is closely related to the diagnosis of cancer, the anticipation by patients of cancer treatment, and the occurrence of anticipatory nausea and vomiting. Since it is known that anxiety can lead to nausea and vomiting in some individuals, it is important to define the extent to which this psychological variable is responsible for anticipatory nausea and vomiting in patients receiving cancer chemotherapy.

Post-chemotherapy emesis

There is a clear relationship between severe emesis induced after application of chemotherapy and the occurrence of anticipatory nausea and vomiting. Poor antiemetic control after chemotherapy is correlated with a major incidence of anticipatory symptoms. The best known prophylactic treatment for anticipatory nausea and vomiting is adequate and effective control of post-chemotherapy induced emesis. It has been shown that patients with anticipatory nausea and vomiting had experienced severe post-treatment emesis from the first cycle of treatment. A sudden increase in chemotherapy-related emesis can be related to the experience of anticipatory symptoms. However, if post-treatment emesis appears after the fourth cycle of chemotherapy, the incidence of anticipatory nausea and vomiting again decreases.

Schedule of cytostatic treatment

There are several studies indicating that patients developing anticipatory nausea and vomiting had generally received chemotherapy for a longer time period than patients without these symptoms, and furthermore that patients with anticipatory nausea and vomiting had also received drug combinations with a higher emetogenic potential.

Susceptibility to motion sickness

As already mentioned, susceptibility to motion sickness is an important prognostic factor for the appearance of post-treatment nausea and vomiting. Since post-treatment symptoms are closely related to the development of anticipatory nausea and vomiting, it seems obvious that susceptibility to motion sickness can also contribute to the development of anticipatory symptoms. In fact, there are some studies indicating a relationship between motion sickness and anticipatory nausea and vomiting, but also other reports where such a correlation could not be found. Therefore it is not yet possible to clearly define the role of motion sickness for the development of anticipatory nausea and vomiting, and perhaps the relationships indicated in some studies are just coincidental.

Age

Besides the known relationships between age and the occurrence of post-chemotherapy nausea and vomiting, there are some studies indicating that age may also play a role in the development of anticipatory nausea and vomiting. Patients below the age of 50 years seem to have a higher incidence of anticipatory symptoms than older patients. There are some possible explanations for this: younger patients may receive more intensive chemotherapeutic treatment in order to achieve a high remission and cure rate, whereas older patients are more frequently exposed only to mild chemotherapeutic regimens with a palliative intention; younger patients are more likely to develop higher anxiety levels, and therefore may experience more often anticipatory nausea and vomiting related to this anxiety. Although these assumptions seem to have a logical basis, recent reports do not support them. Therefore more studies investigating these points are needed.

ALIMENTATION OF PATIENTS WITH CHEMOTHERAPY-RELATED EMESIS

The alimentation of patients receiving chemotherapeutic treatment and experiencing treatment-related nausea and vomiting represents a very difficult issue, despite the progress that has been made with treatment of chemotherapy-induced emesis. In fact, many cancer patients already experience great difficulties with food or liquid ingestion irrespective of the cytostatic treatment. This is for several reasons: in many cases solid tumors, especially those of gastrointestinal origin, may lead to obstruction of the gastrointestinal tract, leading to an inability to swallow food. An altered sense of taste or odor, psychological problems such as depression, stress and anxiety occurring in patients facing a malignant and potentially lethal disease, as well as an altered metabolism, can all contribute to malnutrition.[33-36,42-44]

Decreased or impossible food intake in cancer patients can also result from the mucositis that is frequently caused by intensive cytostatic treatment with certain drugs; furthermore, there may be several gastrointestinal and other secondary complications following chemotherapy, as well as patients' individual aversions to different food components, especially meat.

Nausea and vomiting symptoms related to chemotherapeutic treatment can lead to substantial additional problems.

In many cases, malnutrition of cancer patients caused by the disease itself or the necessary treatment modalities results in the necessity for parenteral nutrition as a last resort.

However, this difficult and demanding issue will not be handled in this chapter.

It is common experience that patients receiving highly emetogenic chemotherapy in many cases are not able to ingest any substantial amount of food on the day chemotherapy is given. Therefore it is recommended that such patients do not eat at least for a 8-hour period after chemotherapy. After this period, a liquid diet may be most appropriate, especially cold sweet drinks, warm tea or iced tea. Light soups, puddings, ice cream and milkshakes are then often best tolerated. Reducing the amount of food in each meal, with small meals taken at shorter periods, can generally help the situation, reducing peptic difficulties with large and heavy meals. Meals and drinks should be taken slowly, and solid food should be chewed well. After eating, a rest period is recommended. Excessively spicy, salty, sour, sweet or fatty foods should be avoided.

Considering the relevance of the nutritional status of the cancer patient for treatment outcome, every effort should be made to effectively treat chemotherapy-induced nausea and vomiting. Aggressive approaches of nutritional support, e.g. total-parenteral nutrition, must be considered in patients where other possibilities of food intake fail and the patient performance status is deteriorating.

REFERENCES

1. Laszlo J, Treatment of nausea and vomiting caused by cancer chemotherapy. *Cancer Treat Rev* 1982; **9**(Suppl B): 3–9.
2. Aapro MS, Prevention of chemotherapy-induced nausea and vomiting in patients with cancer. *Ariz Med* 1981; **38**: 843–5.
3. Seigel LJ, Longo DL, The control of chemotherapy-induced emesis. *Ann Intern Med* 1981; **95**: 352–9.
4. Editorial, Drugs acting on 5-hydroxytryptamine receptors. *Lancet* 1989; **ii**: 717–19.
5. Morrow GR, Chemotherapy-related nausea and vomiting: etiology and management. *CA Cancer J Clin* 1989; **39**: 89–104.
6. Krasnow SH, Problems in antiemetic trial design and interpretation. *Oncology Huntingt* 1989; **3**(8 Suppl): 5–10.
7. Carl PL, Cubeddu LX, Lindley C et al, Do humoral factors mediate cancer chemotherapy-induced emesis? *Drug Metab Rev* 1989; **21**: 319–33.
8. Gralla RJ, An outline of anti-emetic treatment. *Eur J Cancer Clin Oncol* 1989; **25**(Suppl 1): S7–11.
9. Wickham R, Managing chemotherapy-related nausea and vomiting: the state of the art. *Oncol Nurs Forum* 1989; **16**: 563–74.
10. Aitken TJ, Overview of antiemetic use in children receiving chemotherapy. *J Assoc Pediatr Oncol Nurs* 1989; **6**(2): 38.
11. Merrifield KR, Chaffee BJ, Recent advances in

the management of nausea and vomiting caused by antineoplastic agents. *Clin Pharm* 1989; **8**: 187–99.

12. Andrews PL, Rapeport WG, Sanger GJ, Neuropharmacology of emesis induced by anti-cancer therapy. *Trends Pharmacol Sci* 1988; **9**: 334–41.

13. Edwards CM, Chemotherapy induced emesis – mechanisms and treatment: a review. *J R Soc Med* 1988; **81**: 658–62.

14. Gralla RJ, Kris MG, Tyson LB, Clark RA, Controlling emesis in patients receiving cancer chemotherapy. *Recent Results Cancer Res* 1988; **108**: 89–101.

15. Jacobsen PB, Redd WH, The development and management of chemotherapy-related anticipatory nausea and vomiting. *Cancer Invest* 1988; **6**: 329–36.

16. O'Brien ME, Cullen MH, Therapeutic progress – review XXVIII. Are we making progress in the management of cytotoxic drug-induced nausea and vomiting? *J Clin Pharm Ther* 1988; **13**: 19–31.

17. Allan SG, Mechanisms and management of chemotherapy-induced nausea and vomiting. *Blood Rev* 1987; **1**: 50–7.

18. Morrow GR, Dobkin PL, Behavioral approaches for the management of adverse side effects of cancer treatment. *Psychiatr Med* 1987; **5**: 299–314.

19. Triozzi PL, Laszlo J, Optimum management of nausea and vomiting in cancer chemotherapy. *Drugs* 1987; **34**: 136–49.

20. Gralla RJ, Tyson LB, Kris MG, Clark RA, The management of chemotherapy-induced nausea and vomiting. *Med Clin North Am* 1987; **71**: 289–301.

21. Craig JB, Powell BL, The management of nausea and vomiting in clinical oncology. *Am J Med Sci* 1987; **293**: 34–44.

22. Dodds LJ, The control of cancer chemotherapy-induced nausea and vomiting. *J Clin Hosp Pharm* 1985; **10**: 143–66.

23. Yasko JM, Holistic management of nausea and vomiting caused by chemotherapy. *Top Clin Nurs* 1985; **7**: 26–38.

24. Moher D, Arthur AZ, Pater JL, Anticipatory nausea and/or vomiting. *Cancer Treat Rev* 1984; **11**: 257–64.

25. Fiore JJ, Gralla RJ, Pharmacologic treatment of chemotherapy-induced nausea and vomiting. *Cancer Invest* 1984; **2**: 351–61.

26. Pratt A, Lazar RM, Penman D, Holland JC, Psychological parameters of chemotherapy-induced conditioned nausea and vomiting: a review. *Cancer Nurs* 1984; **7**: 483–90.

27. Stoudemire A, Cotanch P, Laszlo J, Recent advances in the pharmacologic and behavioral management of chemotherapy-induced emesis. *Arch Intern Med* 1984; **144**: 1029–33.

28. Sledge GW Jr, Chemotherapy-induced nausea and vomiting. *Curr Opin Oncol* 1990; **2**: 909–14.

29. Pervan V, Practical aspects of dealing with cancer therapy-induced nausea and vomiting. *Semin Oncol Nurs* 1990; **6**(4 Suppl 1): 3–5.

30. Dundee JW, Yang J, The emetic effects of cancer chemotherapy. *Compr Ther* 1990; **16**(11): 58–63.

31. Andrykowski MA, The role of anxiety in the development of anticipatory nausea in cancer chemotherapy: a review and synthesis. *Psychosom Med* 1990; **52**: 458–75.

32. Hockenberry-Eaton M, Benner A, Patterns of nausea and vomiting in children: nursing assessment and intervention. *Oncol Nurs Forum* 1990; **17**: 575–84.

33. Tortorice PV, O'Connell MB, Management of chemotherapy-induced nausea and vomiting. *Pharmacotherapy* 1990; **10**: 129–45.

34. Sobrero A, Guglielmi A, Aschele C, Rosso R, Current strategies to reduce cisplatin toxicity. *J Chemother* 1990; **2**: 3–7.

35. Stewart DJ, Cancer therapy, vomiting, and antiemetics. *Can J Physiol Pharmacol* 1990; **68**: 304–13.

36. Naylor RJ, Rudd JA, Emesis and anti-emesis. *Cancer Surv* 1994; **21**: 117–35.

37. Ettinger DS, Preventing chemotherapy-induced nausea and vomiting: an update and a review of emesis. *Semin Oncol* 1995; **22**(4 Suppl 10): 6–18.

38. Hesketh P, Management of cisplatin-induced delayed emesis. *Oncology* 1996; **53**(Suppl 1): 73–7.

39. Verweij J, de Wit R, de Mulder PH, Optimal control of acute cisplatin-induced emesis. *Oncology* 1996; **53**(Suppl 1): 56–64.

40. Schmoll HJ, Casper J, Management of other non-cisplatin-induced emesis. *Oncology* 1996; **53**(Suppl 1): 51–5.

41. du Bois A, Vach W, Kiechle M et al, Pathophysiology, severity, pattern, and risk factors for carboplatin-induced emesis. *Oncology* 1996; **53**(Suppl 1): 46–50.

42. Morrow GR, Rosenthal SN, Models, mechanisms and management of anticipatory nausea and emesis. *Oncology* 1996; **53**(Suppl 1): 4–7.

43. Martin M, The severity and pattern of emesis following different cytotoxic agents. *Oncology* 1996; **53**(Suppl 1): 26–31.

44. Dicato M, Mechanisms and management of nausea and emesis [editorial]. *Oncology* 1996; **53**(Suppl 1): 1–3.

5

Platinum-induced acute nausea and vomiting

Michael Soukop

INTRODUCTION

Cytotoxic chemotherapy has a reputation with the general population for causing severe and unpleasant side-effects. Those most frequently reported by patients are nausea and vomiting,[1,2] and these are the problems they fear most.[3] Early in the development of chemotherapy, the significance to the patient and the frequency of these side-effects was underestimated. This was particularly true for nausea, which as a purely subjective symptom was often ignored or under-assessed. When nausea and vomiting were recognized, it was often felt that they were inevitable and that little could be done to alleviate them.

The introduction of cisplatin into the clinic, whilst a major advance in the treatment of several tumour types, had profound side-effect consequences. Here was a drug that in standard doses provoked universal nausea and vomiting, and for which, at high doses, emesis was virtually dose-limiting. This resulted in attention to, and strategies for, the relief of chemotherapy-induced emesis.

Whilst the details of assessment and methodology of antiemetic trials are discussed elsewhere, it is important to emphasize that al-though nausea and vomiting have some links, their frequency, severity and duration are separate phenomena.[4] The failure to ameliorate nausea and vomiting for the patient cannot be overemphasized. It influences significantly their quality of life and may lead to refusal to accept chemotherapy.[5] In some reports this may be 20% or more.[6] Fortunately, considerable success has been achieved, especially in the past decade, but more still needs to be done. A recent study has shown that although patients now report vomiting rated as fifth of their concerns, control of nausea is now their priority problem.[7]

Before discussing the results of studies of control of acute nausea and vomiting, it is relevant to outline important variable factors.

CISPLATIN: THE EMETIC CHALLENGE

Cisplatin is regarded as the most emetogenic of all currently used cytotoxic drugs. A recent article proposes a classification of the acute emetogenicity of cancer chemotherapy drugs.[8] Cisplatin is placed in category 5, the most emetogenic agents, in which nearly all

(>90%) patients are expected to vomit. Based on available evidence, cisplatin is placed as the most emetogenic of the level 5 cytotoxics. Cisplatin is one of the few chemotherapy agents in which placebo-controlled results have been reported. In four studies of cisplatin at doses 50–120 mg/m², 47 of 48 patients experienced acute emesis.[9–12]

Emesis has been divided into (a) acute emesis, which occurs within the first 24 hours of chemotherapy, and (b) delayed emesis, which occurs after the first 24 hours. Cisplatin therapy induces emesis with a latency period of about 2–4 hours and a peak incidence of 6–8 hours.[13] This timing clearly falls within the definition of acute emesis. There is a second peak that occurs after 24 hours. Smyth[14] has recently suggested that this separation is too simplistic and arbitrary. He proposed from study data that cisplatin-induced emesis may be triphasic, with an intermediate phase commencing at about 16 hours post therapy and a later phase maximal at 48–72 hours. The available evidence does seem to bear out a physiological difference between early and later emesis after cisplatin therapy. However, the relationship between the acute and delayed phases is complex.[15–17] The presence of early emesis is a strong but not absolute predictor of emesis in the delayed phase.

Equally, delayed emesis from a previous cycle of chemotherapy is a predictor for acute emesis in the subsequent cycle. This latter relationship is not simply explained by the emergence of anticipatory nausea and vomiting. Whilst some of the effect of acute emesis on intermediate- or delayed-phase emesis may be a spill over phenomenon, the major component of the clinical problem is a separate physiological mechanism.[4] The dose of cisplatin also affects the severity of the emetic challenge. Conventionally low-dose cisplatin <50 mg/m² is considered 'moderately' rather than severely emetogenic. The classification by Hesketh et al[8] places cisplatin <50 mg/m² in the level 4 category for agents causing 60–90% emesis. There is evidence of a dose–response effect for cisplatin >50 mg/m², with increasing nausea and vomiting at higher doses.[18]

Patient variability

A considerable variation exists in the susceptibility of patients to nausea and vomiting. These elements are discussed elsewhere in detail; however, it is well recognized that young females may have particular problems with cisplatin chemotherapy.[18–21] The presence of anxiety pre first chemotherapy is also recognized as important. It is of interest that symptoms associated with anxiety such as sweating and agitation may be more predictive for subsequent emesis than mood-related anxiety.[22] Patient perception and expectation as to what they anticipate to happen with their first course of chemotherapy based on their personality type and life experience is also debatably predictive. Patients with poor performance status also experience greater problems with emesis.[20] This may be in part the presence of anorexia, taste changes and pre-chemotherapy nausea, all of which are adverse prognostic factors for emesis with subsequent therapy.[21]

DEFINITIONS OF EMETIC CONTROL

The lack of agreed criteria for estimating the degree of nausea and vomiting presented early researchers with methodological problems. The intensity of emesis and duration that patients could experience with cisplatin resulted in the initial criteria being less rigorous than would have been ideal. In some studies nausea was not reported. With the development of the new serotonin group 3 receptor antagonists and their introduction into clinical practice in 1987, improved criteria were devised. Most studies with ondansetron used the scale shown in Table 5.1(A), with the nausea assessed as a secondary separate endpoint, as shown in Table 5.1(B). Most studies with granisetron used a scale combining vomiting and nausea, as shown in Table 5.1(C). In these scales an emetic episode is defined as one vomit or retch.

Whilst these scales had certain merits at the time, it is now felt that future studies should define complete control as no vomiting and no nausea. Additionally, intertrial comparisons of

Table 5.1 Evaluation scales for emesis	
(A) Measurement of vomiting: ondansetron	
Response	**Emetic Episodes in 24 h**
Complete control	0
Major control	1–2
Minor control	3–5
Failure	5
(B) Measurement of nausea: ondansetron	
None	—
Mild	Does not interfere with normal life
Moderate	Interferes with normal daily life
Severe	Bedridden owing to nausea
(C) Measurement of vomiting/nausea: granisetron	
Response	**Granisetron**
Complete	No vomiting and no or mild nausea
Major	1 emetic episode and/or moderate to severe nausea
Minor	2–4 emetic episodes
Failure	>5 emetic episodes

past studies can be difficult to interpret, depending on the scale used and the way in which the data was reported, i.e. combining percentage responses for complete and major control. Rigorous and uniform definitions of control not only are sensible in order to present accurate results of studies, but also have important practical effects for patients. Whilst most studies of antiemetics examine only the first cycle of chemotherapy in naive patients, the majority of patients receive multiple cycles of therapy. It is well recognized from the clinic that overall antiemetic control tends to diminish with increasing number of treatment cycles,[23] the critical factor for control being the experience of the patient in the previous cycle or cycles. Hence the strongest predictive factors for emesis in a subsequent cycle are found to be severe emesis and severe and prolonged nausea.[22] Therefore we should not ignore the importance of mild nausea or small amounts of vomiting with the first cycle of chemotherapy, since such events may evolve into progressively severe nausea and vomiting with subsequent chemotherapy or even anticipatory problems with multiple treatment cycles. It is ironic to consider that such a patient could have been defined as a complete or major responder in the first cycle of therapy, depending on the scales used.

EMESIS CONTROL WITH DOPAMINE RECEPTOR ANTAGONISTS

This group of compounds includes the substituted benzamide derivatives metoclopramide and alizapride, as well as the phenothiazines and butyrophenones.

The early use of metoclopramide at standard doses indicated that, whilst it had some antiemetic effect for moderately emetogenic chemotherapy, its value in cisplatin chemotherapy was marginal at best. The study reported by Gralla in 1981 of high-dose metoclopramide was revolutionary, both in concept and effect, and can be seen as the commencement of the modern era of antiemetic control.[9]

Gralla administered 10 mg/kg/day of metoclopramide compared with the standard 0.15–0.3 mg/kg/day used previously. The majority of patients experienced amelioration of emesis, and a proportion achieved complete protection. Such a regimen thus rapidly became the gold standard by which to compare further developments in antiemetics for patients receiving cisplatin. It had been assumed that metoclopramide mediated its antiemetic effect through the blockade of peripheral dopamine D2 receptors, as well as those in the chemoreceptor trigger zone. Within five years of Gralla's results, it was found that at high doses metoclopramide exerted its additional benefit by virtue of an affinity for the 5-hydroxytryptamine group 3 receptor (5-HT$_3$ receptor).[25] This resulted in the blockade of the signal transduction through this receptor, giving additional antiemetic protection from high-dose metoclopramide.

The results obtained by Gralla were subsequently confirmed in other studies, and deltarandomized comparisons confirmed the superiority of high-dose metoclopramide (HDM) to prochlorperazine, delta-9-tetrahydrocannabinol, butyrophenones, alizapride and dexamethasone.[24,26] Gralla used an intermittent high dose of 2 mg/kg i.v. and schedule commencing 30 minutes before chemotherapy, and repeated at 1.5, 3.5, 5.5 and 8.5 hours afterwards for a total of five doses.

It was felt by some workers that refinements and modifications to this protocol could be advantageous. Myer et al[27] indicated that a high serum level (>850 ng/ml) was important in obtaining optimum antiemetic control. Other studies emphasized the potential advantage of a prolonged steady state by using an initial bolus followed by a continuous infusion over 8–24 hours.[28] Although these concepts have theoretical advantages, only a few, small studies examined and demonstrated the superiority of metoclopramide 1 mg/kg bolus i.v. followed by 0.5 mg/kg/h infusion for 24 hours over 3–5 boluses of 1 mg/kg i.v. every 2 hours.[29–31] Thus this debate has never been fully resolved, and it can be concluded that in general the benefits of these refinements are relatively minor.[32,33]

Other alterations to the HDM schedule, such as a single 4–6 mg/kg i.v. bolus prechemotherapy compared with a 3 mg/kg i.v. bolus pre-chemotherapy followed by two further doses post-treatment, gave similar results. In two similar studies, the differing HDM schedules were combined with dexamethasone and lorazepam.[33,34] The overall control rates for emesis were similar in all groups, at about 60%. Thus it appears that the initial prechemotherapy antiemetic dose is probably the initial one.

High doses of oral metoclopramide have been tried, and whilst they are reasonably effective for doses of cisplatin up to 60 mg/m^2, they seem overall less beneficial than HDM i.v., and the incidence of extrapyramidal side-effects increases.[35,36] Since HDM i.v. appeared to give complete protection rates from emesis in about 30–40% of patients receiving cisplatin >50 mg/m^2, more progress was needed. The use of combination antiemetics using drugs with different modes of action and sites of activity as well as non-additive toxicities was logical. The most frequent and successful combination is that of HDM with corticosteroids. All randomized studies of such combinations have shown superiority or at least equivalence, with patients' preference in favour of the combination.[37–40]

Dexamethasone is the most commonly selected steroid for combination therapy, usually in doses in the range 8–50 mg.[41] Methylprednisolone has also frequently been studied, using dose ranges of 250–1000 mg.[41] Over these dose ranges there is little evidence that higher steroid doses are superior, or that early repetition of the dose in the first 24 hours post-chemotherapy improves acute emetic control.[42] The mechanism by which steroids exert their antiemetic effect remains uncertain, although a few hypotheses have been proposed:

- Since antineoplastic agents, especially cisplatin, can disrupt the blood–brain barrier and give rise to mild cerebral oedema, steroids may reduce emesis by reversing this.
- The anti-inflammatory effect of steroids may act as an antiemetic by either preventing the release of serotonin in the gut or by interfering with the activation of 5-HT$_3$ receptors in the gastrointestinal tract.

Steroids may act as antiemetics by a combination of these mechanisms or through other pathways that are as yet unclear.

Benzodiazepines were subsequently added to HDM–steroid combinations.[42] Whilst the benzodiazepines have relatively minor antiemetic properties as single agents, the benefits in combination therapy may stem more from their anxiolytic and sedative properties. The impairment of short-term memory may be of practical benefit in patients experiencing distressing nausea and vomiting by reducing perception of the problem and subsequent memory of the events.[33,34,39] This can thus reduce the risks of a conditioned response and the development of anticipatory emesis.

An additional benefit also accrues from the reduction of extrapyramidal side-effects associated with HDM. Therefore the addition of benzodiazepines to inpatient cisplatin regimens can improve patient acceptability and sleep pattern, which is reflected in crossover antiemetic trials as a significant patient preference for the arm containing the benzodiazepine.

However, in patients already well controlled by an HDM–dexamethasone combination the benzodiazepine-induced sedation may not be appreciated, and can engender in patients an unwelcome sense of loss of control and autonomy. It can also preclude the use of such schedules for outpatients.

Interestingly, there is no correlation between the level of sedation and the antiemetic benefit, thus suggesting a true additive benefit. In non-trial routine practice, therefore, benzodiazepines are often kept in reserve for patients in whom standard combinations are inadequate, initially or with subsequent chemotherapy cycles, or when anticipatory problems arise.

Toxicity of high-dose metoclopramide

Whilst extrapyramidal side-effects are rare at normal doses, except in the very young, the incidence increases significantly with HDM. The side-effects are often severe, and include acute dystonia, abnormal postures and muscle spasms. Patients can experience acute torticollis, trismus, laryngeal and pharyngeal spasms, as well as spasms of the tongue and oculogyric crises, opisthotonus and akathisia (restlessness, especially restless legs). Patients experiencing some or a number of the above phenomena are rarely prepared to risk them happening again, even if complete protection from emesis occurred. These extrapyramidal side-effects are related to the dopamine antagonism of metoclopramide.[41] The incidence of this complication is dose- and age-dependent, and also varies with the route of administration. The incidence in patients receiving HDM under 30 years of age was 27% compared with 2% in those over 30 years.[35] Oral metoclopramide increased the incidence of acute dystonic reactions in both age categories to 75% and 8% respectively. Extrapyramidal side-effects can be reversed by i.v. diphenhydramine 50 mg or benzodiazepine.

The use of diphenhydramine prophylactically in combination antiemetic schedules gained popularity but did not afford complete protection. The reduction in extrapyramidal side-effects from lorazepam, HDM and steroids has led to diphenhydramine being omitted from combinations when lorazepam is included.

The diarrhea that can occur secondarily to HDM is rarely a major problem. It has been observed from combination antiemetic studies that its incidence is diminished by corticosteroids.[43]

5-HYDROXYTRYPTAMINE CLASS 3 RECEPTOR ANTAGONISTS

The recognition that HDM's antiemetic effect was the result principally of blockade of the 5-hydroxytryptamine class 3 (5-HT$_3$) receptor together with its major side-effect being attributable to dopamine antagonism led to a number of major pharmacological programmes by several groups.

The characterization of the 5-HT$_3$ receptor led to the discovery of a number of 5-HT$_3$ receptor antagonists. The search was for compounds with a specific and high affinity for the 5-HT$_3$ receptor that would result in a signal blockade of its action. The first clinically reported studies of 5-HT$_3$ receptor antagonists were published in 1987, only six years after the HDM Gralla trials. Thus began a new and exciting chapter in antiemetic control.

The most commonly studied agents of this group are ondansetron (Zofran), granisetron (Kytril) and tropisetron (Navoban), although several other setrons have been produced and tested.

Interestingly, although these compounds differ in their chemical structure and receptor affinity, as well as their metabolism and potency in preclinical models,[44-47] any differences in the clinical setting have been more theoretical than actual.[48] More recent studies of the comparative merits of different 5-HT$_3$ receptor antagonists will be discussed in Chapter 11.

Ondansetron

More has been published on ondansetron alone or in combination schedules than on any other 5-HT$_3$ receptor. Using pharmacodynamic modelling based on plasma concentrations from clinical work, it was suggested that a concentration of 30 ng/ml of drug would be necessary to block all the 5-HT$_3$ receptors. Unlike granisetron, ondansetron was less specific and potent and its half-life in plasma was shorter.[46,47] The dose–response relationship to antiemesis was also nonlinear, with very low doses in preclinical tests being more effective

than slightly higher doses. Still higher doses then produced the best results, without much evidence of a dose–response thereafter. In common with other setrons, the retention time at the receptor may be much more important than the plasma $t_{1/2}$, but little is known of this and whether interpatient variability in receptor retention time exists. Nor is it known if such variability exists or whether this explains some of the clinical failures of 5-HT$_3$ antagonist antiemetics. In view of this lack of knowledge, it was proposed initially that an i.v. bolus dose would be required followed by a 24 mg continuous i.v. infusion over 24 hours. In Europe this regimen was compared in two double-blind randomized crossover studies against HDM using a loading dose of 3 mg/kg followed by 4 mg/kg over 8 hours.[15,16] Both studies demonstrated a superiority of control with ondansetron for nausea and vomiting. No emesis or major control (see Table 5.1) was seen for ondansetron in 75% and 72% of patients in the two studies respectively, compared with 42% and 41% for HDM. The theoretical disadvantage of a 'carry-over effect' between first and second treatment cycles due to the crossover design was not demonstrated in either study.

In the USA, because HDM was given standardly on an intermittent i.v. basis, a similar intermittent 3–6 daily bolus dose schedule for ondansetron was adopted. Superior efficacy was seen with ondansetron doses of 0.12–0.18 mg/kg, with no evidence of improved efficacy at higher doses.[49-52] Thus a schedule of three doses of 0.15 mg/kg every 3–4 hours was selected for the majority of the next series of antiemetic studies.

In a single-blind comparison of this schedule versus HDM (2 mg/kg i.v. × 6) in 307 patients receiving cisplatin at a high dose of ≥ 100 mg/m^2, ondansetron gave complete emetic protection in 40% of patients, compared with 30% for HDM.[53] There was also a higher complete-plus-major response rate and lower rate of failure. The median time to the first emetic episode was longer on ondansetron (20.5 versus 4.3 hours, $p < 0.001$).

A further European study using ondansetron (8 mg i.v. + 24 mg/24 h) compared with HDM

(4 mg/kg i.v. + 3 mg/24 h) in 97 patients receiving cisplatin 80–100 mg/m^2 reported a significantly superior outcome for ondansetron, the complete and major responses being 46% and 29%, compared with 16% and 26% for HDM.[15] In this study it was seen that the complete control rate for nausea (28%) was less satisfactory than that for emesis. This poorer response for the control of nausea has been commonly reported in other studies.

It would thus appear that the schedule of ondansetron administration does not seem to be critical. However, in circumstances in which patients experience acute emesis, despite initial 5-HT$_3$ antagonist prophylaxis, further bolus administration of a 5-HT$_3$ antagonist is frequently effective rescue. It is unknown whether this initial failure followed by rescue is related to 5-HT$_3$ antagonist retention time at the receptor.

There is little evidence that higher doses beyond an 'adequate' amount of a 5-HT$_3$ antagonist improve antiemetic control. A further series of studies explored the relationship of overall dose and schedule to antiemetic response. A large study by Seynaeve et al[54] randomized 535 patients into three antiemetic groups: (a) 8 mg i.v. ondansetron, (b) 32 mg i.v., both pre-chemotherapy, and (c) 8 mg i.v. pre-chemotherapy, followed by 24 mg/24 h infusion. The groups were well balanced for cisplatin dose and gender. There were no significant differences in antiemetic control, complete and major for groups (a) 74%, (b) 78% and (c) 74%. Analysis of the data did show that higher cisplatin doses were more emetogenic: cisplatin <70 mg/m^2, with complete control rates of 65%, versus those receiving >70 mg/m^2, with control rates of 48%. Additionally, females experienced poorer control: 43% compared with 67% for men.

A more recent three-arm study reported by Ruff et al[48] compared (a) 8 mg i.v. ondansetron, (b) 32 mg i.v. ondansetron and (c) 3 mg i.v. granisetron, all given pre-chemotherapy. The complete response rates for all three groups were similar: (a) 59%, (b) 51% and (c) 56%.

In contrast, in a large study in the USA, 699 patients receiving cisplatin, either at 50–70 mg/m^2 or greater than 100 mg/m^2, were randomized to one of three antiemetic arms: (a) 8 mg i.v. ondansetron, (b) 32 mg i.v. ondansetron and (c) 0.15 mg/kg i.v. × 3.[55] In this study 32 mg of ondansetron (b) was found to be significantly superior in emetic control compared with either groups (a) or (c). This was true for both cisplatin treatment levels. The antiemetic arms were comparable for patient prognostic factors. Whilst proportionately more patients in this study received higher-dose cisplatin, the outcome was true for both cisplatin levels. Thus differences between the European and US studies above are difficult to explain, and do not appear to relate to patient factors or cisplatin dose.

Examination of differences in the pattern of emesis in studies by Marty et al[15] and de Mulder et al[16] indicated that emetic failure in the HDM arms had a peak incidence of 6–12 hours. This correlated with the pattern of emesis seen for cisplatin therapy in placebo-treated subjects. In contrast, the pattern of failure in the ondansetron arms was usually delayed till after 16 hours. Work by Cubeddu and colleagues, and others, have demonstrated that 6–12-hour time period also correlated with an increased urinary excretion of 5-hydroxyindoleacetic acid, the main metabolite of 5-HT.[11,56,57] Hainsworth et al[53] suggested that the absence of this emetic pattern in ondansetron treated patients was because of a critical effect of pre-chemotherapy ondansetron on the 5-HT$_3$ receptor. This hypothesis was explored further in a follow-up study in which the total dose of ondansetron was kept the same but was either given as 32 mg i.v. pre-chemotherapy or 8 mg i.v. pre-chemotherapy, followed by 24 mg in a 24-hour infusion. No difference in complete emetic control was seen: 58% and 57% respectively.[58]

Granisetron

Granisetron has been studied at dose ranges from 2 to 300 µg/kg i.v., and been found to have a broad range of efficacy, with loss of activity only occurring at doses below 10 µg/kg.[59–62]

Differences in the scheduling approach and definitions of antiemetic control (see Table 5.1) were adopted for granisetron compared with the ondansetron studies. With granisetron, there was a tendency to a greater reliance on a single pre-chemotherapy i.v. dose, with allowance for two additional doses within the first 24 hours as rescue medication.

Cuppissol et al[12] reported a small randomized study comparing i.v. granisetron 40 μg/kg pre-chemotherapy with placebo in 28 patients receiving a mean cisplatin dose of greater than 80 mg/m². In both groups provision was made for two rescue doses of granisetron 40 μg/kg in the first 24 hours if antiemetic failure occurred.

Control was reported in 93% of the patients receiving granisetron, compared with 7% for the placebo group. Thus 93% of the placebo group required rescue, which resulted in an improvement or resolution of emesis in all patients in minutes. The activity of granisetron was thus clear, and its speed of action is potentially very valuable for patients requiring antiemetic rescue.

A large multicentre, double-blind, randomized study in chemotherapy-naive patients receiving cisplatin (≥50 mg/m²) investigated two doses of granisetron (40 and 160 μg/kg) given as a 5-minute infusion immediately prior to the cisplatin therapy.[60] Two additional rescue doses of 40 μg/kg were allowed in both arms. In the 335-patient study, no difference between the treatment arms was found, with complete control being 57% and 59% for 40 μg/kg and 160 μg/kg granisetron respectively. Hence the 40 μg/kg dose was recommended for subsequent comparative trials.

One such study reported by Chevalier[63] compared this with HDM at a dose of 3 mg/kg i.v., followed by a 4 mg/kg infusion over 8 hours, combined with dexamethasone 12 mg i.v. Seventy-seven chemotherapy-naive patients were randomized, all receiving cisplatin therapy at a minimum dose of 50 mg/m². Similar complete response rates of 70% for granisetron and 68% for the combination were achieved.

A study of similar design reported by Roila et al[64] found significant superiority for granisetron over the same comparator arm of

HDM and dexamethasone. In addition, they indicated that about 70% of patients receiving high-dose cisplatin chemotherapy, given pre-chemotherapy granisetron, are adequately controlled by this single i.v. dose of the 5-HT₃ antagonist.

In order to simplify the antiemetic dosing, 40 μg/kg of granisetron was translated to a standard 3 mg i.v. treatment in future studies. Recent work has demonstrated that this 3 mg dose can be reduced to 1 mg for most patients without loss of antiemetic effect.[62]

Tropisetron

Tropisetron too has been studied over a wide range of doses (5–48 mg/m²), and has been found to be effective and well tolerated at all dose levels.[65] A double-blind study compared three doses of tropisetron 5 mg orally the night before chemotherapy, 5 mg i.v. just prior to chemotherapy, followed by 5 mg orally the morning after chemotherapy, with a rather suboptimal dose of metoclopramide 20 mg/m² i.v. followed by 10 mg/m² orally three times daily together with dexamethasone 10 mg/m² i.v.[66] Perhaps not surprisingly, tropisetron was found to give a significantly superior complete control rate of 76% compared with 39% for the combination. In a follow-up, more conventionally designed study tropisetron was given 5 mg i.v. just prior to chemotherapy, followed by 5 mg orally daily for the three subsequent mornings, compared with HDM 3 mg/kg + 4 mg/kg infusion over 8 hours and 20 mg orally three times daily on days 2–4 post-chemotherapy.[67] The patients given HDM also received dexamethasone 8 mg i.v. pre-chemotherapy, with a further 4 mg i.v. 6 hours later. The combination antiemetic regimen afforded significantly superior complete control: 53% compared with 34% for tropisetron (p = 0.04).

The combined clinical experiences from a number of studies were reviewed by de Bruijn,[68] who reported tropisetron (5 mg i.v. or orally once daily) to be more effective than HDM (4–7 mg/kg) in preventing nausea and vomiting. For patients receiving cisplatin (50–120 mg/m^2), tropisetron was equally effective in controlling acute emesis as a combination of HDM, dexamethasone and either lorazepam or diphenhydramine. However, tropisetron was less successful than the combination in preventing acute nausea.

5-HT$_3$ RECEPTOR ANTAGONISTS IN COMBINATION THERAPY

The strategy of combining HDM and steroids together with the emerging data on 5-HT$_3$ antagonist success naturally led to the idea of 5-HT$_3$ antagonist/steroid combined therapy.

A double-blind, randomized, crossover study was instituted using three doses of ondansetron 0.15 mg/kg i.v. alone, or in combination with dexamethasone 20 mg i.v. pre-chemotherapy. A total of 89 patients completed both antiemetic cycles. Complete protection from emesis was found to be superior for the combination antiemetic regimen: 91% versus 64% ($p = 0.0005$).[69] Similar differences were seen when comparing rates for nausea. A further two studies confirmed the superiority of the combination of ondansetron and dexamethasone. Even though total patient numbers were limited in each of these latter studies, the similar conclusion and degree of difference was persuasive evidence for the validity of the results.

Subsequent studies compared best-combination HDM schedules with a 5-HT$_3$ antagonist combination. One of the first such trials combined HDM + dexamethasone 20 mg i.v. and diphenhydramine prophylactically, to try and reduce extrapyramidal side-effects, and thus improve the acceptability of the regimen, versus ondansetron 0.15 mg/kg × 3 i.v. + dexamethasone 20 mg i.v.[17]

Whilst a superior result for emesis control was achieved (59.6% versus 78.7%, $p < 0.002$) in favour of the ondansetron combination, no such difference was reported for nausea (65.6% versus 77.2% respectively).

An interesting difference also emerged in favour of the 5-HT$_3$ antagonist in that, whilst all patients received identical follow-up antiemetic on days 2, 3 and 4, namely metoclopramide 20 mg orally qid and dexamethasone 8 mg i.m. bid, significantly less vomiting was reported on days 2 and 3 for those receiving the ondansetron combination initially.

A similar study compared ondansetron 8 mg + dexamethasone 20 mg both given i.v. immediately before chemotherapy, followed by an oral ondansetron/dexamethasone combination for days 2–5, versus HDM and dexamethasone as in the previous study together with lorazepam 1.5 mg i.v. pre-chemotherapy, followed by oral metoclopramide/dexamethasone for days 2–5.[70] This double-blind randomized study demonstrated a superiority in favour of complete emetic control in the acute phase on day 1 for the ondansetron combination: 61% versus 40% ($p = 0.002$). These results have been supported by confirmatory studies for ondansetron and granisetron.[71-76] Currently no study of this type has shown an inferior result for a 5-HT$_3$ antagonist/corticosteroid combination. In addition, the side-effect profile in parallel group studies, or from the patient preference in crossover studies, was also in favour of the 5-HT$_3$/steroid combination.

ANTIEMETIC CONTROL WITH MULTIPLE-DAY CISPLATIN REGIMENS

Multiple-day cisplatin regimens are most commonly used in young men with potentially curable testicular germ cell tumours. Such regimens pose particular problems both in terms of the high potential emetogenicity over several days and also because of the age and length of antiemetic requirement of these patients. These factors make the patients very susceptible to extrapyramidal reactions from HDM.

Thus the development of the 5-HT$_3$ receptor antagonists was particularly welcome and potentially beneficial in this group of patients. The initial non-randomized studies confirmed this promise. The antiemetic protection was however, most evident on day 1. A double-blind study was conducted that randomized patients between ondansetron 0.15 mg/kg three times daily or HDM 1 mg/kg three times daily.[77] The failure rate for each 24-hour period (defined as >5 emetic episodes) was significantly more common with HDM than ondansetron: 50% versus 9% respectively ($p = 0.002$). The complete protection rate from emesis was also vastly superior for ondansetron (78% versus 14%, $p < 0.001$) on day 1, but did not achieve significance for days 2–5. The emetic control for ondansetron over progressive chemotherapy days diminished from 78% on day 1 to 57% on day 5. This was in keeping with the data previously reported from the non-randomized trials.[78] HDM conversely gave its best control on day 5, with rates improving from 14% on day 1 to 50% on day 5. Predictably, the reported HDM related extrapyramidal rate was high: 59%.

In keeping with other situations, combination antiemetic schedules of a 5-HT$_3$ antagonist and corticosteroid have further improved results. A small randomized trial by Einhorn et al[79] compared an ondansetron/dexamethasone regimen (ondansetron 0.15 mg/kg × 3 for 4–5 days + dexamethasone 8 mg pre-chemotherapy and 4 mg × 2 q 4-hourly days 1 and 2) against chlorpromizine (orally 50 mg q 4-hourly × 4 for 4–5 days). The reported results indicate a better overall control (defined as <3 emetic episodes in the study period) for the combination regimen: 89% versus 46% ($p = 0.009$). The complete control rates failed to be statistically different for the two groups. However, patient numbers were small.

CONCLUSIONS

The development of 5-HT$_3$ receptor antagonists for the control of chemotherapy-induced emesis represents one of the most significant advances in patient care over the past decade. The rapid translation of basic research to patient application and the concentration of effort on the details of antiemetic trials led to rapid change for patients. Patient perception of the problem has improved, but nausea remains a major concern.[7] The control of emesis acutely in patients receiving cisplatin therapy is best achieved at present by a 5-HT$_3$ receptor antagonist, together with a steroid (see Table 5.2). All 5-HT$_3$ receptor antagonists have a lower threshold. Above a 'standard dose', there is little evidence, overall, for improved control by larger doses. However, a number of studies have demonstrated a trend or occasionally a statistical improvement. Therefore perhaps a small advantage may still exist for a minority of patients from higher-dose 5-HT$_3$ receptor antagonists in situations that are particularly likely to present an emetic challenge, i.e. in the younger female on higher-dose cisplatin (>100 mg/m^2). No study to-date would have been large enough to give significant results for such circumstances. If emesis occurs in the first 24 hours post-cisplatin therapy, there is good evidence for the benefit of 5-HT$_3$ receptor antagonist treatment. Equally, there may be benefit from considering the primary period of control for the pre-chemotherapy antiemetic administration (5-HT$_3$ receptor antagonist + steroid) to be closer to 16 rather than 24 hours. Strategies planned for the complex and difficult problem of delayed emesis should therefore perhaps start then, rather than wait until 16 hours (see Chapter 6).

Patients experiencing problems from a previous cycle of cisplatin chemotherapy, i.e. severe emesis, severe or prolonged nausea, are particularly likely to have recurring and increasing nausea and vomiting with subsequent chemotherapy. In such circumstances, the addition of a benzodiazepine to the 5-HT$_3$ receptor antagonist/steroid combination can be valuable.

A change of 5-HT$_3$ receptor antagonist may also be worth trying, since there is a little evidence to suggest non-cross-resistance, and certainly there are theoretical differences between them.

There should be careful attention to individual factors that may predispose the patient to emesis, and, if possible, these should be addressed. Alternative strategies, such as relaxation techniques, including hypnosis, acupuncture, the additional use of seabands, and changing the time of day chemotherapy is given, have all been shown at times to be beneficial in some patient groups.

Table 5.2 Antiemetic recommendation for cisplatin chemotherapy

Acute period 0–24 hours
    First-line antiemetic immediately prechemotherapy
    Evidence based on 5-HT$_3$ receptor antagonist + steroid

Suggested:	(a)	ondansetron	8 mg i.v., high emetic risk, 32 mg i.v.?
or	(b)	granisetron	1–3 mg i.v., high emetic risk, 3 mg i.v.
or	(c)	tropisetron	5 mg i.v.
plus	(d)	dexamethasone	8–20 mg i.v.
or	(e)	methylpredisolone	250–1000 mg i.v.

Delayed period 24 hours + (see Chapter 6)
    Suggested additional antiemetic if planned at 16 hours

Options:	(a)	metoclopramide orally,	10–20 mg tid
or	(b)	domperidone orally,	10–30 mg tid
or	(c)	5-HT$_3$ receptor antagonist: ondansetron, 8 mg orally bd up to 3 days usually tropisetron, 5 mg orally daily up to 3 days usually granisetron not indicated	
plus	(d)	dexamethasone, orally, varying doses used (e.g. 4 mg tid, 2 days plus 4 mg bd, 3 days)	

Second or subsequent chemotherapy course with previous emetic problems

Suggestions:	(a)	Increase 5-HT$_3$ receptor antagonist dose (e.g. ondansetron, 8–32 mg i.v.)
	(b)	Change 5-HT$_3$ receptor antagonist (e.g. ondansetron to granisetron)
	(c)	Add benzodiazepine (e.g. lorazepam 1–4 mg i.v. pre-chemotherapy, can be repeated) to 5-HT$_3$ receptor antagonist/steroid combination
	(d)	Address risk factors if possible (e.g. consider relaxation therapy, etc.)
	(e)	Methotrimeprazine 25–200 mg i.v. infusion over 24 h

Whilst the majority of patients have acute cisplatin-induced emesis controlled, more trials need to be done. These must, however, be rigorously conducted and a universally adopted assessment of complete control, meaning no vomiting and no nausea, used in future. This would allow easier intertrial comparisons and be a more truthful predictor of emesis control for patients receiving multiple treatment cycles. The development of a new range of NK1 receptor antagonist antiemetics alone, or in combination, is eagerly awaited, and may be another important step in better antiemetic control.

REFERENCES

1. Kaye SB, How should nausea be assessed in patients receiving chemotherapy? *Cancer Treat Rev* 1991; **1**: 85–93.
2. Bakowski MT, Advances in anti-emetic therapy. *Cancer Treat Rev* 1984; **11**: 237–56.
3. Coates A, Abraham S, Kaye SB et al, On receiving end-patient perception of the side-effects of cancer chemotherapy. *Eur J Cancer Clin Oncol* 1983; **19**: 203–8.
4. Morrow GR, The assessment of nausea and vomiting: post problems, current issues and suggestions for future research. *Cancer* 1984; **53**: 2267–78.
5. Hickok JT, Morrow GR, A biobehavioural model of patient reported nausea: implications for clinical practice. *Adv Med Psychother* 1993; **6**: 227–40.
6. Stewart DJ, Cancer therapy, vomiting and antiemetics. *Can J Physiol Pharmacol* 1990; **68**: 304–13.
7. Griffen AM, Butow PN, Coates AS et al, On the receiving end. V: Patient perceptions of the side effects of cancer chemotherapy in 1993. *Ann Oncol* 1996; **7**: 189–95.
8. Hesketh PJ, Kris MG, Grunberg SM et al, Proposal for classifying the acute emetogenicity of cancer chemotherapy. *J Clin Oncol* 1997; **15**: 103–9.
9. Gralla RJ, Itri LM, Pisko SE, Antiemetic efficacy of high-dose metoclopramide: randomised trials with placebo and prochlorperazine in patients with chemotherapy-induced nausea and vomiting. *N Engl J Med* 1981; **305**: 905–9.
10. Homesley HD, Gaincy JM, Jobson VN, Cisplatin chemotherapy and emesis in patients given metoclopramide and controls. *N Engl J Med* 1982; **307**: 250–1.
11. Cubbeddu LX, Hoffman IS, Fuenmayor NT, Finn AL, Efficacy of ondansetron and the role of serotonin in cisplatin-induced nausea and vomiting. *N Engl J Med* 1990; **322**: 810–16.
12. Cupissol DR, Serrou B, Caubel M, The efficacy of granisetron as a prophylactic anti-emetic and intervention agent in high-dose cisplatin-induced emesis. *Eur J Cancer* 1990; **26**: S23–7.
13. Triozzi PL, Laszlo J, Optimum management of nausea and vomiting in cancer chemotherapy. *Drugs* 1987; **2**: 136–49.
14. Smyth J. Delayed emesis after high dose cisplatin – the residual problem. In: *Proceedings of the Satellite Symposium to the XVII Congress of the European Society for Medical Oncology, Lyon, France, 8 November, 1992*: 24–6.
15. Marty M, Pouillart P, Scholl S et al, Comparison of the 5-hydroxytryptamine (serotonin), antagonist ondansetron (GR 38032F) with high-dose metoclopramide in the control of cisplatin-induced emesis. *N Engl J Med* 1990; **322**: 816–21.
16. De Mulder PHM, Seynaeve C, Vermorken JB et al, Ondansetron compared with high-dose metoclopramide in prophylaxis of acute and delayed cisplatin-induced nausea and vomiting. *Ann Intern Med* 1990; **113**: 834–40.
17. Beck TM, Ciociola AA, Jones SE et al, Efficacy of oral ondansetron in the prevention of emesis in outpatients receiving cyclophosphamide-based chemotherapy. *Ann Intern Med* 1993; **118**: 407–13.
18. Seynaeve C, Schuller J, Buser K et al, Comparison of the anti-emetic efficacy of different doses of ondansetron, given as either a continuous infusion or a single intravenous dose in acute cisplatin-induced emesis: A multicentre, double-blind, randomised, parallel group study. *Br J Cancer* 1992; **66**: 192–7.
19. Watson M, Anticipatory nausea and vomiting: broadening the scope of psychological treatments. *Support Care Cancer* 1993; **1**: 171–7.
20. Pollera C, Giannarelli D, Prognostic factors influencing cisplatin-induced emesis. Definition and validation of a predictive logistic model. *Cancer* 1989; **64**: 1117–22.
21. Osoba D, Zee B, Pater J et al, Determinants of post-chemotherapy nausea and vomiting in

patients with cancer. *J Clin Oncol* 1997; **15**: 116–23.

22. Morrow GR, Behavioural factors influencing the development and expression of chemotherapy induced side effects. *Br J Cancer* 1992; **66**(Suppl XIX): S54–61.

23. Roila F, on behalf of the Italian Group for Antiemetic Research, Control of acute cisplatin-induced emesis over repeat courses of chemotherapy. *Oncology* 1996; **53**(Suppl 1): 65–72.

24. Sagar SM, The current role of anti-emetic drugs in oncology: a recent revolution in patient symptom control. *Cancer Treat Rev* 1991; **18**: 95–135.

25. Miner WD, Sanger G, Inhibition of cisplatin-induced vomiting by selective 5-hydroxytryptamine M-receptor antagonism. *Br J Pharmacol* 1986; **88**: 497–9.

26. Craig JB, Powell BL, The management of nausea and vomiting in clinical oncology. *Am J Med Sci* 1987; **293**: 34–44.

27. Meyer BR, Levin M, Draper DE et al, Optimising metoclopramide control of cisplatin induced emesis. *Ann Intern Med* 1984; **100**: 393–5.

28. Kerr PJ, Graham J, McGovern E et al, The relationship between steady state metoclopramide levels and control of emesis during treatment with cisplatin. *Br J Clin Pharm* 1985; **20**: 426–7.

29. Warrington PS, Allan SG, Cornbleet MA et al, Optimising antiemesis in cancer chemotherapy: efficacy of continuous versus intermittent infusion of high-dose metoclopramide in emesis-induced by cisplatin. *Br Med J* 1986; **293**: 1334–7.

30. Agostinucci WA, Gannon RH, Golub GR et al, Continuous infusion of metoclopramide for prevention of chemotherapy-induced emesis. *Clin Pharmacol* 1986; **5**: 150–3.

31. Navari RM. Comparison of intermittent versus continuous infusion metoclopramide in control of acute nausea induced by cisplatin chemotherapy. *J Clin Oncol* 1989; **7**: 943–6.

32. Grunberg SM, McDermed JE, Bernstein L, Cohen JL, Examination of the correlation of serum MCP levels with antiemetic efficacy in patients receiving cisplatin. *Cancer Chemother Pharmacol* 1987; **20**: 332–6.

33. Kris MG, Gralla RJ, Clark RA et al, Antiemetic control and prevention of side effects of anticancer therapy with lorazepam when used in combination with metoclopramide and dexamethasone. *Cancer* 1987; **60**: 2816–22.

34. Clark RA, Gralla RJ, Kris MG, Tyson LB, Exploring very high-dose of MCP (4–6 mg/kg): preservation of efficacy and safety with only one

single dose in a combination anti-emetic regimen. *Proc Am Soc Clin Oncol* 1989; **8**: 330.

35. Tyson LB, Gralla RJ, Kris MG et al, Dose-ranging antiemetic trial of high-dose oral MCP. *Am J Clin Oncol* 1989; **12**: 239–43.

36. Anthony L, Krozeby M, Woodward N et al, Antiemetic efficacy of oral versus intravenous MCP in patients receiving cisplatin. *J Clin Oncol* 1985; **4**: 98–103.

37. Allan SG, Cornbleet MA, Warrington PS et al, Dexamethasone and high-dose metoclopramide: Efficacy in controlling cisplatin-induced nausea and vomiting. *Br Med J* 1984; **289**: 878–9.

38. Rosell R, Abad-Esteve A, Ribas-Munds M, Moreno I, Evaluation of a combination antiemetic regimen including IV high-dose metoclopramide, dexamethasone and diphenhydramine in cisplatin-based chemotherapy regimens. *Cancer Treat Rep* 1985; **69**: 909–10.

39. Roila F, Tonato M, Basurto C et al, Antiemetic activity of high-dose metoclopramide combined with methylprednisolone versus metoclopramide alone in cisplatin-treated cancer patients. *J Clin Oncol* 1987; **5**: 141–9.

40. Cognette F, Carlini P, Pinnaro P et al, Maintenance of antiemetic effect of a MCP/Dex combination during subsequent cisplatin courses. *Oncology* 1986; **43**: 292–4.

41. Seynaeve C, de Mulder PHM, Verweij J, Gralla RJ, Controlling cancer chemotherapy-induced emesis: an update. *Pharm Weekbl (Sci)* 1991; **13**: 189–97.

42. Aapro MS, Present role of corticosteroids as antiemetics. In: *Recent Results in Cancer Research* (Senn HJ, Glaus A, eds). Berlin: Springer-Verlag, 1991: 91–100.

43. Kris MG, Gralla RJ, Tyson LB et al, Improved control of cisplatin-induced emesis with high-dose metoclopramide and with combinations of metoclopramide, dexamethasone and diphenhydramine. *Cancer* 1985; **55**: 527–34.

44. Seynaeve C, Verweij J, de Mulder PHM, 5-HT$_3$ receptor antagonists: a new approach in emesis. A review of ondansetron, granisetron and tropisetron. *Anticancer Drugs* 1991; **2**: 343–55.

45. Tyers MB, Freeman AJ, Mechanism of antiemetic activity of 5-HT$_3$ receptor antagonists. *Oncology* 1992; **49**: 263–8.

46. Andrews PLR, Bhandari P, Davey PT et al, Are all 5-HT$_3$ receptor antagonists the same? *Eur J Cancer* 1992; **28A**(Suppl 1): S2–6.

47. Aapro MS, Setron: are 5-HT$_3$ receptor antagonists different? *Eur J Cancer* 1993; **29A**: 1655.

48. Ruff P, Paska W, Goedhals L et al, Ondansetron compared with granisetron in the prophylaxis of cisplatin-induced acute emesis: a multicentre, double-blind, randomised, parallel-group study. *Oncology* 1994; **51**: 113–18.

49. Grundberg SM, Stevenson LL, Russell CA, McDermed JE, Dose ranging phase I study of the serotonin antagonist GR38032F for prevention of cisplatin-induced nausea and vomiting. *J Clin Oncol* 1989; **7**: 1137–41.

50. Kris MG, Gralla RJ, Clark RA, Tyson LB, Phase II trials of the serotonin antagonist GR38032F for the control of vomiting caused by cisplatin. *J Natl Cancer Inst* 1989; **81**: 42–6.

51. Hesketh PJ, Murphy WK, Lester EP et al, A novel compound effective in the prevention of acute cisplatin-induced emesis. *J Clin Oncol* 1987; **7**: 700–5.

52. Khojasteh A, Sartiano G, Tapazoglou E et al, Ondansetron for the prevention of emesis induced by high-dose cisplatin. *Cancer* 1990; **66**: 1101–5.

53. Hainsworth J, Harvey W, Pendergrass K et al, A single-blind comparison of intravenous ondansetron, a selective serotonin antagonist, with intravenous metoclopramide in the prevention of nausea and vomiting associated with high-dose cisplatin chemotherapy. *J Clin Oncol* 1991; **9**: 721–8.

54. Seynaeve C, Schuller J, Buser K et al, Comparison of the anti-emetic efficacy of different doses of ondansetron, given either as a continuous infusion or as a single intravenous dose, in acute cisplatin-induced emesis. A multicentre, double-blind, randomised, parallel group study. *Br J Cancer* 1992; **66**: 192–7.

55. Beck TM, Hesketh PJ, Madajewicz S et al, Stratified, randomised, double-blind comparison of intravenous ondansetron administered as a multiple-dose regimen versus two single-dose regimens, in the prevention of cisplatin-induced nausea and vomiting. *J Clin Oncol* 1992; **10**: 1969–75.

56. Cubbeddu LX, Hoffman IS, Fuenmayor NT, Malave JJ, Changes in serotonin metabolism in cancer patients: its relationship to nausea and vomiting induced by chemotherapeutic drugs. *Br J Cancer* 1992; **66**: 198–203.

57. Wilder-Smith OHG, Borgeat A, Chappuis P et al, Urinary serotonin metabolite excretion during cisplatin chemotherapy. *Cancer* 1993; **72**: 2239–41.

58. Marty M, D'Allens H, Etude randomisée en double-isu comparant l'efficacité de l'ondansetron selon deux modes d'administration: injec-tion unique et perfusion continué. *Cahiers Cancer* 1990; **2**: 541–6.

59. Kamanabrou D, on behalf of the Granisetron Study Group, Intravenous granisetron. Establishing the optimal dose. *Eur J Cancer* 1992; **28A**(Suppl 1): S6–11.

60. Soukop M, on behalf of the Granisetron Study Group, A comparison of two dose levels of granisetron in patients receiving high-dose cisplatin. *Eur J Cancer* 1990; **29**(Suppl 1): S15–19.

61. Riviere A, on behalf of the Granisetron Study Group, Dose finding study of granisetron in patients receiving high-dose cisplatin chemotherapy. *Br J Cancer* 1994; **69**: 967–71.

62. Navari RM, Kaplan HG, Gralla RJ et al, Efficacy and safety of granisetron, a selective 5-hydroxy-tryptamine-3 receptor antagonist, in the prevention of nausea and vomiting induced by high-dose cisplatin. *J Clin Oncol* 1994; **12**: 2204–10.

63. Chevalier B, on behalf of the Granisetron Study Group, The control of acute cisplatin-induced emesis – a comparative study of granisetron and a combination regimen of high-dose metoclopramide and dexamethasone. *Br J Cancer* 1993; **68**: 176–80.

64. Roila F, Tonato M, Basurto C et al, Protection from nausea and vomiting in cisplatin-treated patients: high-dose metoclopramide combined with methylprednisolone versus metoclopramide combined with dexamethasone and diphenhydramine. *J Clin Oncol* 1989; **7**: 1693–700.

65. Van Belle SJP, Stamatakis L, Bleiberg H et al, Dose-finding study of tropisetron in cisplatin-induced nausea and vomiting. *Ann Oncol* 1994; **5**: 821–5.

66. Krzakowski M, Madaj G, Pawinsky A, A comparative study of the use of ICS 205-930/Navoban. A 5-HT$_3$ antagonist, versus standard anti-emetic regimen of dexamethasone and metoclopramide in the treatment of chemotherapy-induced emesis. *Ann Oncol* 1992; **3**(Suppl 1): 155–9.

67. Kris MG, Tyson LB, Tropisetron (ICS 205-930): a selective 5-hydroxytryptamine antagonist. *Eur J Cancer* 1993; **29A**(Suppl 1): 30–2.

68. de Bruijn KM, Tropisetron: a review of the clinical experience. *Drugs* 1992; **43**(Suppl 3): 11–22.

69. Roila F, Tonato M, Cognetti F et al, Prevention of cisplatin-induced emesis: a double-blind multicentre randomised crossover study comparing ondansetron and ondansetron plus dexamethasone. *J Clin Oncol* 1991; **9**: 675–8.

70. Cunningham D, Hill M, Dicato M et al, Optimal antiemetic therapy for cisplatin-induced emesis over repeated courses. *Proc Am Soc Clin Oncol* 1994; **13**: 449.

71. Italian Group for Antiemetic Research, Ondansetron + dexamethasone vs metoclopramide + dexamethasone + diphenhydramine in prevention of cisplatin-induced emesis. *Lancet* 1992; **340**: 96–9.

72. Hesketh PJ, Harvey WH, Harker WG et al, A randomised, double-blind comparison of intravenous ondansetron alone and in combination with intravenous dexamethasone in the prevention of high-dose cisplatin-induced emesis. *J Clin Oncol* 1994; **12**: 596–600.

73. Smith DB, Newlands ES, Rustin GJS et al, Comparison of ondansetron and ondansetron plus dexamethasone as antiemetic prophylaxis during cisplatin-containing chemotherapy. *Lancet* 1991; **338**: 487–90.

74. Smyth JF, Coleman RJ, Nicolson M et al, Does dexamethasone enhance control of acute cisplatin-induced emesis by ondansetron? *Br Med J* 1991; **303**: 1423–6.

75. Chevalier B, Marty M, Paillarse JM, and the Ondansetron Study Group. Methylprednisolone enhances the efficacy of ondansetron in acute and delayed cisplatin-induced emesis over at least three cycles. *Br J Cancer* 1994; **70**: 1171–5.

76. Heron JF, Goedhals L, Jordaan JP et al, Oral granisetron alone and in combination with dexamethasone: a double-blind randomised comparison against high-dose metoclopramide plus dexamethasone in prevention of cisplatin-induced emesis. *Ann Oncol* 1994; **5**: 579–84.

77. Sledge GW, Einhorn LH, Nagy C, House K, Phase III double-blind comparison of intravenous ondansetron and metoclopramide as an antiemetic therapy for patients receiving multiple-day cisplatin-based chemotherapy. *Cancer* 1992; **70**: 2524–8.

78. Hainsworth JD, The use of ondansetron in patients receiving multiple-day cisplatin regimens. *Semin Oncol* 1992; **19**(Suppl 10): 48–52.

79. Einhorn LH, Nagy C, Werner K, Finn AL, Ondansetron: a new antiemetic for patients receiving cisplatin chemotherapy. *J Clin Oncol* 1990; **8**: 731–5.

6

Platinum-induced delayed emesis

Andreas du Bois

INTRODUCTION

Emesis occurring on the days following the day of cisplatin chemotherapy has commonly been classified as *delayed emesis*. This definition of *acute* and *delayed emesis* has been established based on studies in patients receiving single-day cisplatin-containing chemotherapies who had received antiemetics on the day of chemotherapy only.[1] The investigators observed emesis and nausea in a significant proportion of patients even when good control of acute emesis had been achieved. Acute emesis was defined as emesis occurring within the first 24 hours after cisplatin application (day 1); emesis commencing later than 24 hours following cisplatin has been defined as delayed emesis. Later, the idiom *delayed emesis* has been used for all emesis observed from day 2 of a chemotherapy course on. The application of this idiom was extended to non-cisplatin chemotherapies also, although the original definition was derived from studies in patients with cisplatin-containing chemotherapies only. However, owing to some differences between cisplatin- and non-cisplatin-induced emesis, both groups should be analysed separately.

CISPLATIN-INDUCED DELAYED EMESIS

The pathophysiological mechanisms underlying cisplatin-induced delayed emesis are not yet understood. Serotonin, which plays a major role in the pathomechanism of acute cisplatin-induced emesis, does not seem to play a crucial role as a mediator of delayed emesis. Urinary excretion of 5-hydroxyindoleacetic acid (5-HIAA), the main metabolite of serotonin (5-HT), increases dramatically in the first hours after cisplatin administration, but cannot be demonstrated above baseline levels in the urine collected later than 24 hours in these patients (Figure 6.1, data from our group). The majority of investigators believe that the mechanisms of acute and delayed emesis differ, and some models have been constructed suggesting disturbed gut motility and products of cellular breakdown as etiology for delayed emesis.[2] However, theories remain vague as long as the pathophysiology is not clear. From the clinician's point of view, there is an empirical correlation between acute and delayed emesis: patients in whom acute emesis is controlled completely will develop delayed emesis less frequently than patients with a poor control of acute emesis. This common clinical observation can be interpreted in a twofold way. The first hypothesis is that the occurrence of acute emesis lowers the psychological or physiological thresholds for emesis, or even stimulates the pathomechanisms of delayed emesis. This hypothesis fits well with patients reporting vomiting when brushing teeth in the morning after the chemotherapy day, which implies vomiting induced by a common trigger (mechanical irritation) that normally does not induce vomiting, but does so in a situation when the threshold for vomiting is far lower than under normal circumstances. Contradictory findings are that even patients who had a complete control of acute vomiting can develop delayed emesis. Another possible explanation for delayed emesis is that both forms are completely separate regarding their pathophysiology, and occur coincidentally. A common sensitivity for both triggers for acute and delayed emesis makes one patient very sensitive, whilst another patient is rather refractory against emetogenic stimuli either for acute or delayed emesis. Patients who have a low sensitivity for emetogenic stimuli will then show a complete control of acute emesis and a complete control of delay symptoms in most cases, while patients with a higher sensitivity will vomit on day 1 and will react to the stimuli of delayed emesis in the majority of cases. However, both models have implications for emetic research, especially for studies focusing on delayed emesis. A good control of acute emesis may have an impact on delayed emesis, and may simulate antiemetic efficacy of sub-

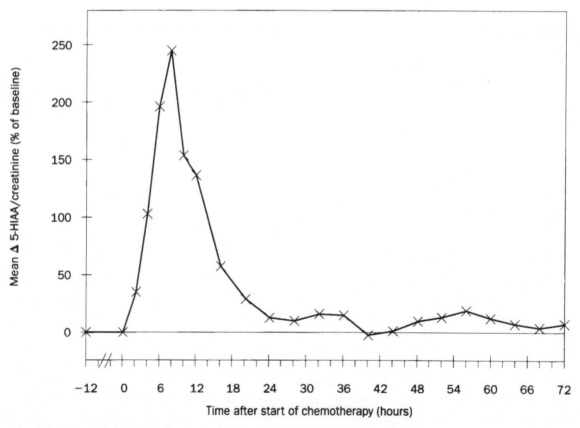

Figure 6.1 Urinary 5-hydroxyindoleacetic acid excretion following cisplatin chemotherapy (5-HIAA corrected for creatinine; values express deviation from baseline values measured before chemotherapy).

stances administered from day 2 on. Furthermore, different antiemetics given on day 1 can interact with delayed emesis in various ways: one substance can act against both delayed and acute emesis, another may only work against acute emesis. Even when acute and delayed emesis are induced by different pathophysiological pathways, the reduction of acute emesis will have an impact on the observation of delayed emesis by changing the cut-off from which on emesis is triggered mainly by the 'delayed-emesis mechanism'. The cut-off of 24 hours has been chosen arbitrarily, and simple mathematical models show the limitations of this fixed cut-off (Figures 6.2 and 6.3). These models show that control of acute emesis put the cut-off between acute and delayed emesis towards earlier hours, even if delayed emesis itself commences unchanged. These obvious difficulties in evaluating a clinical phenomenon without knowledge of its pathophysiological background indicate that all antiemetic studies that focus on delayed emesis should also look at acute emesis, as well as emesis occurring within the whole chemotherapy course.

The 'natural course' of cisplatin-induced delayed emesis

Several studies have reported the 'natural course' of delayed emesis in patients receiving antiemetics on day 1 only.[1,3-8] The curve of the frequency of emesis in these patients shows a peak on day 3, when about half reported delayed emesis (Figure 6.4). The majority of studies observed patients over five days only, although delayed emesis lasts probably for longer than five days. On average, 25% of patients still report emesis on day 5 (Figure 6.4). The analysis of the 'natural course' of delayed emesis has to be interpreted very cautiously, because all these patients have received antiemetics on day 1. There might be an interaction of some antiemetics given on day 1 with delayed emesis. This possibility is confirmed by the observation that different antiemetic regimens given on day 1 have a specific impact on the frequency of delayed emesis, although no

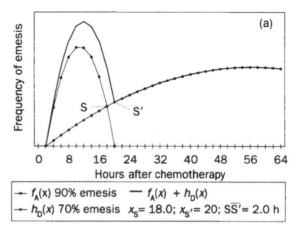

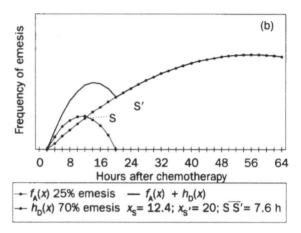

Figure 6.2 Model of acute and delayed emesis A: f_A is acute emesis, which is high (90% emesis considered); h_D is delayed emesis (70% emesis considered), starting together with acute emesis two hours after chemotherapy administration; $f_A + h_D$ is the clinically observed emesis. x_S is the cut-off from which point on emesis is mainly delayed emesis; $x_{S'}$ is the clinically observed 'cut-off' from which point on emesis is defined as delayed emesis. SS' is the distance between the hypothetical pathophysiological and the clinically defined cut-off between acute and delayed emesis. In model (a) no antiemetics are given; in model (b) acute emesis is reduced whilst delayed emesis is not controlled. In model (b) the difference between the observed and the 'true' cut-off is 7.6 hours. Note that in this model the observed 'acute' emesis consists mainly of 'true' delayed emesis.

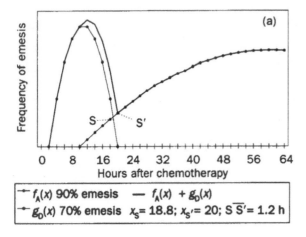

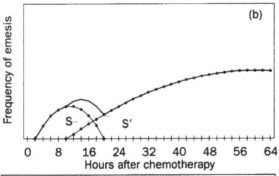

Figure 6.3 Model of acute and delayed emesis D: f_A is acute emesis, which was controlled in 75% of patients (25% acute emesis); g_D is delayed emesis (70% emesis), starting 8 hours later than acute emesis (10 hours after chemotherapy administration); $f_A + g_D$ is the clinically observed emesis. x_S is the cut-off from which point on emesis is mainly delayed emesis; $x_{S'}$ is the clinically observed 'cut-off' from which point on emesis is defined as delayed emesis. SS' is the distance between the hypothetical pathophysiological and the clinically defined cut-off between acute and delayed emesis (in model (b) the difference is 2.8 hours). In model (b) control of acute emesis is simulated.

antiemetics were given on subsequent days (Figure 6.5). Delayed emesis is reported more frequently when the antiemetic regimen on day 1 consists of a combination of metoclopramide and a corticosteroid[3-6,9-12] than in patients receiving single-agent setrons[13-16] or a combination of setrons and corticosteroids for antiemetic prophylaxis on day 1.[7,13,17] The comparison between these three groups based on a retrospective cumulative analysis reveals significantly less emesis in patients treated with a setron–corticosteroid combination on day 1 compared with patients treated with a metoclopramide–corticosteroid combination on day 1. The relative risk for delayed emesis is 0.80 (95% CI 0.68–0.93) in advantage for the setron–corticosteroid combination. Comparison between single-agent setron therapy and the metoclopramide-based combination, as well as the comparison between single-agent setrons with the setron–corticosteroid combination, did not reveal any significant difference (95% CI included 1 in both comparisons).

Management of cisplatin-induced delayed emesis

The cumulative analysis of randomized trials comparing different treatments for cisplatin-induced delayed emesis reveals that both corticosteroids and metoclopramide and single-agent setrons are superior to placebo administration on days 2–5 (Table 6.1). The retrospective analysis of single-agent activity against delayed emesis shows the highest efficacy rates for corticosteroids, followed by single-agent metoclopramide and then setrons (Table 6.2). The latter group proved superior to placebo in two of four studies only. Thus the role of setrons as single-agent treatment for cisplatin-induced delayed emesis should not be regarded as definitively defined. In contrast, setrons combined with corticosteroids have shown activity against delayed emesis exceeding the efficacy reported for single-agent corticosteroids. Generally, combination therapy consisting of either setrons plus corticosteroids or metoclopramide plus corticosteroids seems to produce

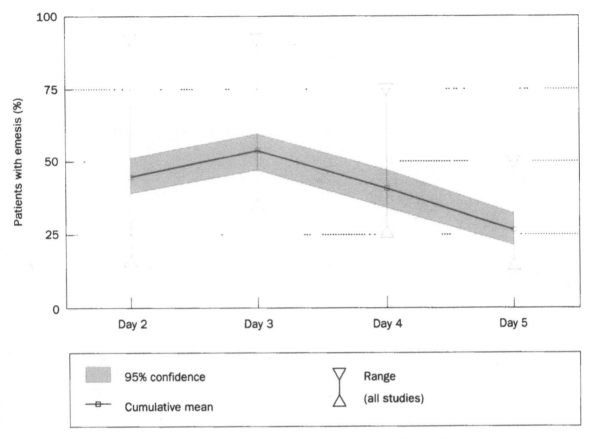

Figure 6.4 Pattern of the 'natural course' of cisplatin-induced delayed emesis in patients receiving any antiemetics on day 1 only. This is a cumulative analysis of eight studies.

superior protection rates from delayed emesis compared with single-agent therapy with each of these antiemetics. The best results are reported for the combination of metoclopramide plus corticosteroids, although significance was failed in two studies comparing this combination with a setron–corticosteroid combination.[18,19] Metoclopramide combined with corticosteroids remains the best treatment when analysis is stratified for the antiemetic treatment on day 1 (Table 6.2). The cumulative analysis of 33 studies stratified for antiemetic treatment on day 1 confirms these results.[3–6,16–18,20–45]

Independently from antiemetic treatment on day 1, single-agent antiemetic treatment on days 2–5 consisting of metoclopramide, corti-

costeroids or setrons shows inferior results regarding delayed emesis when compared with combination antiemetic treatment. Again, retrospective comparison of metoclopramide plus corticosteroids with a setron–corticosteroid combination reveals only borderline significance (RR 1.10; 95% CI 1.00–1.20). The metoclopramide–corticosteroid combination not only shows slightly better results than the setron-based combination, but also leads to a different pattern of delayed emesis. A retrospective analysis of the pattern of cisplatin-induced delayed emesis following each combination is shown in Figure 6.6. All patients had received a setron–corticosteroid prophylaxis on day 1. Consequently, acute emesis was controlled in over 75% of patients. The frequency of

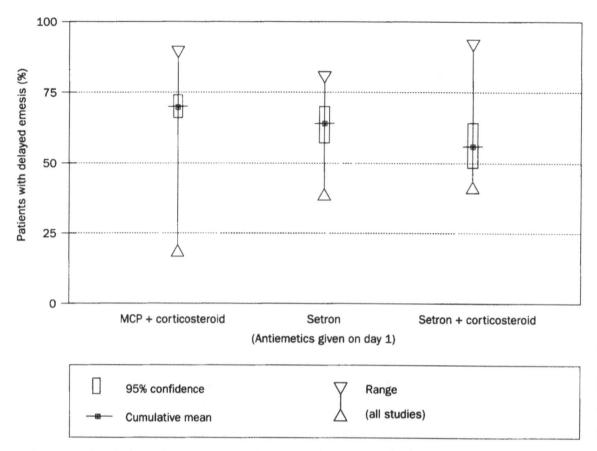

Figure 6.5 Frequency of delayed emesis in patients receiving different antiemetics on day 1 only (MCP = metoclopramide; corticosteroid = dexamethasone or methylprednisolone; setron = ondansetron, granisetron or tropisetron).

delayed emesis showed a linear decline in patients receiving metoclopramide plus corticosteroids from day 2 on, whilst delayed emesis peaked on day 3 in patients receiving a setron–corticosteroid combination as treatment on days 2–5. The shape of the curve in the latter patients looks very similar to the curve showing the natural course of delayed emesis (Figure 6.4), but on a lower level. These observations indicate a beneficial role for the addition of metoclopramide to corticosteroids, especially on days 2–4.

In spite of all limitations inherent in retrospective comparisons, the combination of metoclopramide plus a corticosteroid should be

regarded as the best available treatment for the prophylaxis of cisplatin-induced delayed emesis.

Only a few studies have evaluated the optimal dosage and schedule of metoclopramide plus corticosteroids as antiemetic prophylaxis of cisplatin-induced delayed emesis.[20,29,34] Most studies have used dexamethasone as corticosteroid; only one combined metoclopramide with methylprednisolone. Therefore a statement about the superiority of one corticosteroid over another can not be given. Table 6.3 summarizes the results reported from different metoclopramide–corticosteroid schedules. The cumulative response rate of metoclopramide

Table 6.1 Summary of randomized trials comparing different treatments for cisplatin-induced delayed emesis

Antiemetic treatment for delayed emesis (A versus B)[a]		Studies	Treatment B superior to A	
Treatment A	Treatment B		n (studies)	Significant[b] Number of studies
Placebo	Corticosteroid[3-5]	3	3	2 (3)
	MCP[4]	1	1	1
	Setron[8,16,17,58]	4	4	2
Corticosteroid	MCP[4]	1	1	— (1)
	MCP + corticosteroid[3]	1	1	1
MCP	Setron[28,33]	2	2	1
Setron	MCP[36]	1	1	— (1)
	MCP + corticosteroid[19]	1	1	1
	Setron + corticosteroid[17,19,23,25,27,43]	5	5	1 (3)
	Setron + MCP[43]	1	1	1
Setron + corticosteroid	MCP + corticosteroid[18,19]	2	2	—

[a] MCP = metoclopramide; setron = single-agent ondansetron, granisetron or tropisetron; corticosteroid = dexamethasone or methylprednisolone.
[b] Parentheses indicate that difference reaches significance when nausea ± emesis is considered for comparison.

Table 6.2 Cumulative analysis of different antiemetic regimens for cisplatin-induced delayed emesis stratified for antiemetic treatment on the day of chemotherapy (day 1)[3-6,16-18,20-45]

Antiemetic treatment[a]		Number of patients	Complete response days 2–n[b] (%)
Day 1	Days 2–n[b]		Cumulative mean (95% CI)
MCP + corticosteroid	Corticosteroid	158	53.5 (52–55)
	MCP	271	49.1 (43–55)
	MCP + corticosteroid	210	75.2 (69–81)
Setron	Setron	2240	42.4 (40–45)
Setron + corticosteroid	Setron	530	54.9 (51–59)
	Setron + corticosteroid	269	65.9 (58–70)
	MCP + corticosteroid	1118	71.4 (69–74)

[a] MCP = metoclopramide; setron = single-agent ondansetron, granisetron or tropisetron; corticosteroid = dexamethasone or methylprednisolone.
[b] n = 5 in most studies.

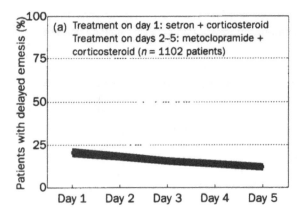

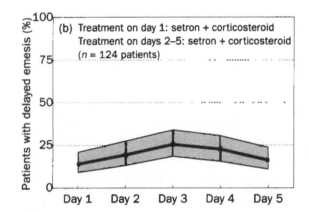

Figure 6.6 The pattern of cisplatin-induced emesis in patients who received a setron–corticosteroid combination from the prophylaxis of acute emesis on day 1, and subsequently received either (a) metoclopramide plus corticosteroids or (b) setrons plus corticosteroids for the prophylaxis of delayed emesis on days 2–5 (retrospective cumulative analysis; means and corresponding 95% confidence intervals are shown).

20 mg orally qid combined with dexamethasone 8 mg bid injected intramuscularly is superior to those of a combination consisting of metoclopramide 40 mg bid and dexamethasone 8 mg per day both administered intravenously (RR for CR days 2–5: 1.85; 95% CI 1.19–2.88). Furthermore, the first schedule is superior to a metoclopramide–methylprednisolone combination (Table 6.3). Obviously, the available data do not allow final conclusions to be drawn about the optimal schedule and dosage producing the best results in the control of cisplatin-induced delayed emesis. However, the best available results are reported for the combination of orally metoclopramide 20 mg qid combined with dexamethasone 8 mg bid given intramuscularly. This schedule should be regarded as the 'standard arm', and should be evaluated in further randomized trials. These future trials should also address the question of treatment duration. There are no data available for a recommendation about how many days treatment should be continued. The retrospective analysis suggests that patients may benefit from a five-day treatment of metoclopramide plus dexamethasone. Risk-factor analysis may help to characterize patients either who need even longer treatment or whose risk for delayed emesis indicates no need for antiemetic treatment from day 1 on. Female gender is one risk factor commonly associated with the risk of delayed emesis. Other, yet not defined, factors may contribute substantially to the risk of developing delayed emesis. Until the pathophysiology of cisplatin-induced delayed emesis is completely understood, clinical studies evaluating such risk factors may contribute to better understanding of this phenomenon.

Further options for the treatment of cisplatin-induced delayed emesis: future aspects

Options for the evaluation of new antiemetic regimens providing improved control of cisplatin-induced delayed emesis are at least threefold:

(i) optimizing schedule and dosage of two-drug combinations containing established substances (i.e. metoclopramide, corticosteroids and, to some extent, setrons);

(ii) evaluating new drug combinations with 'standard' antiemetics;

(iii) introducing new antiemetics as single-agent therapy or adding them to established combinations.

Table 6.3 Cumulative analysis and retrospective comparison of different dosages and schedules of a metoclopramide–corticosteroid combination given as prophylaxis for cisplatin-induced delayed emesis (*Note:* antiemetic treatment on day 1 consisted of single-agent setrons or setrons plus corticosteroids)

Schedule	Antiemetic treatment days 2-n[a,b]	Number of patients	Cumulative mean (95% confidence)	Relative risk (95% confidence)
A	Dexa 2 × 8 mg i.m. + MCP 4 × 20 mg p.o.	1090	71.6 (69–74)	
				A vs B: 1.85 (1.19–2.88)
B	Dexa 1 × 8 mg i.v. + MCP 2 × 40 mg i.v.	31	38.7 (22–58)	
				A vs C: 1.34 (1.11–1.63)
C	MPN 1 × 125 mg i.m. MCP 3 × 0.5 mg/kg i.m.	92	53.3 (43–64)	

[a] All doses are daily doses, treatment was usually continued over five days.
[b] Dexa = dexamethasone; MCP = metoclopramide; MPN = methylprednisolone; i.m. = intramuscular injection; p.o. = oral administration; i.v. = intravenous injection.

As mentioned above, the optimal time schedule for the beginning of antiemetic treatment for delayed emesis is still not completely clear. Re-evaluation of clinical data on the pattern of cisplatin-induced emesis has questioned the arbitrarily definition of a 24-hour cut-off between acute and delayed emesis. Consequently, Gralla and co-workers[46] have started the evaluation of regimens beginning 16 hours after cisplatin with their medication for the prophylaxis of delayed emesis. Antiemetic treatment for delayed emesis consisted of oral ondansetron and oral dexamethasone given for four days, starting 16 hours after cisplatin administration in this study. Treatment for acute emesis represented the golden standard (i.e. a combination of setrons plus corticosteroids). 96 patients were included, and a complete protection rate from delayed emesis was reported in 69% of the patients. These results are encouraging, and should lead to further randomized trials evaluating this schedule of treatment for cisplatin-induced delayed emesis.

The combination of setrons with dopamine (D_2) receptor antagonists might be an alternative to the standard combination of metoclopramide plus corticosteroid. This combination was evaluated in one study,[43] and showed better control of delayed emesis than setron single-agent therapy. A three-drug combination containing a setron, metoclopramide and a corticosteroid has not been evaluated. Each of these drugs possesses at least some activity against cisplatin-induced delayed emesis. Therefore randomized trials should compare a three-drug versus a 'standard' two-drug combination in the setting of cisplatin-induced delayed emesis.

Further attention should be paid to old drugs within a new setting: benzodiazepines, which were frequently combined with metoclopramide and corticosteroid in the late 1980s, may improve efficacy of setron-based combinations. One study combining ondansetron, dexamethasone and lorazepam showed superior efficacy against both acute and delayed emesis associated with cisplatin therapy. The results of the three-drug combination were superior to both setron single-agent therapy and a setron–corticosteroid combination. Unfortunately, only 25 patients per arm were recruited, and significance could not be demonstrated.[23] Larger studies are warranted to evaluate the role of benzodiazepines in combination with setrons.

New insights into the nature and management of chemotherapy-associated emesis have been gained from the introduction of a new class of antiemetics: NK-1 receptor antagonists. These receptors and their ligand substance P are probably involved in the pathomechanisms of emesis, particularly in cisplatin-induced delayed emesis. The first preclinical reports[47] as well as preliminary clinical data[48] indicate a possible role for NK-1 antagonists in the control of emesis. CP-122,721, one of this new class of antiemetics, has shown promising activity against cisplatin-induced delayed emesis. Of 17 patients who received a single dose of CP-122,721 on the day of cisplatin chemotherapy, 14 remained free from delayed emesis (the 95% confidence interval for CR was 57–96%). Further studies evaluating these agents either as monotherapy or in combination regimens are ongoing, and wider experience with these drugs should help to define their role as antiemetics.

CARBOPLATIN-INDUCED DELAYED EMESIS

Despite the similarities in mechanisms of action and cytotoxic efficacy between cisplatin and its second-generation analogue carboplatin, side-effects differ markedly between these two platinum compounds. Carboplatin induces less frequent and less severe emesis than cisplatin.[49] In antiemetic research, carboplatin has been often included in the pool of chemotherapy regimens called 'non-cisplatin chemotherapies'. Consequently, there are only limited data allowing an analysis of carboplatin-induced emesis, and data describing emesis on the days following the day of chemotherapeutic treatment are even rarer.

The 'natural course' of carboplatin-induced emesis

The natural course of carboplatin-induced emesis was analysed in one study including 28 patients.[50] The pattern of emesis showed a monophasic curve, with a peak on day 1 and a duration of emesis of more than 48 hours (Figure 6.7). About 10% of the patients still vomit at the end of day 2. Overall, 82% of patients experienced vomiting, and on average 16 emetic episodes per patient were recorded. In contrast to the pattern of cisplatin-induced emesis, the pattern of carboplatin-induced emesis does not obviously indicate a clear cut-off between acute and delayed emesis. These clinical observations fit well with the experimental data describing the excretion pattern of urinary 5-HIAA. In contrast to cisplatin, carboplatin induces a less dramatic increase in urinary 5-HIAA, but elevated 5-HIAA levels are observed for a longer period (Figure 6.8, data from our group). These data might correspond to different pathophysiological mechanisms involved in the pathways of emesis in both platinum compounds. The so-called 'delayed emesis' following carboplatin might be only a prolongation of acute emesis, and might therefore differ substantially from cisplatin-induced delayed emesis. However, the idiom *delayed emesis*, which was originally reserved for cisplatin-induced emesis, should not be extended uncritically to different forms of emesis. Nevertheless, emesis commencing on the days following day 1 is a clinical problem in a significant proportion of patients.

Management of carboplatin-induced emesis on the days following chemotherapy day

Only three studies have reported results on carboplatin-induced emesis on the days following

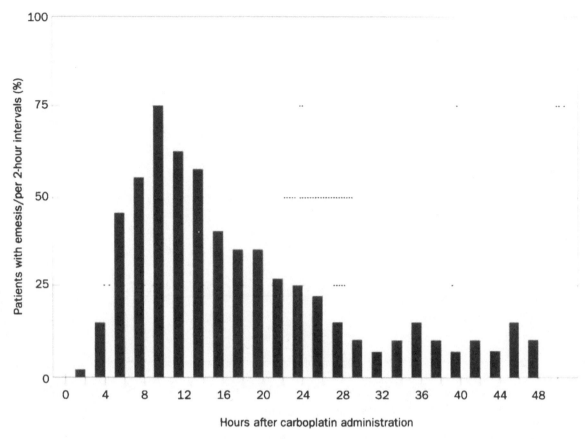

Figure 6.7 The natural course of carboplatin-induced emesis. (Adapted with kind permission from reference 50.)

the chemotherapy day.[51-53] Two studies used single-agent ondansetron as antiemetic prophylaxis on day 1 and the subsequent days. Of 241 included patients, 38.8% showed emesis within days 2–5 (95% CI 32–44%). One study using a setron–corticosteroid combination on day 1 only reported emesis on days 2–5 in 39.4% of 66 patients. The difference regarding treatment on day 1 does not allow a comparison of these studies.

Only a few studies have reported on carboplatin-induced emesis over the whole observation period of 3 or 5 days, including only one randomized trial.[50,52,54-57] Most studies evaluated single-agent setrons given over multiple days. The cumulative analysis of these studies show

61.2% complete response over the whole observation period (95% CI 56–66%) for single-agent setron therapy. The CR rate over days 1–3 increased to 73.7% (95% CI 64–82%) when dexamethasone was added to ondansetron on day 1, followed by single-agent oral ondansetron on days 2–3.[54] The latter regimen was compared randomly with metoclopramide plus dexamethasone on day 1, followed by single-agent metoclopramide on days 2–3. Only 48% of 94 patients remained free from vomiting over days 1–3 when receiving the metoclopramide-based combination. The difference between the setron-based and metoclopramide-based regimens was statistically significant.

Overall, the available data do not allow final

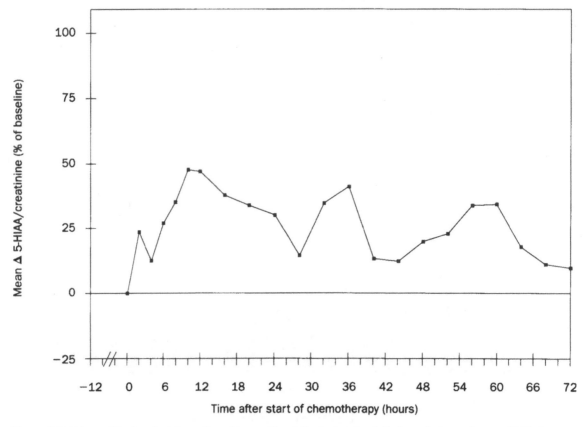

Figure 6.8 Urinary 5-hydroxyindoleacetic acid excretion following carboplatin-based chemotherapy (5-HIAA corrected for creatinine; values express deviation from baseline values measured before chemotherapy).

conclusions to be drawn regarding a standard regimen for carboplatin-induced emesis. There is some evidence that setrons might be efficient on the days following the chemotherapy day, but further studies are warranted. The setron–corticosteroid combination described above should be used as the standard arm in these studies until another regimen has shown superior or at least comparable efficacy.

SUMMARY

Over the last decade, antiemetic research has focused mainly on acute emesis. Tremendous improvements have been achieved in this field. The improved control of acute cisplatin-induced emesis has shifted attention to the control of delayed emesis. In contrast to acute emesis, the pathophysiological mechanisms have not been described, nor has the optimal treatment for delayed emesis been established. A combination of metoclopramide plus dexamethasone should be accepted as the best available treatment for cisplatin-induced emesis today. Recently initiated studies evaluating improved schedules, optimized combinations of established substances and evaluation of new drugs should help to improve the control of this particular form of emesis. Cisplatin is the most widely evaluated cytostatic regarding emesis. The quantity and quality of data reporting antiemetic prophylaxis of carboplatin-induced emesis is far from satisfactory. Only very few data from randomized studies are available. Therefore recommendations regarding the treatment of carboplatin-induced emesis are somewhat arbitrary. The best results are reported for a combination of setrons plus corticosteroids on day 1, followed by single-agent setrons on subsequent days. Further studies are needed before standards can be recommended.

REFERENCES

1. Kris MG, Gralla RJ, Clark RA et al, Incidence, course, and severity of delayed nausea and vomiting following the administration of high-dose cisplatin. *J Clin Oncol* 3: 1379–84.
2. Andrews PLR, Davis CJ, The mechanism of emesis induced by anti-cancer therapies. In: *Emesis in Anti-Cancer Therapy* (Andrews PLR, Sanger GJ, eds). London: Chapman & Hall, 1993: 113–61.
3. Kris MG, Gralla RJ, Tyson LB et al, Controlling delayed vomiting: double-blind, randomized trial comparing placebo, dexamethasone alone, and metoclopramide plus dexamethasone in patients receiving cisplatin. *J Clin Oncol* 1989; 7: 108–14.
4. Roila F, Boschetti E, Tonato M et al, Predictive factors of delayed emesis in cisplatin-treated patients and antiemetic activity and tolerability of metoclopramide or dexamethasone. A randomized single-blind study. *Am J Clin Oncol* 1991; 14: 238–42.
5. Passalaqua R, Cocconi G, Bella M et al, Double-blind, randomized trial for the control of delayed emesis in patients receiving cisplatin: comparison of placebo vs. adrenocorticotropic hormone (ACTH). *Ann Oncol* 1992; 3: 481–5.
6. Shinkai T, Saijo N, Eguchi K et al, Control of cisplatin-induced delayed emesis with metoclopramide and dexamethasone: a randomized controlled trial. *Jap J Clin Oncol* 1989; 19: 40–4.
7. Bresciani G, Böhm S, Oriana S, Control of nausea and vomiting by granisetron in ovarian cancer patients treated with different cisplatin-based regimens. *Tumori* 1994; 80: 344–7.
8. Gandara DR, Harvey WH, Monaghan GG et al, Delayed emesis following high-dose cisplatin: a double-blind randomised comparative trial of ondansetron (GR38032F) versus placebo. *Eur J Cancer* 1993; 29: 35–8.
9. Plezia PM, Alberts DS, Kessler JF et al, Randomized crossover comparison of high-dose intravenous metoclopramide versus a five-drug antiemetic regimen. *J Pain Symptom Manag* 1990; 5: 101–8.
10. Kris MG, Gralla RJ, Clark RA et al, Antiemetic control and prevention of side effects of anti-cancer with lorazepam or diphenhydramine when used in combination with metoclopramide plus dexamethasone. A double-blind, randomized trial. *Cancer* 1987; 60: 2816–22.
11. Grunberg SM, Akerley WL, Krarlo MD et al, Comparison of metoclopramide and metoclopramide plus dexamethasone for complete protection from cisplatinum-induced emesis. *Cancer Invest* 1986; 4: 379–85.
12. Shinkai T, Saijo N, Eguchi K et al, Antiemetic efficacy of high-dose intravenous metoclopramide and dexamethasone in patients receiving cisplatin-based chemotherapy: a randomized controlled trial. *Jap J Clin Oncol* 1986; 16: 279–87.
13. Ohwada M, Suzuki M, Ogawa S et al, Efficacy and tolerability of granisetron with betamethasone, an antiemetic combination, in gynecologic cancer patients receiving cisplatin. *Curr Ther Res* 1995; 56: 1059–65.
14. Marty M, Pouillart P, Scholl S et al, Comparison of the 5-hydroxytryptamine$_3$ (serotonin) antagonist ondansetron (GR38032F) with high-dose metoclopramide in the control of cisplatin-induced emesis. *N Engl J Med* 1990; 322: 816–21.
15. Matsui K, Fukuoka M, Takada M et al, Randomised trial for the prevention of delayed emesis patients receiving high-dose cisplatin. *Br J Cancer* 1996; 73: 217–21.
16. Navari RM, Madajewicz S, Anderson N et al, Oral ondansetron for the control of cisplatin-induced delayed emesis: a large, multicenter, double-blind, randomized comparative trial of ondansetron versus placebo. *J Clin Oncol* 1995; 13: 2408–16.
17. Ossi M, Anderson E, Freeman A, 5-HT$_3$ receptor antagonists in the control of cisplatin-induced delayed emesis. *Oncology* 1996; 53(Suppl): 78–85.
18. Ohmatsu H, Eguchi K, Shinkai T et al, A randomized cross-over study of high-dose metoclopramide plus dexamethasone versus granisetron plus dexamethasone in patients receiving chemotherapy with high-dose cisplatin. *Jap J Cancer* 1994; 85: 1151–8.

19. Gebbia V, Testa A, Valenza R et al, Oral granisetron with or without methylprednisolone versus metoclopramide plus methylprednisolone in the management of delayed nausea and vomiting induced by cisplatin-based chemotherapy. A prospective randomized trial. *Cancer* 1995; 76: 1821–8.

20. Sekine I, Nishiwaki Y, Kakinuma R et al, A randomized cross-over trial of granisetron and dexamethason versus granisetron alone: the role of dexamethasone on day 1 in the control of cisplatin-induced delayed emesis. *Jap J Clin Oncol* 1996; 26: 164–8.

21. Bruntsch U, Drechsler S, Eggert J et al, Prevention of chemotherapy-induced nausea and vomiting by tropisetron (Navoban) alone or in combination with other antiemetic agents. *Semin Oncol* 1994; 21: 7–11.

22. Olver N, Craft PS, Clingan PR et al, An open multicentre study of tropisetron for cisplatin-induced nausea and vomiting. *MJA* 1996; 164: 337–40.

23. Ahn MJ, Lee JS, Lee KH et al, A randomized double blind trial of ondansetron alone versus in combination with dexamethasone versus in combination with dexamethasone and lorazepam in the prevention of emesis due to cisplatin-based chemotherapy. *Am J Clin Oncol* 1991; 17: 150–6.

24. Sorbe B, Högberg T, Himmelmann A et al, Efficacy and tolerability of tropisetron in comparison with a combination of tropisetron and dexamethasone in the control of nausea and vomiting induced by cisplatin-containing chemotherapy. *Eur J Cancer* 1994; 30A: 629–34.

25. Chevallier B, Marty M, Paillarse JM and the Ondansetron Study Group, Methylprednisolone enhances the efficacy of ondansetron in acute and delayed cisplatin-induced emesis over at least three cycles. *Br J Cancer* 1994; 70: 1171–5.

26. Kris MG, Tyson LB, Clark RA, Gralla RJ, Oral ondansetron for the control of delayed emesis after cisplatin. *Cancer* 1992; 70: 1012–16.

27. Joss RA, Bacchi M, Buser K et al, Ondansetron plus dexamethasone is superior to ondansetron alone in the prevention of emesis in chemotherapy-naive and previously treated patients. *Ann Oncol* 1994; 5: 253–8.

28. Heron JF, Goedhals L, Jordaan JP et al, on behalf of the Granisetron Study Group, Oral granisetron alone and in combination with dexamethasone: a double-blind randomized comparison against high-dose metoclopramide plus dexamethasone in prevention of cisplatin-

induced emesis. *Ann Oncol* 1994; 5: 579–84.

29. Italian Group for Antiemetic Research, Ondansetron + dexamethasone vs metoclopramide + dexamethasone + diphenhydramine in prevention of cisplatin-induced emesis. *Lancet* 1992; 340: 96–9.

30. Louvet C, Lorange A, Letendre F et al, Acute and delayed emesis after cisplatin-based regimen: description and prevention. *Oncology* 1991; 48: 392–6.

31. Lim AKH, Haron MR, Yap TM, Ondansetron against metoclopramide/dexamethasone. A comparative study. *Med J Malaysia* 1994; 49: 231–8.

32. Chang T-C, Hsieh F, Lai C-H et al, Comparison of the efficacy of tropisetron versus a metoclopramide cocktail based on the intensity of cisplatin-induced emesis. *Cancer Chemother Pharmacol* 1996; 37: 279–85.

33. Madej G, Krzakowski M, Pawinski A et al, A comparative study of the use of tropisetron (ICS 205-930), a 5-HT$_3$ antagonist, versus a standard antiemetic regimen of dexamethasone and metoclopramide in the treatment of cisplatin-containing chemotherapy. *Drug Invest* 1993; 6: 162–9.

34. Italian Group for Antiemetic Research, Ondansetron versus granisetron, both combined with dexamethasone, in the prevention of cisplatin-induced emesis. *Ann Oncol* 1995; 6: 805–10.

35. Sorbe B, Andersson H, Schmidt M et al, Tropisetron (Navoban) in the prevention of chemotherapy-induced nausea and vomiting – the Nordic experience. *Support Care Cancer* 1994; 2: 393–9.

36. De Mulder PHM, Seynaeve C, Vermorken JB et al, Ondansetron compared with high-dose metoclopramide in prophylaxis of acute and delayed cisplatin-induced nausea and vomiting. A multicenter, randomized, double-blind, crossover study. *Ann Int Med* 1990; 113: 834–40.

37. Tsavaris N, Mylonakis N, Bacoyiannis CH et al, Efficacy of ondansetron treatment with different timing schedules: a randomized double-blind study. *Oncology* 1995; 52: 315–18.

38. Cheirsilpa A, Sinlarat P, Lousoontornsiri W et al, Ondansetron: prevention of nausea and vomiting in cisplatin based chemotherapy. *J Med Assoc Thai* 1994; 77: 201–6.

39. Tsavaris N, Charalambidis G, Pagou M et al, Comparison of ondansetron (GR 38032F) versus ondansetron plus alprazolam as antiemetic prophylaxis during cisplatin-containing chemother-

apy. *Am J Clin Oncol* 1994; **17**: 516–21.

40. Roila F, Bracarda S, Tonato M et al, Ondansetron (GR38032F) in the prophylaxis of acute and delayed cisplatin-induced emesis. *Clin Oncol* 1990; **2**: 268–72.

41. Marty M, Kleisbauer JP, Fournel P et al, Is Navoban R (tropisetron) as effective as Zofran R (ondansetron) in cisplatin-induced emesis? *Anti-Cancer Drugs* 1995; **6**: 15–21.

42. Gebbia V, Cannata G, Testa A et al, Ondansetron versus granisetron in the prevention of chemotherapy-induced nausea and vomiting. Results of a prospective randomized trial. *Cancer* 1994; **74**: 1945–52.

43. Lee CW, Suh CW, Lee JS et al, Ondansetron compared with ondansetron plus metoclopramide in the prevention of cisplatin-induced emesis. *J Korean Med Sci* 1994; **9**: 369–75.

44. De Witt R, Schmitz PIM, Verweij J et al, Analysis of cumulative probabilities shows that the efficacy of 5-HT$_3$ antagonist prophylaxis is not maintained. *J Clin Oncol* 1996; **14**: 644–51.

45. Tsukuda M, Furukawa S, Kokatsu T et al, Comparison of granisetron alone and granisetron plus hydroxyzine hydrochloride for prophylactic treatment of emesis induced by cisplatin chemotherapy. *Eur J Cancer* 1995; **31A**: 1647–9.

46. Gralla RJ, Rittenberg C, Peralta M et al, Cisplatin and emesis: aspects of treatment and a new trial for delayed emesis using oral dexamethasone plus ondansetron beginning at 16 hours after cisplatin. *Oncology* 1996; **53**(Suppl): 86–91.

47. Bountra C, Bunce K, Dale T et al, Anti-emetic profile of a non-peptide neurokinin NK$_1$ receptor antagonist, CP 99,994, in ferrets. *Eur J Pharmacol* 1993; **249**: R3–4.

48. Kris MG, Radford J, Pizo B et al, Dose-ranging antiemetic trial of the NK-1 receptor antagonist CP-122,721: a new approach for acute and delayed emesis following cisplatin. *Proc Am Assoc Clin Oncol* 1996; **15**: 547 (abst 1780).

49. du Bois A, Vach W, Thomssen C et al, Comparison of the emetogenic potential between cisplatin and carboplatin in combination with alkylating agents. *Acta Oncol* 1994; **33**: 531–5.

50. Martin M, Diaz-Rubio E, Sanchez A et al, The natural course of emesis after carboplatin treatment. *Acta Oncol* 1990; **29**: 593–5.

51. Harvey VJ, Evans BD, Mitchell PLR et al, Reduction of carboplatin induced emesis by ondansetron. *Br J Cancer* 1991; **63**: 942–4.

52. du Bois A, Vach W, Cramer-Giraud U et al, Pattern of carboplatin-induced emesis. *Anti-Cancer Drugs* 1995; **6**: 645–51.

53. Pronzato P, Ghio E, Losardo PL et al, Tropisetron–dexamethasone combination for carboplatin-induced emesis. *Oncol Rep* 1996; **3**: 1179–81.

54. du Bois A, McKenna CJ, Andersson H et al, A randomised, double-blind, parallel-group study to compare the efficacy and safety of ondansetron (GR38032F) plus dexamethasone with metoclopramide plus dexamethasone in the prophylaxis of nausea and emesis induced by carboplatin chemotherapy. *Oncology* 1997; **54**: 7–14.

55. Smith DB, Rustin GJS, Howells N et al, A phase II study of ondansetron as antiemetic prophylaxis in patients receiving carboplatin for advanced ovarian cancer. *Ann Oncol* 1991; **2**: 607–8.

56. Gridelli C, Incoronato P, Airoma G et al, Ondansetron in the prophylaxis of nausea and vomiting induced by carboplatin combination chemotherapy. *Eur J Cancer* 1993; **29**: 651–60.

57. Bleiberg H, Spielmann M, Falkson G, Romain D, Antiemetic treatment with oral granisetron in patients receiving moderately emetogenic chemotherapy: a dose-ranging study. *Clin Ther* 1995; **17**: 38–51.

Treatment of moderately emetogenic chemotherapy-induced nausea and vomiting

Fausto Roila, Maurizio Tonato, Albano Del Favero

CONTENTS • Introduction • Prevention of acute emesis induced by moderately emetogenic chemotherapy • Prevention of delayed emesis induced by moderately emetogenic chemotherapy • Conclusions

INTRODUCTION

Nausea and vomiting are among the most distressing side-effects of cancer chemotherapy, and therefore good control of these symptoms is extremely important from the patient's perspective.

In the past few years, with the introduction of the 5-HT$_3$ receptor antagonists in clinical practice, important progress in the prevention of chemotherapy-induced nausea and vomiting has been made. This chapter will summarize the results of comparative studies of various antiemetic regimens in the prevention of acute and delayed emesis induced by moderately emetogenic chemotherapy. A unanimous consensus on what a moderately emetogenic chemotherapy regimen is does not exist, but, generally, intravenous cyclophosphamide, doxorubicin, epirubicin and carboplatin, used alone or in some combination, are consistently considered moderately emetogenic chemotherapeutic drugs.

The pattern of emesis after their administration is characteristic.[1] In fact, cyclophosphamide induces a late onset of emesis (about 10–12 hours after its administration). When cyclophosphamide is combined with doxorubicin, a shorter time to onset of vomiting is shown (6–8 hours). Carboplatin induces a pattern of emesis similar to that induced by cyclophosphamide (emesis begins about 6–7 hours after its administration).

PREVENTION OF ACUTE EMESIS INDUCED BY MODERATELY EMETOGENIC CHEMOTHERAPY

Before the introduction of 5-HT$_3$ receptor antagonists

Relatively few studies were conducted on patients undergoing chemotherapy with moderately emetogenic chemotherapy before the introduction of 5-HT$_3$ receptor antagonists.

Although a wide range of antiemetic drugs has been employed (including phenothiazines, butyrophenones, benzamides and corticosteroids), we shall limit our review to the most recent and interesting studies, which have most frequently evaluated metoclopramide and corticosteroids.

Chemotherapeutic regimens containing doxorubicin, alone or in combination with cyclophosphamide and vincristine (CAV) or with fluorouracil and cyclophosphamide (FAC), are reported to produce vomiting in about 60% of patients. Contrasting data have been published regarding the efficacy of metoclopramide in preventing emesis due to doxorubicin, while corticosteroids seem to offer a better treatment.[2-4] Two double-blind trials have shown a high rate of complete protection with intravenous dexamethasone (20 mg immediately before chemotherapy followed by 10 mg × 4 doses orally every 6 hours) as well as with intravenous methylprednisolone (125 mg × 3 doses every 6 hours).[2,5] Compared with meto-

clopramide, methylprednisolone also seems to have lower toxicity.[2]

The intravenous combination of cyclophosphamide, methotrexate and fluorouracil (CMF), frequently used to treat breast cancer, induces emesis in 70–90% of patients. Again, contrasting results have been reported on the efficacy of metoclopramide. In fact, this compound, at standard oral or high intravenous doses, similar to those administered to cisplatin-treated patients, has been shown to be no more efficacious than placebo in some studies,[6,7] while better efficacy has been reported in others by using

---

Table 7.1 5-HT$_3$ receptor antagonists vs metoclopramide

Study[a]	Number of patients	Chemotherapy[b]	Antiemetics (first dose)[c]	MR[d] (%)	Results[b]	Ref
DB XO	65	FU + DOX + CTX or FU + EPI + CTX	OND 4 mg i.v. +4 mg orally	86	OND > MTC Preference OND	15
			MTC 60 mg i.v. +20 mg orally	42		
DB	93	CTX + DOX or CTX + EPI	OND 8 mg i.v.	80	OND ≥ MTC	16
			MTC 60 mg i.v.	62		
DB	122	CTX + DOX or CTX + EPI	OND 8 mg orally	72	OND > MTC	17
			MTC 60 mg i.v.	61		
DB	187	CTX-containing chemotherapy	OND 8 mg i.v. + DEX 16 mg i.v.	91[e]	OND + DEX > MTC + DEX	18
			MTC 60 mg i.v. + DEX 16 mg i.v.	60[e]		

[a] DB = double-blind; XO = crossover.
[b] MTC = metoclopramide; OND = ondansetron; DEX = dexamethasone; CTX = cyclophosphamide; DOX = doxorubicin; EPI = epirubicin; FU = fluorouracil.
[c] Subsequent oral doses: OND 8 mg every 8 hours; MTC 20 mg every 8 hours.
[d] MR = major response (≤2 emetic episodes).   [e] Complete protection from acute vomiting.

intravenous or intramuscular metoclopramide 20 mg × 5 or 3 doses every 3 or 6 hours respectively.[8-10] Again, intravenous or intramuscular methylprednisolone (40–125 mg × 3 doses every 6 hours) or dexamethasone (8 mg intravenously before chemotherapy plus 4 mg intramuscularly 24 and 12 hours before and 6 and 12 hours after chemotherapy) seems to provide better control of emesis, since they induce complete protection from vomiting in about 50–80% of patients according to different studies.[9,11,12]

However, the dose and schedule of corticosteroids seem important to guarantee good efficacy. In fact, in patients submitted to CMF chemotherapy, a single 125 mg intravenous dose or two 125 mg intravenous doses of methylprednisolone before chemotherapy did not seem to have good efficacy, since complete protection from vomiting and nausea was obtained in two studies in only 11% and 34% of patients respectively.[13,14]

It appears clear from these data that corticosteroids, used at high and repeated doses, are the most efficacious and well-tolerated antiemetic treatment for acute emesis induced by some of the most widely utilized chemotherapeutic regimens, such as those containing doxorubicin and/or cyclophosphamide.

After the introduction of 5-HT₃ receptor antagonists

A number of studies have been published on the efficacy of 5-HT$_3$ receptor antagonists in the prevention of acute emesis induced by moderately emetogenic chemotherapy. The 5-HT$_3$ receptor antagonists alone or in combination with steroids have been compared with several antiemetic compounds, such as metoclopramide, alizapride, phenothiazines and corticosteroids, and generally they have shown good efficacy, inducing complete protection from acute vomiting in 60–80% of patients treated with a variety of regimens of moderately emetogenic chemotherapy.

Seven studies have compared a 5-HT$_3$ receptor antagonist with metoclopramide (Tables 7.1

and 7.2). In three studies, ondansetron has been shown to be of superior or equal efficacy compared with metoclopramide, and always to be less toxic (Table 7.1).[15-17] Another study comparing the same drugs, both combined with dexamethasone, showed better efficacy and lower toxicity of ondansetron-containing regimens (Table 7.1).[18] In a randomized open study, tropisetron demonstrated superior antiemetic activity compared with metoclopramide combined with lorazepam (Table 7.2).[19] Finally, two studies evaluated the antiemetic activity of a 5-HT$_3$ receptor antagonist with respect to high-dose metoclopramide (Table 7.2). In the first, two different single doses of intravenous dolasetron (1.2 and 1.8 mg/kg) showed similar antiemetic efficacy to a 2 mg/kg loading dose of metoclopramide followed by a 3 mg/kg 8-hour continuous infusion. In the second, a randomized open study, oral ondansetron plus dexamethasone was compared with a combination of high-dose metoclopramide plus dexamethasone and orphenadrine.[21] Ondansetron was significantly superior to the metoclopramide regimen.

Two studies compared a 5-HT$_3$ receptor antagonist with alizapride (Table 7.3). In the first, oral ondansetron was compared with alizapride. Complete protection from acute vomiting with ondansetron was significantly superior compared with alizapride.[22] In the second, a small open randomized study, even tropisetron was shown to be more efficacious than alizapride.[23]

Three studies, all evaluating granisetron, compared it with a phenothiazine (Table 7.4). In one double-blind study, the superiority of granisetron compared with prochlorperazine in 230 patients was clearly shown.[24] In the other two studies, granisetron was shown to be more efficacious and less toxic than the combination of dexamethasone plus a phenothiazine (chlorpromazine and prochlorperazine).[25,26] However, in both these studies, dexamethasone was administered as a single intravenous dose before chemotherapy, a schedule that is open to criticism, and its combination with phenothiazines can also be criticized, since the efficacy of phenothiazines in the prevention of acute eme-

Table 7.2 5-HT₃ receptor antagonists vs metoclopramide

Study[a]	Number of patients	Chemotherapy[b]	Antiemetics[b]	CP[c] (%)	Results[b]	Ref
O	102	DOX, CBDCA + CTX, CBDCA + IFO, etc.	TROP 5 mg i.v. MTC 20–100 mg i.v. + 20 mg orally every 4–6 hours + LOR 2–4 mg i.v.	45 22	TROP > MTC	19
DB	309	CTX, DOX, etc.	DOL 1.2 mg i.v. DOL 1.8 mg i.v. MTC 2 mg/kg loading dose + 3 mg/kg as 8 hour c.i.[d]	56 64 53	1.2 mg/kg = 1.8 mg/kg DOL = MTC	20
O	64	FU + DOX + CTX or FU + EPI + CTX	OND 8 mg orally every 8 hours + DEX 20 mg i.v. MTC 3 mg/kg × 2 + 40 mg orally every 3 hours × 4 doses + DEX 20 mg i.v. + ORP 40 mg i.m.	74 44	OND + DEX > MTC + DEX + ORP	21

[a] O = open; DB = double-blind.
[b] MTC = metoclopramide; OND = ondansetron; TROP = tropisetron; DOL = dolasetron; LOR = lorazepam; DEX = dexamethasone; ORP = orphenadrine; CTX = cyclophosphamide; DOX = doxorubicin; EPI = epirubicin; FU = fluorouracil; CBDCA = carboplatin; IFO = ifosfamide.
[c] CP = complete protection from acute vomiting.
[d] c.i. = continuous infusion.

sis induced by moderately emetogenic drugs is far from being proven.

On the basis of the results of these studies, we can draw the conclusion that 5-HT₃ receptor antagonists have superior antiemetic activity to metoclopramide, alizapride or phenothiazines, but before they can be considered the first choice antiemetic prophylaxis for the prevention of acute emesis induced by moderately emetogenic chemotherapy, they have to be compared with high and repeated doses of corticosteroids.

The first study comparing a 5-HT₃ receptor antagonist (ondansetron) with dexamethasone used at high and repeated doses found the two antiemetic drugs to be equally efficacious in the control of acute nausea and vomiting, but dexamethasone was superior in the control of delayed nausea (Table 7.5).[27]

Moreover, two studies clearly demonstrated

Study[a]	Number of patients	Chemotherapy[b]	Antiemetics[b]	CP[c] (%)	Results[b]	Ref
DB	259	FU + DOX + CTX or FU + EPI + CTX	OND 8 mg orally every 8–12 hours	57	OND > ALZ	22
			ALZ 150 mg i.v. + + 50 mg orally every 8–12 hours	31		
O	30	CTX-containing chemotherapy	TROP 5 mg i.v.	93[d]	TROP > ALZ	23
			ALZ 100 mg i.v.	60[d]		

Table 7.3 5-HT$_3$ receptor antagonists vs alizapride

[a] DB = double-blind; O = open.
[b] OND = ondansetron; TROP = tropisetron; ALZ = alizapride; CTX = cyclophosphamide; DOX = doxorubicin; EPI = epirubicin; FU = fluorouracil.
[c] CP = complete protection from acute vomiting.
[d] ≤2 emetic episodes.

that a combination of a 5-HT$_3$ receptor antagonist with dexamethasone can further improve the control of acute vomiting and nausea (Table 7.6). In fact, in one double-blind study, the addition of a corticosteroid (also in this case a single intravenous dose of 12 mg dexamethasone was used) to tropisetron was able to improve the efficacy compared with the 5-HT$_3$ receptor antagonist used alone.[28]

A second large prospective multicentre double-blind study added further evidence to support the advantage of using a combination of a corticosteroid with a 5-HT$_3$ receptor antagonist. Patients scheduled to receive moderately emetogenic chemotherapy were randomized to receive granisetron alone or dexamethasone alone, or the combination of dexamethasone and granisetron at the same doses and schedules (Table 7.6).[29] Patients were followed up to four days after chemotherapy without further antiemetic prophylaxis. Complete protection from acute vomiting, nausea and both nausea and vomiting was found to be significantly

superior with the dexamethasone plus granisetron combination (93%, 72% and 70%) compared with dexamethasone alone (71%, 55% and 49%) and granisetron alone (72%, 48% and 43%).[29]

The good protection obtained from acute emesis was also responsible for the better protection from delayed emesis (while patients were not receiving any antiemetic prophylaxis) in patients receiving dexamethasone plus granisetron (81%) or dexamethasone alone (86%) compared with granisetron alone (72%), confirming the results of a previous study.[26]

Another interesting aspect of this study is that patients were followed for three consecutive cycles in a double-blind manner.[30] In all three cycles, the combination of dexamethasone plus granisetron induced significantly greater complete protection from vomiting, nausea and both nausea and vomiting compared with granisetron alone. Instead, compared with dexamethasone alone, complete protection from vomiting was significantly superior in the first and second

Table 7.4 5-HT₃ receptor antagonists vs phenothlazines

Study[a]	Number of patients	Chemotherapy[b]	Antiemetics[b]	CP[c] (%)	Results[b]	Ref
DB	230	NS	GRAN 1 mg orally every 12 hours	74	GRAN > PCP	24
			PCP 10 mg orally every 12 hours	41		
SB	228	CBDCA, CTX, DOX, EPI etc.	GRAN 40 µg/kg i.v.	70	GRAN > CPZ + DEX	25
			CPZ 25 mg i.v. or i.m. and 25–50 mg orally every 4–6 hours + DEX 12 mg i.v.	49	<sedation with GRAN	
DB	152	DOX- and CTX- containing chemotherapy	GRAN 80 µg/kg i.v.	70	GRAN >PCP + DEX	26
			PCP 10 mg i.v. + DEX 10 mg i.v.	34		

[a] DB = double-blind; SB = single-blind.
[b] GRAN = granisetron; CPZ = chlorpromazine; PCP = prochlorperazine; DEX = dexamethasone; CTX = cyclophosphamide; DOX = doxorubicin; EPI = epirubicin; CBDCA = carboplatin; NS = not specified.
[c] CP = complete protection from acute vomiting.

Table 7.5 5-HT₃ receptor antagonists vs dexamethasone

Study[a]	Number of patients	Chemotherapy[b]	Antiemetics[b]	CP[c] (%)	Results[b]	Ref
DB XO	112	CTX ± DOX ± VP16	OND 4 mg i.v. + 4 mg orally every 6 hours	73	OND = DEX	27
			DEX 8 mg i.v. + 4 mg orally every 6 hours	66		

[a] DB = double-blind; XO = crossover.
[b] OND = ondansetron; DEX = dexamethasone; CTX = cyclophosphamide; DOX = doxorubicin; VP16 = etoposide.
[c] CP = complete protection from acute vomiting.

Table 7.6 5-HT$_3$ receptor antagonists + dexamethasone vs 5-HT$_3$ receptor antagonists or dexamethasone alone

Study[a]	Number of patients	Chemotherapy[b]	Antiemetics[b]	CP[c] (%)	Results[b]	Ref
DB	126	CBDCA- or CTX-containing chemotherapy	TROP 5 mg i.v. + DEX 12 mg i.v.	89	TROP + DEX > TROP	28
			TROP 5 mg i.v.	75		
DB	428	CBDCA or CTX or DOX or EPI	GRAN 3 mg i.v.	72	GRAN + DEX > GRAN and DEX	29
			DEX 8 mg i.v. + 4 mg orally every 6 hours	71		
			GRAN + DEX as above	93		

[a] DB = double-blind.
[b] TROP = tropisetron; GRAN = granisetron; DEX = dexamethasone; CTX = cyclophosphamide; CBDCA = carboplatin; DOX = doxorubicin; EPI = epirubicin.
[c] CP = complete protection from acute vomiting.

cycle, while complete protection from nausea was superior only in the first cycle.[30]

In conclusion, it seems from these studies that in the prevention of acute emesis induced by moderately emetogenic chemotherapy, a combination of a 5-HT$_3$ receptor antagonist plus high and repeated doses of dexamethasone is the most efficacious antiemetic treatment.

The advantage of using a combination of an antiemetic with a 5-HT$_3$ receptor antagonist has also been found recently with metopimazine. In fact, a double-blind crossover study compared oral ondansetron (8 mg twice a day) plus oral metopimazine (30 mg four times a day) with ondansetron alone.[31] In 30 patients, who had vomited during the previous cycle of chemotherapy, 63.3% obtained complete protection from acute vomiting with the combination, compared with 46.6% with ondansetron alone.

Prevention of emesis induced by oral CMF chemotherapy

The control of nausea and vomiting induced by 14-day oral cyclophosphamide at doses of 100 mg/m^2 per day, as used in the standard CMF regimen in breast cancer patients, has only recently been evaluated.

In a randomized, double-blind placebo-controlled trial in 82 patients, oral ondansetron (8 mg 3 times daily for 15 days) gave significantly greater complete protection from vomiting (60%) compared with placebo (35%).[32] A double-blind, randomized study in 165 patients compared ondansetron (8 mg 3 times daily orally for 7 days) with dexamethasone (10 mg single dose intravenously) plus metoclopramide (10 mg 3 times daily orally for 7 days).[33] There was no statistically significant difference in efficacy between the regimens, except for significantly less nausea during the first 24 hours after chemotherapy in patients receiving the metoclopramide combination regimen.

What is the optimal oral dose of a 5-HT₃ receptor antagonist?

Recently, the problem of optimal dose and schedule of 5-HT₃ receptor antagonists has been re-examined because of its important implications from a clinical and economic point of view. Unfortunately, the available data did not always clearly indicate the most efficacious, suitable and cost-effective antiemetic dose for each compound.

Oral administration of 5-HT₃ receptor antagonists has been used most frequently in the prevention of emesis induced by moderately emetogenic chemotherapy.

At first, the approved oral dose of ondansetron was 8 mg every 8 hours. In fact, a non-blinded study, carried out in 60 patients submitted to doxorubicin and cyclophosphamide, which compared oral doses of 1, 4 and 8 mg three times daily, showed that ondansetron efficacy was dose-related, with an 8 mg dose inducing complete protection from vomiting in 85% of patients.[34] However, contrasting results came from other trials.

One study, involving 349 patients submitted for the first time to cyclophosphamide plus methotrexate or doxorubicin therapy, compared oral doses of 1, 4 and 8 mg of ondansetron three times daily to placebo.[35] Similar complete protection from vomiting was obtained in patients receiving the three doses of ondansetron (57%, 65% and 66% respectively) even if the protection was statistically superior to those obtained with placebo (19%).

Different results were obtained in another study involving 324 patients in which the same oral doses of ondansetron were again compared with placebo.[36] Complete protection from acute vomiting was always superior compared with placebo, but higher doses were more efficacious than lower doses (64% with 4 mg and 66% with 8 mg versus 37% with 1 mg versus 12% with placebo).

More recently, three large double-blind trials have been published.[37-39] Two of these, performed in 324 patients and 402 patients respectively, receiving cyclophosphamide, doxorubicin or epirubicin plus other non-cisplatin cytostatics, compared ondansetron 8 mg intravenously before chemotherapy followed by 8 mg orally two or three times daily. Both the two- and three-times daily schedules provided similar good control of nausea and vomiting and were well tolerated.[37,38]

In the third study, carried out on 302 patients, a single oral dose of 16 mg before chemotherapy was shown to be as efficacious as a dose of 8 mg twice daily.[39]

Therefore it can be concluded from these studies that a 16 mg single oral dose or an 8 mg twice daily oral regimen of ondansetron could be a good and convenient choice in the prevention of emesis in outpatient treatment with moderately emetogenic chemotherapy. However, the efficacy of such lower doses should also be further studied.

The first double-blind dose-ranging study with granisetron evaluated two different single intravenous doses (40 and 160 µg/kg) in 443 patients. Complete protection from vomiting was obtained in 76% and 81% of patients respectively.[40]

Subsequently, pilot studies have suggested that the optimal oral dose of granisetron is between 0.25 and 2.5 mg twice daily, and two large double-blind studies evaluated different oral doses of granisetron.[41,42] The first, performed in 930 patients submitted to moderately emetogenic chemotherapy, compared the antiemetic activity and tolerability of four doses of granisetron: 0.25 mg, 0.5 mg, 1 mg and 2 mg twice daily.[41] The study showed a dose–response relationship up to the dose of 1 mg twice daily. The dose of 2 mg twice daily did not give superior results. More recently, in a study performed in 697 patients submitted to moderately emetogenic chemotherapy, a comparison of oral granisetron 1 mg twice daily with a 2 mg single oral dose before chemotherapy has been made.[42] Complete protection from vomiting in the first 24 hours after chemotherapy was very similar between the two antiemetic regimens (81.9% versus 76.7% respectively).

Therefore a single oral dose of 2 mg or 1 mg twice daily is the optimal granisetron dose for the prevention of emesis induced by moderately emetogenic chemotherapy.

Three double-blind studies, published only as abstracts, evaluated the optimal oral dose of dolasetron in patients submitted to moderately emetogenic chemotherapy.[43-45]

In the first, 319 patients were randomized to receive one of the following single oral doses of dolasetron before chemotherapy with doxorubicin and/or cyclophosphamide: 25 mg, 50 mg, 100 mg and 200 mg.[43] At 24 hours, a linear trend across the four doses was significant for complete protection from vomiting (31%, 41%, 61% and 59% respectively). As there was no difference between the response obtained with 100 and 200 mg, the first was considered the optimal dose.

These results were not confirmed in other two trials, however. In one, 307 patients receiving carboplatin or low-dose cisplatin were randomized to receive the same doses of dolasetron.[44] The dose response for complete protection from acute vomiting across the four oral doses was 33% with 25 mg, 49% with 50 mg, 62% with 100 mg and 70% with 200 mg, with the 200 mg single dose giving the best results.

In the other study, 398 cancer patients submitted to cyclophosphamide, doxorubicin or carboplatin were randomized to receive the same four doses of dolasetron or oral ondansetron (8 mg × 3 or × 4 doses).[45] A statistically significant linear trend was observed across the 25 mg, 50 mg, 100 mg and 200 mg doses (complete protection from acute vomiting in 45%, 49.4%, 60.5% and 76.3% respectively). Complete protection obtained with the 200 mg dose was similar to that obtained with ondansetron (72.3%). Therefore, the optimal single oral dose seems to be 100 or 200 mg.

As far as oral tropisetron dosage is concerned, only one double-blind, dose-ranging study has been published.[46] In 152 chemotherapy-naive patients submitted to low-dose cisplatin or non-cisplatin chemotherapy, two different single oral doses of tropisetron were compared (2 mg versus 5 mg). Complete control of acute vomiting was significantly superior with the 5 mg dose (73% versus 55%), although headache was significantly more frequent with the higher dose.

Are there any differences among 5-HT$_3$ receptor antagonists?

Four double-blind studies have been carried out in patients submitted to moderately emetogenic chemotherapy, with contrasting results (Table 7.7).[47-50]

Unfortunately, only one study has been published in full,[47] and therefore the reasons for the different results found in these studies are difficult to understand. All these studies enrolled an adequate number of patients.

Stewart's study compared two different schedules of ondansetron administered for five days with a single i.v. dose of granisetron on the first day of chemotherapy. It showed similar complete protection from acute vomiting, but, as expected, more nausea was reported by granisetron-treated patients on days 2–5, and, furthermore, these patients required rescue medication more frequently.[47]

In Perez's crossover study, 32 mg i.v. ondansetron gave similar complete protection from acute vomiting, but inferior complete protection from acute nausea compared with 10 µg/kg i.v. of granisetron.[48] The abstract contains only the results obtained in the first cycle of chemotherapy, and the results of the analysis of the crossover design have not yet been published. Therefore these results cannot be considered as definitive.

In contrast, Pion's study showed that oral granisetron 1 mg b.i.d. was superior to 8 mg oral ondansetron b.i.d.[49] However, the statistical analysis, as reported in the abstract, is inconclusive, because neither the cycle effect nor the carry-over effect were investigated, and, moreover, the study does not seem to have sufficient power to detect significant differences.

Finally, Lofters' study comparing 32 mg i.v. ondansetron with 2.4 mg/kg i.v. dolasetron in

Table 7.7 Comparative studies among 5-HT$_3$ antagonists in patients submitted to moderately emetogenic chemotherapy

Study[a]	Number of patients	Antiemetics[b]	CP[c] (%)	Results[b]	Ref
DB	514	OND 8 mg i.v. + 8 mg orally every 12 hours for 5 days	78.0		
		OND 8 mg orally every 12 hours for 5 days	78.0	OND = GRAN > nausea, > rescue with GRAN on days 2–5	47
		GRAN 3 mg i.v.	81.0		
DB XO	623	OND 32 mg i.v. ± DEX i.v.	62.0	OND = GRAN OND > GRAN for nausea	48
		GRAN 10 µg/kg i.v. ± DEX i.v.	58.0		
DB XO	188	GRAN 1 mg orally every 12 hours	73.3[d]	GRAN ⩾OND especially in 2nd cycle	49
		OND 8 mg orally every 12 hours	68.5[d]		
DB XO	703	OND 32 mg i.v. ± DEX i.v.	67.0	OND > DOL DEX increase efficacy	50
		DOL 2.4 mg/kg i.v. ± DEX i.v.	57.0		

[a] DB = double-blind; XO = crossover.
[b] OND = ondansetron; GRAN = granisetron; DOL = dolasetron; DEX = dexamethasone.
[c] CP = complete protection from acute vomiting.
[d] Results in first cycle of chemotherapy.

703 patients showed that complete protection from acute vomiting was significantly superior with ondansetron.[50]

In conclusion, although more studies should be carried out to further investigate possible differences among 5-HT$_3$ receptor antagonists in this group of patients, it is unlikely that major differences exist among different compounds.

PREVENTION OF DELAYED EMESIS INDUCED BY MODERATELY EMETOGENIC CHEMOTHERAPY

Delayed emesis has been studied mainly in cis-platin-treated patients, but it also occurs with moderately emetogenic chemotherapy, especially carboplatin and cyclophosphamide. The incidence and characteristics of delayed emesis differ among patients receiving cisplatin-based or moderately emetogenic chemotherapy.

The onset of emesis after carboplatin and cyclophosphamide occurs with a latency period of 6–12 hours. Symptoms are most intense in the first 24 hours, but nausea and vomiting can persist over a 24–36 hour period. In a study in which 31 breast cancer patients treated with 5-fluorouracil, doxorubicin and cyclophosphamide were observed for four consecutive days without receiving any antiemetic prophylaxis, most of them experienced vomiting for two or more days.[51]

In another study, performed on 28 patients treated with carboplatin, peak intensity of emesis occurred between 8 and 12 hours after chemotherapy, and, although symptoms subsided significantly within 24 hours, some patients (11%) continued to have emesis during the subsequent 48 hours.[52]

Until recently, the problem of delayed emesis due to moderately emetogenic chemotherapy has received little attention. Most of the published studies had as primary objective the evaluation of different antiemetic drugs in the prevention of acute emesis. In some of these studies, the same drugs were continued in the subsequent days to analyse their efficacy on delayed emesis as well. These studies will not be taken into consideration, because to find the superiority of one drug with respect to another in the prophylaxis of delayed emesis could mean either that the drug is really superior or that the superiority is simply due to better results obtained with this drug in the control of acute emesis during the first 24 hours (the so-called dependence effect). To discriminate between these two effects, a multifactorial analysis comparing the results obtained in the prevention of delayed emesis adjusted for those obtained in the prevention of acute emesis must be carried out, but unfortunately this analysis was not performed in these studies, making their interpretation difficult.

So far, only two comparative studies have been specifically planned to evaluate different antiemetic drugs in the prevention of delayed emesis induced by moderately emetogenic chemotherapy.[39,53]

In the first, carried out on 302 patients receiving a combination of single-dose i.v. dexamethasone plus ondansetron in the first 24 hours, patients were randomized to receive on days 2–5 after chemotherapy oral ondansetron (8 mg every 12 hours) or placebo. Complete protection from delayed vomiting was significantly superior with ondansetron compared with placebo (60% versus 42%), as well as complete protection from delayed nausea.[39]

The second was an open study carried out in 98 patients receiving single-dose i.v. dexa-

Table 7.8 Incidence of delayed vomiting in patients submitted to moderately emetogenic chemotherapy[a]		
Cycle	Acute vomiting (%)	No acute vomiting (%)
1	14.7	80.0
2	10.5	66.7
3	16.5	72.7

[a] For prophylaxis of acute emesis; granisetron 3 mg i.v. + dexamethasone 8 mg i.v. + 4 mg orally every 6 hours for 4 doses, starting contemporarily with chemotherapy.

Table 7.9 Incidence of delayed moderate–severe nausea in patients submitted to moderately emetogenic chemotherapy[a]		
Cycle	No acute nausea or mild nausea (%)	Acute moderate–severe nausea (%)
1	14.5	66.7
2	14.1	76.5
3	21.6	70.6

[a] For prophylaxis of acute emesis: granisetron 3 mg i.v. + dexamethasone 8 mg i.v. + 4 mg orally every 6 hours for 4 doses starting contemporarily with chemotherapy.

methasone plus granisetron for the prophylaxis of acute emesis. At 24 hours, patients were randomized between oral dexamethasone (4 mg every 12 hours on days 2–5) or no therapy.[53] Complete protection from delayed vomiting was significantly superior in patients submitted to dexamethasone (57% versus 33%). No data on complete protection from delayed nausea were reported.

One drawback of these studies could be the fact that patients did not receive the best treatment for acute emesis (high and repeated doses of dexamethasone plus a 5-HT$_3$ receptor antagonist) during the first 24 hours. If adopted, this treatment would determine a greater percentage of complete protection from acute emesis that would significantly reduce the incidence of delayed emesis. A recent study by the Italian Group for Antiemetic Research showed that patients obtaining complete protection from acute vomiting and nausea because treated with granisetron (3 mg i.v.) plus dexamethasone (8 mg i.v. plus 4 mg orally 4 times every 6 hours, starting contemporarily with chemotherapy) have a very low incidence of delayed vomiting or moderate–severe nausea (Tables 7.8 and 7.9).[54] Therefore, on the basis of these data, patients having no acute vomiting or no acute moderate–severe nausea do not require antiemetic prophylaxis. These patients can be treated with a rescue antiemetic if delayed emesis occurs. However, patients who have suffered from acute vomiting or acute moderate–severe nausea should always be treated with an antiemetic prophylaxis for delayed emesis. Although further studies are necessary to identify the optimal treatment in this subgroup of patients, dexamethasone or a 5-HT$_3$ receptor antagonist may be efficacious.

CONCLUSIONS

With the introduction of 5-HT$_3$ receptor antagonists, significant progress in the prevention of acute emesis induced by moderately emetogenic chemotherapy has been made. In fact, a combination of a 5-HT$_3$ receptor antagonist plus high and repeated doses of dexamethasone induces complete protection from acute vomiting in over 90% of patients. This antiemetic activity is maintained during the subsequent cycles of chemotherapy. Which 5-HT$_3$ receptor antagonist should be considered the best choice is a matter of opinion. Contrasting results have been observed in the four double-blind trials comparing different 5-HT$_3$ receptor antagonists in the prevention of acute emesis induced by moderately emetogenic chemotherapy. Considering that the studies for the prevention of high-dose cisplatin-induced acute emesis have shown similar efficacy and toxicity among various compounds, those with a lower acquisition cost in each country should be chosen.

Delayed emesis induced by moderately emetogenic chemotherapy has been a little-studied phenomenon. In this case, patients having no acute vomiting or no acute moderate–severe nausea do not seem to require antiemetic prophylaxis. These patients can be treated with a rescue antiemetic if delayed emesis occurs. However, patients with acute vomiting or acute moderate–severe nausea should always be treated with antiemetic prophylaxis for delayed emesis. Although further studies are necessary to identify the optimal treatment in this subgroup of patients, dexamethasone or a 5-HT$_3$ receptor antagonist may be efficacious.

In the prevention of emesis induced by oral CMF chemotherapy, a combination of dexamethasone plus metoclopramide showed efficacy similar to that of a 5-HT$_3$ receptor antagonist, and should be considered the treatment of choice because of its lower cost. In this case, the addition of dexamethasone to a 5-HT$_3$ receptor antagonist should be compared with the dexamethasone and metoclopramide combination in well-conducted double-blind studies.

REFERENCES

1. Martin M, The severity and pattern of emesis following different cytotoxic agents. *Oncology* 1996; **53**(Suppl 1): 26–31.
2. Basurto C, Roila F, Bracarda S et al, A double-blind trial comparing antiemetic efficacy and toxicity of metoclopramide versus methylprednisolone versus domperidone in patients receiving doxorubicin chemotherapy alone or in combination with other antiblastic agents. *Am J Clin Oncol* 1988; **11**: 594–6.
3. Edge SB, Funkhouser WK, Berman A et al, High-dose oral and intravenous metoclopramide in doxorubicin/cyclophosphamide-induced emesis. A randomized double-blind study. *Am J Clin Oncol* 1987; **10**: 257–63.
4. Mellink WA, Blijham GH, Van Deyk WA, Amitriptyline plus fluphenazine to prevent chemotherapy-induced emesis in cancer patients: a double-blind randomized cross-over study. *Eur J Cancer Clin Oncol* 1984; **20**: 1147–50.
5. Markman M, Sheidler V, Ettinger DS et al, Antiemetic efficacy of dexamethasone. Randomized, double-blind, crossover study with prochlorperazine in patients receiving cancer chemotherapy. *N Engl J Med* 1984; **311**: 549–52.
6. Morran C, Smith DC, Anderson DA, McArdle CS, Incidence of nausea and vomiting with cytotoxic chemotherapy. A prospective randomised trial of antiemetics. *Br Med J* 1979; **1**: 1323–4.
7. David M, Durand M, Chauvergne J et al, Cyclophosphamide, methotrexate, and 5-FU (CMF)-induced nausea and vomiting: a controlled study with high-dose metoclopramide. *Cancer Treat Rep* 1984; **68**: 921–2.
8. Chiara S, Scarsi P, Campora E et al, Low-dose metoclopramide versus methylprednisolone in controlling chemotherapy induced nausea and vomiting. *Chemioterapia* 1984; **3**: 333–6.
9. Roila F, Tonato M, Basurto C et al, Double-blind controlled trial of the antiemetic efficacy and toxicity of methylprednisolone (MP), metoclopramide (MTC) and domperidone (DMP) in breast cancer patients treated with i.v. CMF. *Eur J Cancer Clin Oncol* 1987; **23**: 615–17.
10. Roila F, Basurto C, Minotti V et al, Methylprednisolone vs metoclopramide for prevention of nausea and vomiting in breast cancer patients treated with intravenous cyclophosphamide, methotrexate, 5-fluorouracil: a double-blind randomized study. *Oncology* 1988; **45**: 346–9.
11. Chiara S, Campora E, Lionetto R et al, Methylprednisolone for the control of CMF-induced emesis. *Am J Clin Oncol* 1987; **10**: 264–7.
12. Pollera CF, Nardi M, Marolla P et al, Effective control of CMF-related emesis with high-dose dexamethasone: results of a double-blind, crossover trial with metoclopramide and placebo. *Am J Clin Oncol* 1989; **12**: 524–9.
13. Gez E, Sulkes A, Ochayon L et al, Methylprednisolone versus metoclopramide as antiemetic treatment in patients receiving adjuvant cyclophosphamide, methotrexate, 5-fluorouracil (CMF) chemotherapy: a randomized crossover blind study. *J Chemother* 1989; **1**: 365–8.
14. Gez E, Strauss N, Vitzhaki N et al, Methylprednisolone as antiemetic treatment in breast-cancer patients receiving cyclophosphamide, methotrexate, and 5-fluorouracil: a prospective, crossover, randomized blind study comparing two different dose schedules. *Cancer Chemother Pharmacol* 1992; **30**: 229–32.
15. Bonneterre J, Chevallier B, Metz R et al, A randomized double-blind comparison of ondansetron and metoclopramide in the prophylaxis of emesis induced by cyclophosphamide, fluorouracil and doxorubicin or epirubicin chemotherapy. *J Clin Oncol* 1990; **8**: 1063–9.
16. Kaasa S, Kvaloy S, Dicato MA et al, A comparison of ondansetron with metoclopramide in the prophylaxis of chemotherapy-induced nausea and vomiting: a randomized, double-blind study. *Eur J Cancer* 1990; **26**: 311–14.
17. Marschner NW, Adler M, Nagel GA et al, Double-blind randomised trial of the antiemetic efficacy and safety of ondansetron and metoclopramide in advanced breast cancer patients treated with epirubicin and cyclophosphamide. *Eur J Cancer* 1991; **27**: 1137–40.
18. Soukop M, McQuade B, Hunter E et al, Ondansetron compared with metoclopramide in the control of emesis and quality of life during repeated chemotherapy for breast cancer. *Oncology* 1992; **49**: 295–304.
19. Anderson H, Thatcher N, Howell A et al, Tropisetron compared with a metoclopramide-based regimen in the prevention of chemotherapy-induced nausea and vomiting. *Eur J Cancer* 1994; **30A**: 610–15.
20. Fauser A, Bleiberg H, Chevallier B et al, A double-blind randomized comparative trial of iv dolasetron vs iv metoclopramide in prevention

of emesis in moderately emetogenic chemotherapy. *Proc Am Soc Clin Oncol* 1995; **14**: 530 (abst).

21. Campora E, Giudici S, Merlini L et al, Ondansetron and dexamethasone versus standard combination antiemetic therapy. *Am J Clin Oncol* 1994; **17**: 522–6.

22. Clavel M, Bonneterre J, d'Allens H, Paillarse JM and the French Ondansetron Study Group, Oral ondansetron in the prevention of chemotherapy-induced emesis in breast cancer patients. *Eur J Cancer* 1995; **31A**: 15–19.

23. De Nigris A, Paladini G, Giosa F et al, Tropisetron (Navoban) compared with alizapride in the control of emesis induced by cyclophosphamide-containing regimens. *Eur J Cancer* 1994; **30A**: 1902–3.

24. Palmer R, Moriconi W, Cohn J et al, A double-blind comparison of the efficacy and safety of oral granisetron with oral prochlorperazine in preventing nausea and emesis in patients receiving moderately emetogenic chemotherapy. *Proc Am Soc Clin Oncol* 1995; **14**: 528 (abst).

25. Marty M, on behalf of the Granisetron Study Group, A comparative study of the use of granisetron, a selective 5-HT$_3$ antagonist, versus a standard anti-emetic regimen of chlorpromazine plus dexamethasone in the treatment of cytostatic-induced emesis. *Eur J Cancer* 1990; **26**(Suppl 1): 28–32.

26. Warr D, Willan A, Fine S et al, Superiority of granisetron to dexamethasone plus prochlorperazine in the prevention of chemotherapy-induced emesis. *J Natl Cancer Inst* 1991; **83**: 1169–73.

27. Jones AL, Hill AS, Soukop M et al, Comparison of ondansetron and dexamethasone in the prophylaxis of emesis induced by moderately emetogenic chemotherapy. *Lancet* 1991; **338**: 483–7.

28. Adams M, Soukop M, Barley V et al, Tropisetron alone or in combination with dexamethasone for the prevention and treatment of emesis induced by non-cisplatin chemotherapy: a randomized trial. *Anti-Cancer Drugs* 1995; **6**: 514–21.

29. The Italian Group for Antiemetic Research, Dexamethasone, granisetron, or both for the prevention of nausea and vomiting during chemotherapy for cancer. *N Engl J Med* 1995; **332**: 1–5.

30. The Italian Group for Antiemetic Research, Persistence of efficacy of three antiemetic regimens and prognostic factors in patients undergoing moderately emetogenic chemotherapy. *J Clin Oncol* 1995; **13**: 2417–26.

31. Herrstedt J, Sigsgaard T, Boesgaard M et al, Ondansetron plus metopimazine compared with ondansetron alone in patients receiving moderately emetogenic chemotherapy. *N Engl J Med* 1993; **328**: 1076–80.

32. Buser KS, Joss RA, Piquet D et al, Oral ondansetron in the prophylaxis of nausea and vomiting induced by cyclophosphamide, methotrexate and 5-fluorouracil (CMF) in women with breast cancer. Results of a prospective, randomized, double-blind, placebo-controlled study. *Ann Oncol* 1993; **4**: 475–9.

33. Levitt M, Warr D, Yell L et al, Ondansetron compared with dexamethasone and metoclopramide as antiemetics in the chemotherapy of breast cancer with cyclophosphamide, methotrexate and fluorouracil. *N Engl J Med* 1993; **328**: 1081–4.

34. Fraschini G, Ciociola A, Esparza L et al, Evaluation of three oral dosages of ondansetron in the prevention of nausea and emesis associated with cyclophosphamide–doxorubicin chemotherapy. *J Clin Oncol* 1991; **9**: 1268–74.

35. Beck TM, Ciociola AA, Jones SE et al, Efficacy of oral ondansetron in the prevention of emesis in outpatients receiving cyclophosphamide-based chemotherapy. *Ann Intern Med* 1993; **118**: 407–13.

36. Cubeddu LX, Pendergrass K, Ryan T et al, Efficacy of oral ondansetron, a selective antagonist of 5-HT$_3$ receptors, in the treatment of nausea and vomiting associated with cyclophosphamide-based chemotherapies. *Am J Clin Oncol* 1994; **17**: 137–46.

37. Dicato M, Oral treatment with ondansetron in an outpatient setting. *Eur J Cancer* 1991; **27**(Suppl 1): 518–19.

38. Beck T, York M, Chang A et al, Oral ondansetron 8 mg bid is as effective as 8 mg tid in the prevention of nausea and vomiting associated with cyclophosphamide-based chemotherapy. *Proc Am Soc Clin Oncol* 1995; **14**: 538 (abst).

39. Kaizer L, Warr D, Hoskins P et al, Effect of schedule and maintenance on the antiemetic efficacy of ondansetron combined with dexamethasone in acute and delayed nausea and emesis in patients receiving moderately emetogenic chemotherapy: a phase III trial by the National Cancer Institute of Canada Clinical Trials Group. *J Clin Oncol* 1994; **12**: 1050–7.

40. Smith IE, on behalf of the Granisetron Study Group, A comparison of two dose levels of granisetron in patients receiving moderately emetogenic cytostatic chemotherapy. *Eur J Cancer* 1990; **26**(Suppl 1): 19–23.

41. Hacking A, on behalf of the Granisetron Study Group, Oral granisetron – simple and effective: a preliminary report. *Eur J Cancer* 1992; **28A** (Suppl 1): 28–32.

42. Ettinger DS, Eisenberg PD, Fitts D et al, A double-blind comparison of the efficacy of two dose regimens of oral granisetron in preventing acute emesis in patients receiving moderately emetogenic chemotherapy. *Cancer* 1996; **78**: 144–51.

43. Rubenstein E, Kalman J, Hainsworth J et al, Dose–response trial across 4 oral doses of dolasetron for emesis prevention after moderately emetogenic chemotherapy. *Proc Am Soc Clin Oncol* 1995; **14**: 527 (abst).

44. Grote T, Pineda L, Modiano M et al, Dose–response trial across four oral doses of dolasetron mesylate for prevention of acute nausea and vomiting after platinum-containing moderately emetogenic chemotherapy. *Proc Am Soc Clin Oncol* 1996; **15**: 533 (abst).

45. Del Favero A, Bergerat J, Chemaissani A, Dressler H, Single oral doses of dolasetron versus multiple dose of ondansetron in preventing emesis after moderately emetogenic chemotherapy. *Support Care Cancer* 1995; **3**: 337 (abst).

46. Wymenga ANM, van der Graaf WTA, Wils JA et al, A randomized, double-blind, multicentre study comparing daily 2 and 5 mg of tropisetron for the control of nausea and vomiting induced by low-dose cisplatin- or non-cisplatin-containing chemotherapy. *Ann Oncol* 1996; **7**: 505–10.

47. Stewart A, McQuade B, Cronje JDE et al, Ondansetron compared with granisetron in the prophylaxis of cyclophosphamide-induced emesis in out-patients: a multicentre, double-blind, double-dummy, randomised, parallel-group study. *Oncology* 1995; **52**: 202–10.

48. Perez EA, Lembersky B, Kaywin P et al, Intravenous granisetron vs ondansetron in the prevention of cyclophosphamide-doxorubicin-induced emesis in breast cancer patients: a double-blind crossover study. *Proc Am Soc Clin Oncol* 1996; **15**: 543 (abst).

49. Pion JM, Fournier C, Darloy F et al, Oral granisetron vs oral ondansetron, a comparative double-blind cross-over multicenter study of preventive anti-emetic in moderately emetogenic chemotherapy, by the French Northern Oncology Group (FNOG). *Proc Am Soc Clin Oncol* 1996; **15**: 530 (abst).

50. Lofters WS, Zee B, for the Symptom Control Committee of the National Cancer Institute of Canada Clinical Trials Group, Dolasetron vs ondansetron with and without dexamethasone in the prevention of nausea and vomiting in patients receiving moderately emetogenic chemotherapy. *Support Care Cancer* 1995; **3**: 338 (abst).

51. Martin Jimenez M, Diaz-Rubio E, Blazquer Encinar JC et al, Tolerancia, toxicidad y aceptación del tratamiento quimioterapico adiuvante FAC (5-fluorouracilo, adriamicina y ciclofosfamida) en el cancer de mama. Analisi de 100 paciences consecutivas. *Neoplasia (Barc)* 1988; **5**: 8–14.

52. Martin M, Diaz-Rubio E, Sanchez A et al, The natural course of carboplatin-induced emesis. *Acta Oncol* 1990; **29**: 593–5.

53. Koo WH, Ang PT, Role of maintenance oral dexamethasone in prophylaxis of delayed emesis caused by moderately emetogenic chemotherapy. *Ann Oncol* 1996; **7**: 71–4.

54. De Angelis V, Roila F, Campora E et al, Incidence and pattern of delayed emesis induced by moderately emetogenic chemotherapy. *Tumori* 1996; **82**(Suppl): 110 (abst).

8

Treatment of radiotherapy-induced nausea and vomiting

Petra Feyer, Otto J Titlbach

INTRODUCTION

Cancer is the second most common cause of death after heart and circulatory diseases. The established treatments involve surgery, radiotherapy and chemotherapy, and new approaches are under development. Radiotherapy and surgery are locally limited, in contrast to chemotherapy. They have an effect exclusively at the place of application, and can be curative only in localized disease.

Localized disease can be found in approximately 55% of patients, about two-thirds of whom have a possibility of cure: about one-third with surgery alone, about one-third with radiotherapy alone and 1–2% with chemotherapy alone. Thus about 50% of curative cancer treatment is realized by radiotherapy alone. There remains one-third of localized disease with no cure at present. Such disease is currently the subject of research into new methods and combined modalities. At the time of diagnosis, 45% of patients have metastatic disease (Figure 8.1).

In summary, about 60% of all cancer patients are incurable at the time of diagnosis.[1] Approximately 70% of incurable cancer patients receive radiotherapy at some point during their disease as a palliative treatment, while 50% receive chemotherapy.

The therapeutic concept in radiotherapy takes into consideration the possibilities of cure. In the planning of treatment efficacy–risk analysis is of great importance. The therapeutic benefit defines the extent of tolerable side-effects. When a cure is possible, a temporary increase in side-effects is tolerable, but in palliative treatment any reduction in the quality of life caused by the therapy is unacceptable.

Quality of life is one of the most important parameters in oncology, and there are numerous assessment scales that are helpful in daily clinical practice and for comparison in scientific evaluation. In clinical practice this means improvement of prognosis and quality of life – the therapeutic aims in oncology.

Importance of gastrointestinal side-effects in radiotherapy

Gastrointestinal side-effects complicate the course of curative or palliative radiotherapy. Nausea and vomiting are among the most distressing side-effects for patients, influencing their quality of life.[2]

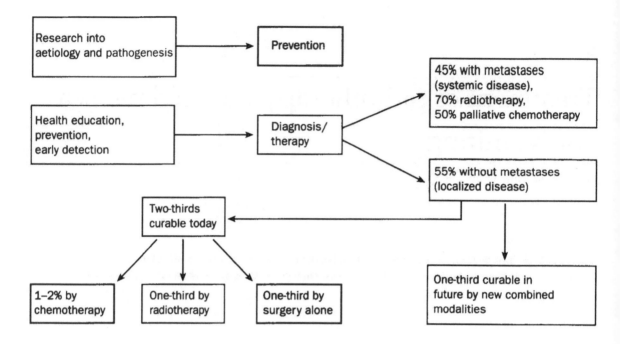

Figure 8.1 The cancer problem (modified from reference 1).

In curative treatment the recovery of the patient may be put at risk by any interruption of the therapy necessitated by the severity of these side-effects. There is evidence that breaks in treatment have unfavourable effects on tumour control.[3,4] Effective control of symptoms is necessary in order to complete the required radiotherapy without interruption.

In the case of palliative treatment untreated gastrointestinal side-effects cause stress to the patient and further reduce the quality of life.[5] Emesis and nutritional problems involving body-weight loss, electrolyte disturbance and reduced quality of life develop.[6] Side-effects like nausea and emesis often require hospitalization even when outpatient treatment would be possible in their absence.

It is important to recall that the distress to the patient during fractionated irradiation may be particularly pronounced, since the treatment can comprise up to 40 sessions. However, since a course of radiation may involve up to 30–40 fractions given over a period of 6–8 weeks, the potential for distress to the patient due to the sickness continuing for that length of time is considerable.[7]

If untreated, emesis may persist throughout this period and cause physiological changes, such as dehydration, electrolyte imbalance and/or malnutrition, which in turn can hamper the quality of life and the final goal of the treatment.[8]

These connections demonstrate the important role of antiemetic therapy in the treatment of cancer patients.

Incidence of nausea and vomiting in radiotherapy

The intensity and severity of emesis are related to a large number of parameters, including the site treated, the dose and size of the irradiated field, biological events following irradiation, and clinical considerations, including prior surgery, exposure to cytotoxic drugs, and the psychological and metabolic status of the patient. In general, the severity of emesis and nausea in patients receiving radiotherapy is lower than associated with more aggressive chemotherapy treatments.[9]

The incidence, severity and onset of radiation-induced emesis may vary with the site of irradiation, the dose per fraction and the field size.

Total-body irradiation and irradiation of the upper parts of the abdomen are the most strongly emetogenic regimens in radiotherapy, and are associated with nausea, vomiting, anorexia and diarrhoea. The irradiation of whole-abdominal fields in the treatment of cancer is also associated with these severe side-effects.

Emesis can occur two to three weeks after the onset of treatment in approximately 50% of patients receiving conventionally fractionated radiation (1.8–2.0 Gy) to the upper abdomen. Previous reports have indicated that emesis occurs in approximately 50% of patients receiving fractionated radiotherapy to the whole abdomen[10] and in over 80% when single treatments are given[11]. During irradiation of the pelvic region alone, nausea and vomiting are not frequent clinical problems.[12] An analysis of the management of nausea and vomiting in fractionated radiotherapy between thorax and pelvis with mild to moderate risk for emesis, including 1387 patients from 11 radiotherapy centres from 5 countries, reported that approximately 40% of the patients with no antiemetic prophylaxis experienced nausea and vomiting.[13]

Franzen et al[14] reported on 109 patients irradiated to the abdomen and pelvis, fractionated daily, 55% of whom without antiemetic prophylaxis experienced emesis.

Sommer et al[15] performed a study of acute and late toxicity of radiation therapy for testicular seminoma, with the radiation field including the paraaortal and parailiacal region, and found an incidence of mild to moderate nausea and vomiting and increased bowel frequency of 87%. However, emesis can be more acute when patients receive treatment with larger fields (e.g. total-body irradiation (TBI) or half-body irradiation (HBI) with doses >5 Gy).

Coccia et al[16] reported an incidence of 95% mild to moderate and 5% severe nausea and vomiting in patients who received 12 Gy TBI (2 Gy/fraction twice a day × 3 days) following cytosine arabinoside. Danjoux et al[11] reported an 83% incidence of radiation-induced emesis following >5 Gy delivered to the upper half of the body (from the umbilicus up to and including the head), but only 39% incidence after lower HBI.

Emesis usually occurred within 40–90 minutes following upper HBI without benefit of antiemetic preparations, which included prochlorperazine, diazepam and metoclopramide.

Henriksson et al[8] emphasized that up to 80% of patients receiving radiotherapy with high single fractions develop nausea and vomiting. Currently available antiemetics (e.g. metoclopramide or nabilone) have been shown to control these problems in about 50% of patients during prolonged radiotherapy courses.[17]

Tiley et al[18] discussed nausea and vomiting during TBI as the most significant side-effects, and assumed that they can be very distressing for the patient. Particular problems are associated with nausea in the context of single-fraction low-dose-rate TBI as used in their centre. The patient is isolated in the radiotherapy unit for 5–7 hours. A study of emesis performed in the TBI unit found that 50% of patients vomit during TBI,[19] despite the current prophylaxis with phenobarbitone and hydrocortisone. Westbrook et al[19] noted that in single dose TBI emesis usually begins after a dose of 2–3 Gy, and may persist up to 12 hours from the start of treatment. There can be a recurrence of vomiting after 2–5 days.

Hunter et al[20] reported their experiences with TBI in the Royal Free Hospital, London. In their unit TBI is delivered as a single fraction at a fast dose rate (0.15 ± 0.02 Gy/min) up to a total dose of approximately 7.5 Gy. This has consistently induced emesis in more than 95% of patients, despite the use of combination antiemetic therapy. During TBI, patients

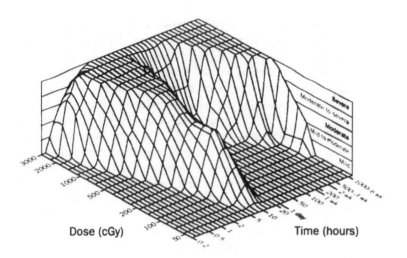

Figure 8.2 Three-dimensional plot of the relationship of radiation dose, time and severity of 'upper gastrointestinal symptoms' (modified from references 21 and 29).

Dose (cGy)

Time (hours)

develop abdominal cramps, nausea, sweating and vomiting approximately 35 minutes after starting treatment (the estimated dose received is 3.5–4.0 Gy). Symptoms may be so severe that treatment has to be interrupted, and these symptoms may last for 24 hours or longer.

A study of the 1986 reactor accident at Chernobyl has demonstrated that the latency before onset of emesis is in inverse correlation to the dose (Figures 8.2 and 8.3).[21]

critical organs responsible for radiation-induced emesis are in the upper abdomen, and the underlying mechanism may be related to a toxin released by degradation of tumour proteins. The production of a second messenger resulting from radiation-associated cellular damage has been considered.

Radiation-induced nausea: pathomechanism

The mechanism of emesis after irradiation is a complex multifactorial clinical event defined by different factors (site of irradiation, dose per fraction and field size), as well as by psychological and physiological variables.

The pattern of symptoms following a single high dose of irradiation was described in 1953 by Court-Brown.[22] The pattern consisted of three phases: a latent period, a period of acute disturbances and a recovery phase. Danjoux et al[11] described symptoms following half-body irradiation. The incidence of radiation-induced emesis was higher after mid and upper half-body irradiation. These observations by Court-Brown[22] and by Danjoux et al[11] suggest that the

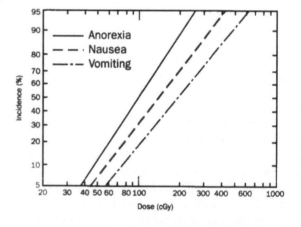

Figure 8.3 Relationship of prodromal symptoms (incidence of anorexia, nausea and vomiting) and radiation dose. Probit analysis of the data of Langham[100] and Lushbaugh[101,102] from Harding et al.[29]

The effects and side-effects of radiotherapy are based on the same damage mechanism. In general, proliferating cell populations are the most at risk from the lethal effects of ionizing radiation. We know a great deal about the lethal effects of radiation on cells and tissues.[23,24] However, the pathological mechanism of radiation-induced emesis remains only partially understood.

The effect of irradiation depends on the extent of cell death, and is influenced by proliferation, differentation of the tissue and repair capacity. Furthermore, the cell-cycle phase is of importance, and different tissues have different radiosensitivies. Mammalian cells are most radiosensitive during the mitotic phase of the cell cycle.

Cell death can occur quickly and in the absence of failure of mitosis. Apoptosis or active cell death has been invoked to explain the selective and rapid death seen following irradiation of certain cells near the bases of the intestinal crypts.[25] In man there is no ED100 for radiation-induced emesis: even with the most emetogenic radiotherapy, only about 80–90% of patients can be expected to vomit in the absence of antiemetic therapy.[26] Davis et al[27] have described vomiting in terms of a hierarchically organized toxin defence system in which the irradiated individual responds in a stereotypical manner to a perceived toxin and in this way tries to protect itself from damage. Vomiting is an important post-irradiation symptom. Other effects, such as post-irradiation fatigue and weakness, have also been widely reported in the literature, but they are less well understood and more difficult to quantify than radiation-induced vomiting. The work of Anno et al[21] also highlights the involvement of other gastrointestinal symptoms, such as dysmotility and diarrhoea, as both early and later responses to radiation exposure.

The LD50 for man (assuming no medical intervention) has recently been placed at a dose of approximately 2.9 Gy delivered to the bone marrow (Table 8.1).[28]

Investigations using radioprotective substances do not show any reduction in radiation-induced emesis. Thus there is no evidence to

Table 8.1 Ionizing radiation: emetic sensitivity, latency and LD$_{50}$ (from reference 32)

Species	Latency (min)	Dose (cGy108) ED$_{50}$	LD$_{50}$
Human	60–90	200	290
Dog	80–90	230	260
Ferret	30	100	<200
Rhesus monkey	45	450	550

Latency = time to first emetic episode; ED$_{50}$ = dose of radiation required to cause emesis in 50% of the subject population; LD$_{50}$ = dose of radiation required to kill 50% of the subject population. In humans, the value is reported as an LD$_{50/60}$, the dose calculated to kill 50% of subjects within 60 days. In animals, the assessment period is 30 days, and the value is reported as LD$_{50/30}$.

suggest that radioprotective compounds will reduce the incidence of radiation-induced vomiting. The relationship between radiation and the majority of cell-death episodes and vomiting does not prove the hypothesis that cell death is the major acute emetic stimulus. However, it has been speculated that the use of radioprotective compounds should lead to a reduction in prodromal symptoms such as vomiting, because toxicity will then be confined to a smaller population of cells.[29]

Irritation of the local gastrointestinal mucosa is a potent emetic stimulus,[30] and inflammation may constitute the irritant emetic stimulus following irradiation. Inflammation can lead to further tissue damage and exacerbate the destruction due to radiation-induced cell death alone. Therefore radiotherapy may also be considered in terms of a series of inflammatory insults.[31] The post-irradiation inflammatory reaction complicates the recovery of tissues and contributes to the histopathologies seen in the days following irradiation. Vomiting in the first day may be viewed as a pathophysiological effect, while delayed vomiting is perhaps more closely related to histopathological effects, and may involve additional mechanisms. In all animals with an emetic response to radiation, the latency period seen before the onset of emesis implies that emesis is not induced directly by radiation exposure.

Some second-order mechanisms are probably necessary following the deposition of radiation in tissues. Release of serotonin (5-hydroxytryptamine, 5-HT) from enterochromaffin-like cells located in the bowel mucosa is a likely arbiter of the emetic process. It is not clear how radiation or other emetics accomplish this release. We do know that free radicals are released into tissues and cells immediately following irradiation. Typically, it is the lethal cytotoxic effects of radiation that have been studied and cited as the major explanation for the symptomatology. However, emesis may be induced by sublethal doses of radiation. The emetic dose of radiation is well below that which would lead to appreciable somatic cell death, and emesis occurs well before failure at mitosis accounts for the death of actively dividing cell types.

It is believed that apoptosis – actively induced cell death – may be a potentially important contributor.[32] Potten[25] has shown that there is a sensitive subpopulation of stem cells in the crypts, which undergo morphologically distinct stages of cell death. In summary, apoptosis is a very radiation-sensitive rapid reaction, and is maximal at low doses (1 Gy). The sensitive crypt cells that undergo apoptosis immediately following irradiation, and some of the equally sensitive intra-epithelial lymphocytes, are located proximal to the enteochromaffin-like cells. Could these dying cells contribute to the stimulus for 5-HT release?

Hypothetically, there can be two different pathophysiological mechanisms working together in inducing emesis:

1. a passive cell damage mechanism (histopathological effect), in the sense of a release reaction of transmitters that induce or contain emesis;

2. an active functional defence mechanism (pathophysiological effect) through the release of mediators by functioning cells.

Free radicals are released immediately after irradiation in the tissues and cells. Furthermore, an inflammatory reaction has been described: irradiation-induced inflammation. Buell and Harding[31] described an accumulation of neutrophils in the rat intestinal mucosa in the acute period following exposure to 10 Gy. This and other data[33,34] are consistent with a post-irradiation inflammatory response.

The inflammatory reaction possibly leads to the release of histamines and other transmitters affecting emesis.

Enterochromaffin cells of the mucosa are important. They have a high serotonin (5-hydroxytryptamine, 5-HT) content.[35] Damage of the enterochromaffin cells by toxins and/or irradiation leads to the release of serotonin, which is stored in the granula and to the stimulation of serotonin receptors of subtype 3 (5-HT$_3$ receptors) in the ends of afferent vagal fibres. Neuronal impulses reach the central area postrema and the nucleolus region, which is located in the floor of the fourth ventricle, and the chemoreceptor trigger zone (CTZ).[36-39]

In the CTZ there also exist other transmitter systems (employing carrier substances and their specific receptors, like dopamine, histamine, acetylcholine, adrenaline and noradrenaline as well as morphine). These can be stimulated by serotonin circulating in the blood or by other transmitter substances. In the emesis centre the impulses of the area postrema, CTZ, cerebellum, diencephalon and cerebral hemisphere are integrated. These control the efferent impulses, and in this complex way induce the vomiting reflex.

Various neurotransmitter systems are localized in the area postrema, and therefore a number of different receptor blocking substances have been investigated in order to get an antiemetic effect through inhibition of these neurotransmitter systems. Serotonin may mediate emesis through mechanisms involving 5-HT$_3$ receptors and activation of the CTZ through visceral afferent pathways. The correlation of radiation-induced emesis and 5-hydroxyindoleacetic acid (5-HIAA) levels strongly suggests that the mechanism of radiation-induced emesis is related to serotonin

release. The increase in 5-HIAA after upper and mid half-body irradiation and the fact that serotonin is found in high concentrations in the upper abdomen support a model for radiation-induced emesis in which serotonin stimulates the afferent fibres and the CTZ.[40]

A possible classification scheme for emesis is given in Table 8.2.

FACTORS AFFECTING INCIDENCE AND SEVERITY OF RADIATION-INDUCED EMESIS

There are numerous factors influencing the incidence and severity of nausea and vomiting during radiotherapy. Some are specific to radiotherapy (e.g. physical factors), but there are also factors in common with other causes of emesis, as well as individual risk factors. Radiation-induced emesis and chemotherapy-induced emesis involve some common basic factors. The most important factors influencing radiation-induced emesis are summarized in Table 8.3. In the following sections we go into the details of the most important of these.

Physical factors influencing radiation-induced emesis

Energy and beam quality
Emesis may vary as a function of the type of the radiation as well as of the radiation dose. Thus

---

Table 8.2 Classification of emesis

(A) By cause
- Toxins/vagal stimulation
- Radiation
- Anticipatory
- Psychogenic
- Sensory-reactive

(B) By time course
- Acute (1–2 hours after treatment)
- Delayed (>24 hours after treatment)
- Intermittent
- Persistent

(C) By severity
(1) *Verbal scale/visual analogue scale*
   Mild–moderate–severe
(2) *Differentiation by WHO criteria*
   Nausea:
   - 0   none
   - 1   mild (normal nutrition possible)
   - 2   moderate (nutritional intake reduced)
   - 3   severe (no oral nutrition possible)
   Vomiting:
   - 0   none
   - 1   mild (1 episode per day)
   - 2   moderate (2–5 episodes per day)
   - 3   severe (6–10 episodes per day)
   - 4   life-threatening (>10 episodes per day or parenteral nutrition necessary)

Table 8.3 Factors influencing radiation-induced emesis

- Single and total dose
- Fractionation
- Irradiated volume
- Organs included in the radiation field
- Radiation technique and beam energy
- Previous or simultaneous therapy
- General health of the patient

linear energy transfer is important, as well as the energy of the beams used. The higher linear energy transfer, the higher is the probability of emesis, which means that the ED50 is reduced. These are the same basic principles that apply in radiobiology when considering the biological effects of ionizing radiation.[41]

For example, the results of Rabin et al[41] showed that the mean effective doses for iron ions (0.35 Gy) and neutrons (0.40 Gy) were similar. High-energy electrons were the least effective form of radiation, with a ED50 of 1.38 Gy. Gamma rays, with a ED50 of 0.95 Gy, showed an intermediate effectiveness. These results suggest that the relative effectiveness of the different types of radiation in general increases with increasing linear energy transfer (LET), although the latter is not completely predictive of relative behaviourial effectiveness. Thus energy and beam quality are of importance for emesis. A similar relationship can be established for the radiation energy: the higher the energy, the deeper the radiation can penetrate and the higher is emetic potential, because emetic-sensitive structures are localized in the depth of the mid-body (upper abdomen, first parts of the small intestine, and vagal afferent fibres).

Site of irradiation: organs included in the irradiation field

The target volume and irradiated volume can affect emesis. Bremer[42] proposed a relationship between the probability of emesis and the site and volume of radiotherapy: the larger the irradiated volume, the higher is the risk of emesis and the upper abdomen is the most critical region. The site and volume dependencies of radiotherapy-induced emesis are summarized in Figure 8.4 and Table 8.4.[43]

A number of factors influencing likelihood of radiation-induced emesis have been identified. Radiotherapy to the upper abdomen is the most likely to produce nausea and vomiting. Animal studies have shown that such exposure causes the release of emetic substances from the first part of the small bowel. Stimulation of the chemoreceptor trigger zone via vagal afferent fibres from the upper gastrointestinal tract has

Table 8.4 Emetogenic potential of radiotherapy: site aspects

Severe	Moderate
• Total-body irradiation	• Lower thorax region
• Upper half-body irradiation	• Upper abdominal region
• Total nodal irradiation	• Pelvis
• Abdominal bath	• Lower half-body irradiation

Low

• Head and neck
• Extremities

also been implicated.[44] Danjoux et al[11] reported an 83% incidence of radiation-induced emesis after doses of >5 Gy in upper or mid half-body irradiation, and 39% after lower half-body irradiation. Scarantino et al[45] reported an 85% incidence after upper and mid half-body irradiation and only 15% after lower half-body irradiation. Cubeddu et al[46] observed increases in urinary excretion of 5-HIAA and plasma levels parallel to the onset and development of emesis. Direct correlation of emesis and serotonin after half-body irradiation suggests a direct role of serotonin as a mediator for radiation-induced emesis. Although theoretical pathways exist to explain the mechanism by which upper abdominal irradiation causes emesis, it remains the case that a small but significant proportion of patients receiving radiotherapy to other sites may also experience considerable emesis.[7]

Field size

The greater the volume of tissue irradiated, the greater is the risk of nausea and vomiting.

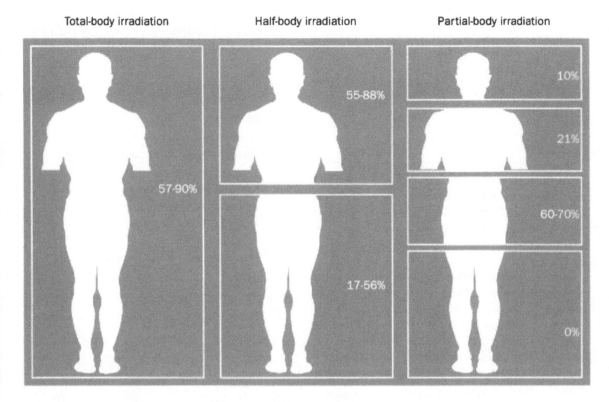

Figure 8.4 Emetogenicity of irradiation: site dependence.

Total-body irradiation therefore presents the greatest emetic challenge. Coccia et al[16] reported 95% incidence of mild to moderate and a 5% incidence of severe emesis after 12 Gy TBI (2 Gy per fraction twice a day for three days). The field size should be tailored exactly to the target volume in order to limit the irradiated body volume (individual satellites and blocks) and to minimize side-effects during irradiation.[5,43]

Dose per fraction

The greater the dose of irradiation given in each treatment, the greater is the risk of emesis. Emesis can occur two to three weeks after the onset of irradiation in 30–50% of patients receiving conventional fractionated irradiation (1.8–2 Gy) to the upper abdomen. However, emesis can be more acute and more consistent in patients receive higher single doses (>5 Gy) to larger fields (total- or half-body irradiation).[45]

Palliative radiotherapy may be given with single exposures of 8–15 Gy, greatly increasing the risk of emesis for the patient. Patients receiving more than 8 Gy as a single dose are more likely to experience emesis than those receiving smaller doses of approximately 2 Gy as in fractionated radiotherapy.[7] There is also evidence to suggest that emesis occurs following a cumulative dosing threshold of more than 3 Gy.[19,47]

In summary, the frequency and intensity of emesis vary depending on the dose schedule and the irradiated volume as well as the site of treatment. Approximately 80% of patients receiving single-high-dose abdominal radiotherapy of more than 6 Gy develop nausea and vomiting, whereas only 50% of patients with daily fractionated doses of more than 1.8 Gy are affected.[10,11]

Dose rate

There are only a few data concerning the influence of dose rate. Westbrook et al[19] described the onset of emesis in TBI using a low dose rate of 0.02–0.04 Gy/min above doses of 2–3 Gy. Similar results were found by Feyer.[47]

Patient positioning

There is some evidence that motion can affect emesis. There are data by Westbrook et al[19] indicating a lower incidence of emesis if the patient is not moved in TBI: there is a difference between irradiation with one source or two sources. The incidence of emesis is reduced by limitation of patient movement during irradiation.

Combined modalities

Cytotoxic drugs used simultaneously with radiotherapy may potentiate nausea and vomiting through their own emetogenicity.[5]

A summary of the characteristics of radiation-induced vomiting in man is given in Table 8.5.[29]

Individual risk factors

Age, gender, alcohol consumption and previous experiences of emesis are in general considered as risk factors for emetogenic therapies. They can be summarized in an emesis-risk score.[5] Physical factors that influence the incidence and severity of radiation-induced emesis are taken partially into consideration in the course of treatment planning. In contrast to this, individual risk factors are rarely taken into consideration for treatment planning. However, there are numerous reports in the literature concerning the importance of individual risk factors for treatment-induced emesis. These are

Table 8.5 Characteristics of radiation-induced vomiting in humans (from reference 29)

- Low threshold, about 1 Gy
- ED50 ≤ 2 Gy
- No ED100
- Dose rate less important than actual accumulated dose (at >2 cGy/min)
- Vomiting usually seen in the second hour following accumulation of emetic dose
- Emetic episodes last for several hours
- Emesis typically less severe than with some cytotoxics
- Upper abdomen = most-emetic radiation site

summarized in the following with the help of available data.

Bremer[42] established a risk score with the following factors. The risk of emesis is high for female patients, for those younger than 50 years and for those who are not regular consumers of (low amounts of) alcohol, as well as for those with previous experience of nausea and vomiting. In males older than 50 years, as well as in those with an alcohol consumption of more than 100 g per day, there is a significantly lower incidence of nausea and vomiting.[35,48,49]

Therefore an individual risk score can be defined for every patient, taking these individual factors into consideration (Table 8.6).

Age

Children younger than 3 years are less sensitive.[50,51] Adolescents are most sensitive between the ages of 11 and 14 years.[51-53] Antiemetic therapy with metoclopramide in these patients is not so effective as in older patients. Cannabinoids are more effective antiemetics in younger patients than in older patients.[54,55] The

Table 8.6 Definition of individual emesis risk by prognostic factors (modified from reference 42)

Emesis – risk factor	Score
Age:	
>50 years	1
<50 years	2
Sex	
Male	1
Female	2
Alcohol consumption:	
Yes	1
No	2
Experience of nausea and emesis:	
No	1
Yes	2

Individual score ≤ 5: normal individual emetogenic risk; ≥6: high individual emetogenic risk.

incidence of side-effects is also age-dependent. There is a higher incidence of Parkinsonism-like side-effects in younger patients.[56]

Compared with the effects of chemotherapy, where children are more likely to experience emesis, there is some evidence to suggest that they are less susceptible to radiation-induced emesis than adults, particularly during TBI.[7]

Westbrook et al[19] also defined age-specific differences. They found that younger children have little appreciation of the significance of their treatment. The maximum incidence of problems arises in the 10–20 age group, who understand the life-threatening nature of their disease and treatment, but who are perhaps less able to cope with it than older patients undergoing transplantation. Furthermore, patients with a poor understanding of English also showed higher levels of anxiety, and vomited more frequently.

Gender and hormonal status

There is evidence of sexual differences. The most sensitive patients seem to be pre-menopausal women.[57–59] The role of chorionic gonadotropin has been discussed. Antiemetic therapy seems to be less effective in women.[60] The antiemetic effect of droperidol is reduced in women during the first 9 days after the onset of the menstrual cycle.[61]

Alcohol consumption

In chronic alcohol abuse (daily alcohol use of more than 100 g) there is less sensitivity to emetogenic stimuli.[62–64]

Obesity

Overweight patients seem to be more susceptible to nausea and vomiting.[56]

Anxiety

As with chemotherapy, there are suggestions that anxiety and apprehension may increase the likelihood of sickness in patients receiving radiotherapy.[7] Westbrook et al[19] found that the incidence of emesis is related to anxiety. Also, Waldvogel[56] suggested that anxious or stressed patients may vomit more frequently because of central adrenergic stimulation. Antiemetic prophylaxis and treatment seem to be more effective in an oncological first-treatment (naive group) than after repeated treatments (non-naive group).

Conditioning

Repeated experiences of emesis may cause a psychogenic conditioning, resulting in a so-called anticipatory nausea and vomiting complex.

Predisposition

Patients with high susceptibility to induced nausea and vomiting as well as patients with motion sickness[65] seem to have increased nausea and vomiting if they are exposed to emetic stimuli.[66]

Dizziness

Patients who suffer from dizziness are more susceptible to emesis.[65,67] Westbrook et al[19] demonstrated a reduction in the incidence of emesis with comfortable positioning of the patient during irradiation. Then, with reduced psychological strain and elimination of movement, there was an improved tolerance of radiotherapy. Westbrook et al[19] also showed that movement of the head probably precipitates vomiting by activating the vestibular apparatus, as will rotation of a sleeping patient.

Pain

Insufficient treatment of pain can promote nausea and vomiting.[56] An increased emetogenic risk also exists in patients with reduced general condition, for example that caused by the advanced stages of cancer.[39]

Summary

The intensity and severity of emesis are related to a great number of parameters, including the site treated, the dose and size of the irradiated field, biological events following irradiation, and clinical considerations, including prior surgery, exposure to cytotoxic drugs, and the psychological and metabolic status of the patient.[68]

APPROACHES TO THE PREVENTION OF RADIATION-INDUCED EMESIS

Primary prevention

This means the prevention of nausea and vomiting by eliminating the possibility of emetogenic risk.

If possible, one should prevent the risk of emesis by taking into consideration the physical factors, i.e. minimizing the emetogenicity of irradiation. In daily irradiation planning recent innovations in radiotherapy (3-D treatment planning, multileaf collimators, dose–volume histograms) should be used in order to reduce the irradiated volume.[43] As small a target volume as possible should be chosen, taking into consideration the basical principles of treatment planning. It is important to obtain good definitions of tumour volume, clinical target volume, planning target volume, and consequently the irradiated and treated volumes. This can be done with improved imaging methods. It is necessary to achieve reproducible positioning of the patient every day in fractionated radiotherapy in order to minimize deviations in the definitions of these volumes. Furthermore, if it is necessary to irradiate critical regions, low single doses should be chosen whenever possible.

There are recent results concerning chronobiological effects indicating that the sensitivity of the gastrointestinal tract to toxins varies with the time of day. An investigation by Gagnon and Kuettel[69] showed that the gastrointestinal tract is more sensitive to damage in the late morning than in the afternoon. Therefore if it is necessary to irradiate critical regions of the gastrointestinal tract, this should be done in the afternoon.

Secondary prevention

This means the prevention of nausea and vomiting by the use of prophylactic antiemetic therapy. It is necessary if the irradiation of a critical region cannot be avoided, if the irradiation carries a moderate or high emetogenic risk, and the patient is at risk from nausea and vomiting without prophylaxis. Risk-adapted medication should be administered, taking into consideration the emetogenicity of the irradiation as well as the individual risk profile of the patient.

Rescue medication

If a patient has experienced nausea and vomiting, it is necessary to give the most potent drug at the right time in an adequate dosage, perhaps in combination with other drugs. Morrow et al[70] showed with the help of a mathematical model that if nausea and vomiting persist, it is possible with an optimal treatment only to control 50% of patients. In conclusion, treatment should not be delayed until the onset of symptoms.

Antiemetics in radiotherapy

Drugs used for nausea are mostly neuroleptics, antihistamines, anticholinergics, benzodiazepines, glucocorticoids, cannabinoids, benzamides or 5-HT$_3$ receptor antagonists. A summary is given in Table 8.7. The common principle involved is the blocking of dopamine receptors. In order to avoid the application of high toxic single doses of antiemetics, if possible a combination of low doses of different antiemetics with the same or different points of action should be used. Bremer[42] described the different points of action of antiemetics. It is possible to improve the antiemetic effect using glucocorticoids.[38,39]

In daily practice the most commonly used antiemetics are benzamides (e.g. metoclopramide and alizapride), usually in combination with neuroleptics (e.g. haloperidol) or benzodiazepines (e.g. lorazepam and diazepam). The 5-HT$_3$ antagonists $\pm$ glucocorticoids are used mostly in the highly emetogenic regimens of radiotherapy (e.g. in TBI). There are some results concerning the effects of dopamine antagonists (butyrophenones) in radiotherapy as well as those of opiate receptor antagonists (cannabinoids).

Dopamine antagonists: domperidone (butyrophenone)
Domperidone acts on dopamine receptors, and has been shown to increase the gastric emptying rate in human studies. Reyntjens[71] reported on the effect of domperidone on radiation-induced emesis in 30 patients. Field size could be assumed in only the 6 patients who received TBI. The data from the remaining 24 patients remains unclear. Of the patients,[19] (6 TBI, 13 abdomen or thoracic) received 10 mg domperidone orally, and 11 (abdomen or thoracic) received 20 mg domperidone. Emesis was controlled in 14 and was present in 17 patients. There was no difference between the two levels of domperidone.

Cannabinoid derivatives: levonantradol and nabilone
Lucraft and Palmer[72] compared the antiemetic effects of chlorpromazine (25 mg every day) with levonantradol given at two doses of 0.5 and 0.75 mg in patients receiving palliative radiotherapy. Forty-three patients were randomized, and received single-fraction irradiation of 10 Gy (1 patient), 12.5 Gy (17 patients) or 15 Gy (25 patients) to the lower thoracic and/or lumbar spine (41 patients) and hypochondrium (2 patients); there was no specification of field size. The frequency of emesis was similar in the three treatment groups, and was reported as 50% (7 of 14 patients) after chlorpromazine and 64% and 53% after 0.5 and 0.75 mg levonantradol respectively. The number of patients was too small for any statistical analysis. Priestman and Priestman[10] reported on the effects of nabilone, a dibenzopyrene cannabinoid, in 30 patients given fractionated radiotherapy to the upper abdomen. All patients had a minimum field size of 200 cm^2 with a daily dose of 2 Gy five days a week for a minimum of three weeks. Patients with nausea received metoclopramide 10 mg three times a day initially, and those who did not respond were then given nabilone 1 mg twice daily. Fourteen patients (46%) did not require antiemetics. Of the remaining 54% of patients, metoclopramide controlled symptoms in 10 patients who experienced nausea and vomiting on average 3.5 days after starting irradiation. Six patients needed nabilone, which was started two days after radiotherapy. The investigators suggested that there may be a place for cannabinoids as antiemetics if conventional agents fail. It is important to note that there was only a 54% incidence of emesis.[68] Henriksson et al[73] reported on the protective effect of sulcralfate in patients with irradiation in the pelvis, and observed less nausea and vomiting. Sulcralfate is a cytoprotective complex of saccharose, octyl sulfate and polyaluminium hydroxide, which gives a protective shield to the gastrointestinal mucosa. It has adsorbent properties, and stimulates the synthesis of prostaglandin, the release of epidermal growth factors, the activation of macrophages and cell proliferation.[8,74]

The results of studies by Lucraft and Palmer,[72] Priestman and Priestman,[10] and Reyntjens[71] suggest that conventional antiemetics are

Table 8.7 Antiemetic drugs and dosages (modified from reference 103)

Substance	Dosage
Substituted benzamides	
• Metoclopramide	1–3 mg/kg; i.v., p.o.; every 2–4 h
• Alizapride	100 mg; i.v., i.m., p.o.; every 4–8 h. 300–500 mg; i.v., over 24 h
Neuroleptics	
• Chlorpromazine	25 mg; i.v.; i.m.; every 4–6 h. 25–50 mg; p.o.; every 2–4 h
• Triflupromazine	10–20 mg; i.v., i.m., p.o., rectal; every 8 h
• Levomepromazine	10–25 mg; (i.v.), i.m., p.o.; every 8 h
• Haloperidol	1–3 mg; i.v.; every 2–6 h. 1–2 mg; i.m., p.o.; every 3–6 h
• Droperidol	5–15 mg; i.v., i.m.; every 4–6 h
Benzodiazepine	
• Lorazepam	1–2 mg/m²; i.v.; every 4 h. 1–2.5 mg; p.o.; every 8 h
• Diazepam	5–10 mg; i.v., i.m., p.o., rectal; every 4 h
Anticholinergics	
• Scopolamine	1.5 mg; s.c.; every 12–72 h
Antihistamines	
• Diphenhydramine	150 mg; p.o.; every 4–8 h
• Promethazine	50 mg; i.v., i.m., p.o., rectal; every 6–12 h
Corticoids	
• Dexamethasone	4–20 mg; i.v., p.o.; every 4–24 h
• Methylprednisone	200–500 mg; i.v.; every 4–24 h
Opiate-receptor antagonists/cannabinoids	
• Nabilone	1 mg every 12 h
• Levonantradol	0.5 mg every 24 h or 0.75 mg
5-HT₃ antagonists	
• Ondansetrone	32 mg; i.v., cont or every 24 h. 8 mg; i.v., p.o.; every 8–12 h
• Granisetrone	3–9 mg; i.v., p.o., every 8–24 h
• Tropisetrone	5–10 mg; i.v., p.o., every 24 h

inadequate in cases of moderate or severe radiation-induced emesis, especially in single-dose irradiation. However, marked improvements in the control of emesis have been obtained with 5-HT$_3$ receptor antagonists. In ferrets ondansetron prevented emesis associated with irradiation,[75] and the first studies of 5-HT$_3$ antagonists in preventing radiation-induced emesis in humans were described by Priestman[76] in 1989. In the following we shall review the most important studies of the use of 5-HT$_3$ antagonists in radiotherapy.

Effect of 5-HT$_3$ antagonists in radiation-induced emesis

Single high-dose irradiation of the upper abdomen

Priestman[76] demonstrated in a non-randomized study with ondansetron that doses of 4 mg four times a day or 8 mg three times a day achieved complete or substantial control of vomiting in 77–91% of patients, and mild or absent nausea in 72–77% following single-exposure high-dose (8–10 Gy) radiotherapy to the upper abdomen. This was followed by a double-blind prospective randomized trial comparing ondansetron 8 mg three times a day with metoclopromide 10 mg three times a day in the prevention of emesis in single radiation doses of 8–10 Gy to the upper abdomen. On the day of radiotherapy, ondansetron achieved significantly greater control of vomiting and retching ($p > 0.001$) and nausea ($p = 0.001$) than metoclopramide. An advantage was also seen for ondansetron on days two and three after irradiation, although this did not reach a statistically significant level. In 1990 Priestman et al[77] described further results from a randomized double-blind comparative study of ondansetron and metoclopramide in the prevention of nausea and vomiting following high-dose upper-abdominal irradiation, and in 1991 Collis et al[78] gave the final assessment of this study. There was complete control of emesis in 50% of patients with metoclopramide and in 75% with ondansetron.

It is interesting that on the days following radiotherapy there is no longer a statistically significant difference between ondansetron and metoclopramide, which may be related to a reduced emetic effect of the radiation dose on days 2–5. There is also evidence that nausea is less well controlled than vomiting.

Half-body irradiation-induced emesis

Roberts and Priestman[7] started a pilot study in the regional radiotherapy centre in Newcastle using a premedication with a combination of ondansetron 8 mg and dexamethasone 8 mg. They evaluated 11 patients with upper half-body irradiation at a dose of 8 Gy and 1 patient with lower half-body irradiation with 6 Gy, and achieved 86% complete control of emesis with ondansetron. Nausea with or without vomiting

became apparent 27–72 hours after the single dose of radiation in 6 patients. The technique of half- (or hemi-) body irradiation was first introduced by Fitzpatrick and Rider[79] in 1976. Danjoux et al[11] did not observe a significant decrease in emesis following pretreatment with several antiemetics, including prochlorperazine, diazepam and metoclopramide. Salazar et al[80] introduced a comprehensive premedication that included glucocorticosteroids, and reported minimal emesis following the treatment. Scarantino et al[81] suggested in 1988 a more abbreviated schedule of antiemetics including glucocorticosteroids, and eliminated the need for hospitalization. In 1992 Scarantino et al[68] demonstrated good control of emesis with ondansetron in upper and mid half-body irradiation. Scarantino et al[45] suggested a relation between 5-HIAA release and emesis: the observation of an increase in 5-HIAA levels associated with a parallel increase in emesis suggests a role for serotonin as a mediator in radiation-induced emesis. Logue et al[82] conducted a pilot study in 22 patients receiving lower half-body radiotherapy of 8 Gy in a single exposure for multiple metastases. Patients were treated by the injection of two different doses of granisetron one hour prior to radiotherapy. Complete response was observed in 9 of 13 and 6 of 9 in the 20 µg/kg and 40 µg/kg groups respectively. The results are difficult to assess, because there is a lower incidence of emesis in lower half-body irradiation of only up to 40%.

Total-body irradiation

There are numerous studies concerning TBI-induced emesis because this is the most emetogenic radiotherapeutic regimen.

Despite the use of conventional antiemetics such as metoclopramide, nausea and vomiting are almost universal after TBI, and are equally prevalent whether treatment is given as a single dose or in a fractionated course with daily doses as low as 1.2 Gy[19]. Westbrook et al[19] evaluated 305 patients undergoing total-body irradiation before bone-marrow transplantation, and used an antiemetic therapy with hydrocortisone and phenobarbitone, and diazepam if necessary for additional sedation. With this antiemetic treatment, control of symptoms was achieved in 50% of patients. Prentice et al[83] investigated 30 patients receiving highly emetogenic fast-dose-rate single-fraction total-body irradiation prior to bone-marrow transplantation. Patients were randomized into one of two groups, receiving either granisetron or a combination of metoclopramide, dexamethasone phosphate and lorazepam to assess the comparative efficacy of the two regimens in the control of radiation-induced nausea and vomiting. After 24 hours, 8 patients (53%) treated with granisetron showed a complete response, compared with 2 patients (13%) in the comparison group. The control of vomiting by granisetron over both 24-hour and 7-day periods was significantly better than that seen with the comparison, and required significantly fewer rescue doses.

Belkacémi et al[84] investigated 36 patients receiving single-dose TBI before bone-marrow transplantation. The patients received granisetron before TBI, with two different modalities: a total dose of 3 mg as a 5-minute intravenous infusion, or the same treatment plus 3 mg granisetron as a 24-hour continuous i.v. infusion (total dose 6 mg). During TBI, 50% of patients were scored as a complete response, 3% as major responders, 25% as minor responders and 22% as non-responders. In a univariate analysis it was found that the 12-hour probability of emesis was significantly higher in patients undergoing hyperdiuresis (63% vs 30%) and in patients older than 45 years.

Gibbs and Cassoni[85] examined the duration of the antiemetic effect of granisetron in a pilot study of patients ($n = 26$) undergoing a standard emetogenic stimulus in the form of TBI fractionated over three or four days in a randomized comparison with twice-daily ondansetron. A single intravenous dose of granisetron at the onset of therapy was effective over the entire follow-up period in 50% (6/12) of patients, compared with 77% (10/13) prescribed twice-daily oral ondansetron for three or four days. The response rate within the first 24 hours from the start of irradiation was 67% for granisetron and 77% for ondansetron.

Granisetron and ondansetron were therefore of similar efficacy within the first 24-hour period, but granisetron was less efficacious more than 24 hours after the onset of the therapy. Patients who required a second dose of granisetron did so at intervals of 12, 42, 47 and 48 hours following the first fraction of radiotherapy.

Croockewit[86] investigated 21 patients in a study of the control of emesis during TBI after high-dose cyclophosphamide. Patients were treated with ondansetron 8 mg i.v. three times a day. Complete or substantial control of emesis was achieved in 71–95% during TBI and 82–95% in the five days following TBI. Control of emesis was a little bit poorer on the first day of irradiation compared with the second day. Patients received 6 Gy for two days, and the control of nausea was not so good as that of vomiting.

Kaasa et al[87] gave a TBI with 1.3 Gy two fractions a day over a period of five days followed by high-dose cyclophosphamide. They achieved 50–80% good control of nausea and vomiting during TBI with ondansetron, and 55–80% of patients reported nausea as absent or mild on each day.

Spitzer et al[88] reported a retrospective analysis of about 29 patients of the Georgetown University Medical Center, who received 13.2 Gy of TBI in 11 fractions over four days prior to high-dose chemotherapy. All patients experienced vomiting despite the use of aggressive antiemetic therapy. The peak number of emetic episodes occurred during the first day of TBI. The median number of emetic episodes was five (range 1–32) over the four days of therapy.

In 1994 Spitzer et al[89] performed a randomized double-blind placebo-controlled evaluation of oral ondansetron in the prevention of nausea and vomiting associated with fractionated TBI. Twenty patients who received four days of TBI as part of their preparative regimen before bone-marrow transplantation were randomized to receive either 8 mg oral doses of ondansetron or placebo. Initial rescue therapy consisted of intravenous ondansetron 0.15 mg/kg following two or more emetic episodes between successive fractions of TBI or five total emetic episodes during the four days of therapy. Patients who received oral ondansetron had significantly fewer emetic episodes than those who received placebo ($p = 0.005$) over the entire four-day study period. Oral ondansetron was also significantly superior to placebo with respect to the time of onset of emesis or rescue ($p = 0.003$). Six of 10 patients treated with oral ondansetron completed the study without additional antiemetic therapy, while none of 10 patients who received placebo completed the study without rescue antiemetic therapy. Six placebo patients who received initial rescue therapy with i.v. ondansetron required no additional antiemetics.

A pharmacokinetic analysis was also performed, and revealed no relationship between peak ondansetron concentration or the area under the concentration-versus-time curve and number of emetic episodes. Significantly higher levels of urinary 5-HIAA excretion were observed in the placebo group, suggesting that ondansetron interfered with TBI-induced serotonin synthesis or release.[90] A summary is given in Table 8.8.

Conventional daily fractionated radiotherapy in the abdominal region

Several studies have compared the safety and efficacy of 5-HT$_3$ antagonists and conventional antiemetics. One study has been conducted to compare the safety and efficacy of ondansetron and prochlorperazine in patients receiving multiple daily fractions of radiotherapy to the upper abdomen.[7,94,95] A prospective double-blind randomized trial comparing ondansetron and prochlorperazine involved a total of 192 patients. In this multicentre international double-blind trial patients were randomized to receive either oral ondansetron 8 mg three times a day or oral prochlorperazine 10 mg three times a day throughout their radiation course in order to try to prevent nausea and vomiting. 61% of patients prescribed ondansetron and 35% of those given prochlorperazine had a complete response with no emetic episodes throughout their treatment course ($p = 0.002$). There was no significant dif-

ference between the two groups with the respect to the incidence and severity of nausea. 24% of the patients on ondansetron and 29% of those given prochlorperazine were treatment failures, experiencing more than five emetic episodes on their worst day during the study. When emesis control was evaluated according to the number of fractions of radiotherapy received, ondansetron provided complete control in a greater proportion of patients than prochlorperazine, irrespective of the length of fractionated treatment. Furthermore, a significantly greater proportion of emesis-free days was observed in the ondansetron-treated patients than in those receiving prochlorperazine ($p = 0.05$).

Sorbe et al[6] evaluated tropisetron as antiemetic prophylaxis during postoperative abdominal irradiation of ovarian cancer patients. Twenty women with stages I–III (FIGO) epithelial ovarian carinomas were included, twelve of whom received a whole abdominal field with 1 Gy per fraction during six weeks and eight of whom were irradiated on the lower abdomino-pelvic fields, 1.7 Gy per fraction during five weeks. Nausea was generally mild and of short duration, increasing from the start (30%) to the end (54%) of radiotherapy. Nausea was more pronounced in patients receiving whole abdominal irradiation than in those with abdomino-pelvic irradiation. Episodes were few in number, occurring in 10% of cases. The efficacy of tropisetron was rated as excellent or good in 80% of cases. The overall ratings for quality of life were excellent or good in 75–85% of the cases.

In 1996 Franzen et al[14] performed a randomized placebo-controlled study with ondansetron in patients undergoing fractionated radiotherapy. The study involved 111 patients who were to commence a course of 10 or more daily fractionated radiotherapy including the abdomen. 67% of patients given ondansetron had complete control of emesis compared with 45% of patients with placebo ($p < 0.05$). The number of emetic episodes recorded on the worst day was 1.4 for the ondansetron group and 3.1 for the placebo group ($p < 0.01$). Patients given ondansetron had fewer days

Table 8.8 5-HT₃ receptor antagonist trials for TBI-induced emesis (modified from reference 98)

Reference	Centre	Trial design	No. of patients	Conditioning regimen	Drug	Dosage	Outcome
91	Hospital for Sick Children, Bristol, UK	RET	15	CY 120 mg/kg → TBI 1.8 cGy b.d. at 0.2 cGy/min × 4 days	OND	5 mg/m² i.v. q8h × 7 days	93% CR or MR
20	Royal Free Hospital, London, UK	RET	32	TBI 7.5 cGy at 0.5 ± 0.02 cGy/min	GRA	40 µg/kg prior to TBI	97% CR or MR
92	Universität Kinderklinik Münster	RET	15	NS	OND	2, 4 or 8 mg i.v. t.d.s.	57% CR (vomiting) 86% CR or MR (nausea) on 'worst' TBI day
93	Berlin	RET	25	TBI 2.0 cGy b.d. or 4.0 cGy q.d.s. × 3 days	OND	5 mg/m² before TBI (additional 2 doses as required)	
18	Royal Marsden Hospital, London	PRO	20	MEL 110 mg/m² TBI 10.5 cGy at 0.04 cGy/min	Phenobarbitone + corticosteroids ±OND	8 mg i.v. before TBI	Fewer emetic episodes (p = 0.029) compared with placebo
89	Georgetown, Washington, DC	PRO	20	TBI 13.2 cGy at 0.22 cGy/min in 11 fractions over 4 days	OND (versus placebo)	8 mg p.o. before each TBI dose	Fewer emetic episodes (p = 0.005), delayed time of onset (p = 0.003) compared with placebo
47	Universität Leipzig	RET	59 (35 vs 24)	FTBI (2.0 Gy b.c. × 3 days) CY 60 mg/m² (2 days)	OND	8 mg i.v. before TBI + 8 mg dexamethasone	90–97% CR, MR
					MCP		54% CR, MR

RET, retrospective; PRO, prospective; CY, cyclophosphamide; OND, ondansetron; GRA, granisetron; TBI, total-body irradiation; CR, complete response; MR, major response; MEL, melphalan; NS, not specified.

with nausea and vomiting than those given placebo ($p < 0.05$), and the mean sum score of patients' weekly grading of symptoms showed that the ondansetron group experienced less inconvenience than the placebo group ($p < 0.05$). This difference persisted during the first three weeks, but not thereafter. Similarly, some quality-of-life measurements showed significant differences in favour of the ondansetron group. In this study patients given ondansetron reported better general functioning, quality of life and lower symptom levels at week 2 evaluated by the QLQ-C30, indicating a more favourable effect of ondansetron in com-

parison with placebo. Many of these aspects, such as sleep disturbance and appetite, are important for patients during a radiotherapy course. This is one of the few studies that have considered quality of life, and displayed an increased quality of life with the use of 5-HT$_3$ receptor antagonists during radiotherapy (Figure 8.5).

Mirabell et al[96] performed a prospective trial to better assess the risk of nausea and vomiting and the rescue value of tropisetron in 88 patients undergoing fractionated radiotherapy to the abdomen or to large supradiaphragmatic fields and failing a first antiemetic trial with

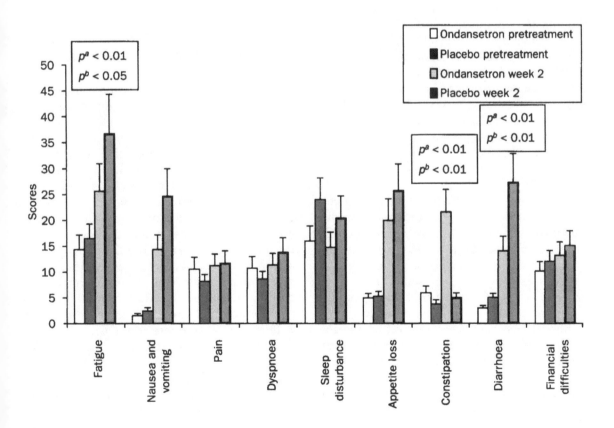

Figure 8.5 EORTC QLQ C-30 symptom scales and items. Mean standard error at pre-treatment and week 2 (higher score = greater degree of symptoms) (from reference 14).

metoclopramide. Nausea requiring antiemetics more than grade 2 was present in 64% of patients. Metoclopramide was able to control nausea (<grade 1) in 45% who developed >grade 2 nausea during radiation treatment, 34 patients required tropisetron, and 31 experienced immediate relief. Nausea recurred in 7 patients from one to three weeks after starting tropisetron. Only 24/88 patients vomited after starting radiotherapy. Metoclopramide helped to eliminate emesis in one third of these patients. Tropisetron controlled vomiting in 73% of the salvaged patients. This time-dependent nausea recurrence could reflect either a weakening of the antiemetic effect over time or a non-admitted lack of compliance. So the possibility of loss of efficacy over time should be kept in mind, especially for long radiotherapy treatments. In a short communication in 1992 Rosenthal et al[97] reported on the effective use of oral ondansetron in patients receiving whole abdominal radiotherapy with symptoms that were refractory to conventional antiemetic agents. They gave a case report on two patients, and concluded that ondansetron should be used as rescue medication but not as a first-line antiemetic therapy because of the high cost. This could be considered as controversial, if we take into consideration the data of Morrow et al[70] that showed lower effectiveness of ondansetron in patients who had vomited before.

Henriksson et al[8] reported on 33 patients receiving fractionated upper abdominal irradiation (field larger than 100 cm^2, dose 1.8–4 Gy daily) for a mean of 13 days. These patients were treated with ondansetron 8 mg t.d.s. p.o. Emesis was completely controlled in 26 of 33 patients, that is, 79% of patients throughout the radiation course on 94% of treatment days. An additional possible beneficial effect in preventing diarrhoea was found, but this must be evaluated further. Data are summarized in Table 8.9.

A recently completed study reported that about approximately 40% of patients without antiemetic prophylaxis experienced nausea and vomiting when undergoing fractionated radiotherapy between thorax and pelvis. In a sub-group of patients given an antiemetic prophylaxis because of a high risk of developing symptoms, there was control in only approximately 50% when using conventional antiemetics (mostly metoclopramide). It is therefore necessary to recommend a tailored antiemetic prophylactic therapy based on the emetogenic potential of the radiotherapy and the individual risk profile of the patient.[13]

Further investigations by Feyer[43] reported on about 94 patients with moderate emetogenic risk from radiotherapy (upper abdominal region) and prophylactic antiemetic treatment with ondansetron. There was complete control in 84%, 2–5 emetic episodes in 16%, and no response, with >5 emetic episodes in 24 hours, in 6%. A comparable patient group with conventional antiemetics (most metoclopramide) showed 43% complete control. This demonstrates an enhancement of approximately 50% of the control rate by ondansetron.[43]

CONCLUSIONS AND FUTURE DIRECTIONS

The introduction of 5-HT$_3$ receptor antagonists has resulted in a dramatic improvement in the control of emetogenic cancer therapies, including radiotherapy, especially highly emetogenic schemes like TBI. The use of 5-HT$_3$ receptor antagonists is likely to improve the quality of life in patients receiving emetogenic radiation therapy. These agents have shown marked efficacy in the prevention of nausea and vomiting associated with other highly emetogenic treatments such as half-body irradiation and upper abdominal irradiation. However, despite the great advances, several questions remain regarding the antiemetic efficacy and the mechanism of action of these new antiemetic agents. Is there a dose–response relationship for 5-HT$_3$ receptor antagonists? Response rates of 60–97% have been observed with these agents, confirming the importance of 5-HT$_3$ receptors in the mechanism of TBI-induced emesis.[98] But the data also show that protection is incomplete. In TBI, for example, up to 40% of ondansetron-treated patients experienced nausea and vomiting requiring rescue therapy.[43,98]

Table 8.9 Effect of antiemetics on radiation-induced emesis (modified from reference 68)

Reference	Field size (cm²)	Site	Dose (Gy) (Fraction/Total)	Drug	Response (%)
Non-5-HT₃ antagonists					
71		TBI	NS	Domp	82
72	Small	T–L spine	10–15/–	Chlorp Lev	50
10	≥200	Upper abdomen	2/30	Met Nabilone	58
5-HT₃ antagonists					
6	>1000	Whole abdomen, pelvis	1.0–1.7/20–40	Trop	83
77	100	T–L spine, abdomen; pelvis	8–10/–	Ondan Met	97 45
91		TBI	1.8/14	Ondan	93
68	>1500	Mid-upper HBI	5–8/–	None Other Ondan	19 43 100

T–L, thoracic–lumbar; NS, normal saline; Domp, domperidone; Chlorp, chlorpromazine; Lev, levonantradol; Met, metoclopramide; Trop, tropisetron; Ondan, ondansetron.

The data by Spitzer[98] demonstrated on a small patient population (10 patients) that it was possible to improve the antiemetic effect of 5-HT₃ antagonists with higher doses. There has been complete antiemetic protection in approximately 80% of patients receiving TBI, suggesting that dose or perhaps route of administration (oral or intravenous) may be important in optimal antiemetic control. Furthermore, the role of combination antiemetic therapy also requires further investigation. It is necessary to define the potentiating role of glucocorticoids in antiemetic efficacy. First results have been given by Roberts and Priestman,[7] and by a randomized trial by the Italian Group for Antiemetic Research[99] showing the superiority of a combination of granisetron and dexamethasone for the control of chemotherapy-induced emesis. The first data on prevention of TBI-induced emesis with a combination of 5-HT₃ receptor antagonists and dexamethasone show the same trends. Further definition of the mechanism of action of 5-HT₃ receptor antagonists in the prevention of radiation-induced emesis will be helpful in optimizing the design of future antiemetic treatment strategies. Understanding the complex interaction of drugs and their receptors, as well as the impact of drugs on the synthesis and release of important mediators of nausea and vomiting, will probably lead to more effective strategies for the complete prevention of immediate and delayed nausea and vomiting.[98] However, because of the significant variations in the efficacy of 5-HT$_3$ antagonists among individual patients, we need more detailed comparative studies concentrating on those patients who actually develop nausea and vomiting.[14] The optimal dosage of 5-HT$_3$ receptor antagonists in radiation-induced emesis has not been sufficiently clarified nor has the role of combination therapy.

Roberts and Priestman[7] demonstrated the efficacy of ondansetron in radiation-induced emesis as a rescue therapy. Effective antiemesis reduces the morbidity of radiotherapy, especially in fractionated radiotherapy given over some weeks. It also allows radiotherapy to be administered on an outpatient basis. Furthermore, routine prophylaxis with ondansetron should allow the use of fewer larger fractions of radiation for the palliation of, for example, metastases in the skeletal system. To avoid overtreating patients who may never need antiemetics, future trials in patients treated by radiotherapy should be confined to those who actually require treatment for nausea and vomiting.[96]

Morrow et al[70] demonstrated reduced efficacy of 5-HT$_3$ antagonists in patients with pre-vious experience of emesis. Furthermore, the question of dosage two times 8 mg versus three times 8 mg orally or intravenously, and the combination with glucocorticoids, as well as the question of sedation, should be discussed with regard to radiation-induced emesis.

Bremer[42] proposed a risk-adapted step-by-step antiemetic therapy. Feyer[43] developed a treatment schedule that takes into consideration the emetogenic risk of the therapy as well as the individual risk profile of the patient, and proposed an adapted prophylactic treatment.

Proposals for therapeutic strategies in radiation-induced emesis must take into consideration the emetogenic potential of the irradiated volume (region and dose). In low-risk cases treatment can be started with metoclopramide, alizapride, dexamethasone or a benzodiazepine. If nausea and vomiting still continue or in high-risk cases 5-HT$_3$ receptor antagonists should be used. If necessary these should be combined with dexamethasone. Benzodiazepines can be used in the evening with good effect. A summary of indications for antiemetic therapy is given in Table 8.10.

Conventional, cheaper, antiemetics should be

Table 8.10 Indications for the use of antiemetics, depending on the emetogenic risk during radiotherapy

Emetogenic potential radiotherapy	Risk profile of patient	Antiemetic prophylaxis
Mild	Normal	None
	High	None
Moderate	Normal	None
	High	Non 5-HT$_3$ antagonists or 5-HT$_3$ antagonists (p.o.)
Severe	Normal	5-HT$_3$ antagonists (p.o.)/(i.v.)
	High	or 5-HT$_3$ antagonists + dexamethasone (i.v.) ± sedation

used in cases of low emetogenic risk. There exist a number of therapeutic strategies for chemotherapy-induced emesis, but up to now there is no consensus for radiation-induced emesis.

In cases of high emetogenic risk it should be discussed whether it is useful to use metoclopramide up to five times a day. This has no greater cost–benefit advantage in comparison with 5-HT$_3$ antagonists given twice a day.[42]

There is a need for more effective strategies for the complete prevention of immediate and delayed radiation-induced nausea and vomiting. It is necessary to take into consideration antiemetic prophylaxis and therapy as an established part of supportive therapy, and make it an integral part of radiotherapy, especially in order to improve the quality of life of patients.

REFERENCES

1. Sauer R, *Strahlentherapie und Onkologie, 2 Aufl.* München: Urban & Schwarzenberg, 1993.
2. Coutes A, Abraham SK, Kaye SB, On the receiving and patient perception of the side effects of cancer chemotherapy. *Eur J Cancer Clin Oncol* 1983; **19**: 203.
3. Fowler J, Lindstrom M, Loss of local control with prolongation in radiotherapy. *Int J Radiat Oncol Biol Phys* 1992; **23**: 457–67.
4. Robertson A, Robertson C, Symonds R, Effect of varying schedules on carcinoma of the larynx. *Eur J Cancer* 1993; **29**: 501–10.
5. Paulsen F, Hoffmann W, Kortmann RD et al, Acute gastrointestinal side effects of radiotherapy – What can be called 'State of the Art'? *Strahlenther Onkol* 1996; **2**: 53–63.
6. Sorbe B, Berglind AM, de Bruijn K, Tropisetron, a new 5-HT$_3$-receptor antagonist, in the prevention of radiation-induced emesis. *Radiother Oncol* 1992; **2**: 131–2.
7. Roberts JT, Priestman TJ, A review of ondansetron in the management of radiotherapy induced emesis. *Oncology* 1993; **50**: 173–9.
8. Henriksson R, Lomberg H, Isrealsson G et al, The effect of ondansetron on radiation-induced emesis and diarrhoea. *Acta Oncol* 1992; **317**: 767–9.
9. Priestman T, Challoner T, Butcher M, Priestman S, Control of radiation-induced emesis with GR 38032 F. *Proc Am Soc Clin Oncol* 1988; **7**: 281.
10. Priestman FJ, Priestman SG, An initial evaluation of nabilone in the control of radiotherapy induced nausea and vomiting. *Clin Radiol* 1984; **35**: 265–6.
11. Danjoux E, Rider WD, Fitzpatrick PJ, The acute radiation syndrome. *Clin Radiol* 1979; **30**: 581–4.
12. Krook JE, Moertel CG, Gunderson LL, Effective surgical adjuvant therapy for high risk rectal carcinoma. *N Engl J Med* 1991; **324**: 709.
13. Feyer PC, Incidence of emesis and nausea in fractionated radiotherapy patients. In: *Advances in Optimising the Control of Emesis ESMO Satellite Symposium, Lisbon, 1994.*
14. Franzen L, Nyman I, Hagberg H et al, A randomised placebo controlled study with ondansetron in patients undergoing fractionated radiotherapy. *Am Oncol* 1996; **7**: 587–92.
15. Sommer K, Brockmann WP, Hübener KH, Treatment results and acute and late toxicity of radiation therapy for testicular seminoma. *Cancer* 1990; **66**: 259–63.
16. Coccia PF, Strandjord SE, Warkentin PI, High dose cytosine arabinoside and fractionated total body irradiation: an important preparation regimen for bone marrow transplantation of children with acute lymphoblastic leukemia in remission. *Blood* 1988; **71**: 888–93.
17. Priestman FJ, Priestman SG, Canney PA, A double-blind randomized cross-over comparison nabilone and metoclopramide in the control of radiation induced nausea. *Clin Radiol* 1987; **38**: 543–4.
18. Tiley C, Powles R, Caatalano J et al, Results of a double blind placebo controlled study of ondansetron as an antiemetic during total body irradiation in patients undergoing bone marrow transplantation. *Leuk Lymphoma* 1992; **7**: 317–21.
19. Westbrook C, Glasholm J, Barrett A, Vomiting associated with whole body irradiation. *Clin Radiol* 1987; **38**: 263–6.
20. Hunter AE, Prentice HG, Pothecary K, Granisetron, a selective 5-HT$_3$-receptor antago-

nist for the prevention of radiation induced emesis during total body irradiation. *Bone Marrow Transplant* 1991; 7: 439–41.

21. Anno GH, Baum SJ, Withers HR, Young RW, Symptomatology of acute radiation effects in humans after exposure to doses of 0.5–30 Gy. *Health Phys* 1989; 56: 821–38.

22. Court-Brown WM, Symptomatic disturbance after single therapeutic dose of x-rays. *Br J Med* 1953; 1: 802–5.

23. Hall EJ, *Radiobiology for the Radiologist*, 3rd edn. Philadelphia: JB Lippincott, 1988.

24. Haskell CM, *Cancer Treatment*, 3rd edn. Philadelphia: WB Saunders, 1990.

25. Potten CS, Extreme sensitivity of some intestinal crypt cells to x- and gamma irradiation. *Nature* 1977; 269: 518–21.

26. Barret A, Total body irradiation (TBI) before bone marrow transplantation in leukaemia: a cooperative study from the European Group for Bone Marrow Transplantation. *Br J Radiol* 1982; 55: 562–70.

27. Davis CJ, Harding RK, Leslie RA, Andrews PLR, The organization of vomiting as a protective reflex. In: *Nausea and Vomiting: Mechanisms and Treatment* (Davis CJ, Lake-Bakaar GV, Grahame-Smith DG, eds). Berlin: Springer-Verlag, 1986: 65–75.

28. Levin SG, Young RW, Stohler RL, Estimates of the median human lethal radiation dose, computed from data on occupants and architecture, of two reinforced concrete structures in Nagasaki, Japan. *Health Phys* 1992; 63: 522–31.

29. Harding RK, Young RW, Anno GH, Radiotherapy-induced emesis. In: *Emesis in Anticancer Therapy: Mechanisms and Treatment* (Andrews PLR, Sanger GJ, eds). London: Chapman & Hall, 1993: 163–78.

30. Andrews PLR, Rapeport WG, Sanger GJ, Neuropharmacology of emesis induced by anti-cancer therapy. *Trends Pharmacol Sci* 1988; 9: 334–41.

31. Buell MG, Harding RK, Pro-inflammatory effects of local irradiation on the rat gastrointestinal tract. *Dig Dis Sci* 1989; 34: 390–9.

32. Harding RK, 5-HT$_3$ receptor antagonists and radiation-induced emesis: preclinical data. In: *Serotonin and the Scientific Basis of Antiemetic therapy* (Reynolds DJM, Andrews PLR, Davis CJ, eds). Oxford: Oxford Clinical Communications, 1995: 127–33.

33. Harding RK, Leach KE, Prud'homme-Lalonde L, Ferrarotto CL, Release of inflammatory mediators from irradiated gastrointestinal tissues. *Gastroentrerology* 1991; 98: A285.

34. Harding RK, Morris GP, Prud'homme-Lalonde L, Leach KE, Acute effects of 5 Gy ionizing irradiation on mast cell populations in the ferret jejunum. *Gastroenterology* 1992; 102: A635.

35. Blower PR, The role of specific 5-HT$_3$-receptor antagonism in the control of cytostatic drug-induced emesis. *Eur J Cancer* 1990; 26(Suppl 1): 8–11.

36. Cubeddu LX, Hofmann IS, Fuenmayor NT, Finn AL, Efficacy of ondansetron (GR-38032F) and the role of serotonin in cisplatin-induced nausea and vomiting. *N Engl J Med* 1990; 322: 821–5.

37. Göthert M, Antiemetische Therapie. *Krankenhausarzt* 1992; 65(Sonderheft): 12–15.

38. Gralla RJ, An outline of anti-emetic treatment. *Eur J Cancer Clin Oncol* 1989; 25(Suppl 1): 7–11.

39. Joss RA, Brand BC, Buser KS, Cerny T, The symptomatic control of cytostatic drug-induced emesis. A recent history and review. *Eur J Cancer* 1990; 26(Suppl 1): 2–8.

40. Scarantino CW, Ornitz RD, Hoffman LG, Anderson RF, On the mechanism of radiation induced emesis. The role of serotonin. *Int J Radiat Oncol Biol Phys* 1993; 27(Suppl 1): 159.

41. Rabin BM, Hunt WA, Wilson ME, Joseph JA, Emesis in ferrets following exposure to different types of radiation: a dose–response study. *Aviat Space Environ Med* 1992; 63: 702–5.

42. Bremer K, Individuelle risikoadaptierte antiemetische Stufentherapie. *Dtsch Med Wschr* 1994; 119: 598–604.

43. Feyer P, Ondanestron in radiotherapy-induced emesis. *J Pharmacol Ther* 1995; 4: 112–13.

44. Harding RK, Prodromal effects of radiation: pathways, models and protection by antiemetics. *Pharmacol Ther* 1988; 39: 335–45.

45. Scarantino CW, Ornitz RD, Hoffman LG, Anderson RF, On the mechanism of radiation induced emesis: the role of serotonin. *Int J Radiat Oncol Biol Phys* 1994; 30: 825–30.

46. Cubeddu LX, Hoffman IS, Fuenmayor NT, Malave JJ, Changes in serotonin metabolism in cancer patients: its relationship to nausea and vomiting induced by chemotherapeutic drugs. *Br J Cancer* 1992; 66: 198–203.

47. Feyer P, Investigations comparing acute reactions and late effects of different conditioning regimens prior to bone marrow transplantation. Thesis, University of Leipzig, 1994.

48. Blijham GH, Does granisetron remain effective

over multiple cycles? *Eur J Cancer* 1992; **28**(Suppl 1): 17–21.

49. Bremer K, on behalf of the Granisetron Study Groups, A single-blind study of the efficacy and safety of intravenous granisetron compared with alizapride plus dexamethasone in the prophylaxis and control of emesis in patients receiving 5-day cytostatic therapy. *Eur J Cancer* 1992; **28**: 1018–22.

50. Khalil SN, Berry JM, Howard G et al, The antiemetic effect of lorazepam after outpatient strabismus surgery in children. *Anesthesiology* 1992; **77**: 915–19.

51. Rowley MP, Brown TC, Postoperative vomiting in children. *Anaesth Intensive Care* 1982; **10**: 309–13.

52. Cohen MM, Cameron CB, Cuncan PG, Pediatric anesthesia morbidity and mortality in the perioperative period. *Anesth Analg* 1990; **70**: 160–7.

53. Roila F, Tonato M, Basurto C et al, Protection from nausea and vomiting in cisplatin-treated patients: high-dose metoclopramide combined with methylprednisolone versus metoclopramide combined with dexamethasone and diphenhydramine: a study of the Italian Oncology Group for Clinical Research. *J Clin Oncol* 1989; **7**: 1693–1700.

54. Pollera CF, Giannerelli D, Prognostic factors influencing cisplatin-induced emesis. Definition and validation of a predictive logistic model. *Cancer* 1989; **64**: 1117–22.

55. Sallan SE, Zinberg NE, Frei E, Antiemetic effect of delta-9-tetrahydrocannabinol in patients receiving cancer chemotherapy. *N Engl J Med* 1975; **293**: 795–7.

56. Waldvogel HH, *Antiemetische Prophylaxe und Therapie*. Stuttgart: G Thieme Verlag, 1995.

57. Beattie WS, Lindblad T, Buckley DN, Forrest JB, The incidence of postoperative nausea and vomiting in women undergoing laparoscopy is influenced by the day of menstrual cycle. *Can J Anaesth* 1991; **38**: 298–302.

58. Honkavaara P, Lehtinen AM, Hovorka J, Korttila K, Nausea and vomiting after gynaecological laparoscopy depends upon the phase of the menstrual cycle. *Can J Anaesth* 1991; **38**: 876–9.

59. Roila F, Basurto C, Minotti V et al, Methylprednisolone versus metoclopramide for prevention of nausea and vomiting in breast cancer patients treated with intravenous cyclophosphamide–methotrexate–5-fluorouracil:

a double-blind randomized study. *Oncology* 1988; **45**: 346–9.

60. Tonato M, Roila F, Del-Favero A, Methodology of antiemetic trials: a review. *Ann Oncol* 1991; **2**: 107–14.

61. Lindblad T, Beattie WS, Forrest JB, Buckley DN, Loss of the antiemetic effect of droperidol in menstruating women. *Can J Anaesth* 1990; **37**: 139.

62. Hesketh PJ, Comparative trials on ondansetron versus metoclopramide in the prevention acute cisplatin-induced emesis. *Semin Oncol* 1992; **19**(Suppl 10): 33–40.

63. Spiess JL, Adelstein DJ, Hines JD, Evaluation of ethanol as an antiemetic in patients receiving cisplatin. *Clin Ther* 1987; **9**: 400–4.

64. Sullivan JR, Leyden MJ, Bell R, Decreased cisplatin-induced nausea and vomiting with chronic alcohol ingestion. *N Engl J Med* 1983; **309**: 796.

65. Morrow GR. The effect of a susceptibility to motion sickness in the side effects of cancer chemotherapy. *Cancer* 1985; **55**: 2766–70.

66. Palazzo MG, Strunin L, Anaesthesia and emesis. I: Etiology. *Can Anaesth Soc J* 1984; **31**: 178–87.

67. Meyer BR, O'Mara V, Reidenberg MM, A controlled clinical trial of the addition of transdermal scopolamine to a standard metoclopramide and dexamethasone antiemetic regimen. *J Clin Oncol* 1987; **5**: 1994–7.

68. Scarantino CW, Ornitz RD, Hoffmann LG, Anderson RF, Radiation-induced emesis: effects of ondansetron. *Semin Oncol* 1992; **6**(Suppl 15): 38–43.

69. Gagnon GJ, Kuettel M, Diurnal variation in acute GI-toxicity from prostate cancer radiotherapy. *Proc Am Soc Ther Radiol Oncol* 1994; **1018**: 253.

70. Morrow GR, Soukop M, Richard A, Maximising control of emesis over repeat courses. In: *Advances in Optimising the Control of Emesis. ESMO Satellite Symposium, Lisbon, 1994.*

71. Reyntjens R, Domperidone as an anti-emetic: summary of research reports. *Postgrad Med J* 1979; **55**: 50–4.

72. Lucraft HH, Palmer MK, Randomized clinical trial of levonantradol and chlorpromazine in prevention of radiotherapy-induced vomiting. *Clin Radiol* 1982; **33**: 621–2.

73. Henriksson R, Arevarn M, Ranzen L et al, Beneficial effects of sucralfate in radiation induced diarrhoea. An open randomized study

in gynecological cancer patients. *Eur J Gynaec Oncol* 1990; **11**: 299–302.

74. Sur RK, Hochhar R, Singh DP, Oral sucralfate in acute radiation esophagitis. *Acta Oncol* 1994; **33**: 61–3.

75. Tyers MB, Bunce KT, Humphrey PPA, Pharmacological and antiemetic properties of ondansetron. *Eur J Cancer Clin Oncol* 1989; **25**(Suppl 1): 15–19.

76. Priestman TJ, Clinical studies with ondansetron in the control of radiation-induced emesis. *Eur J Cancer Clin Oncol* 1989; **25**: 29–33.

77. Priestman TJ, Roberts JT, Lucraft H et al, Results of a randomized, double-blind comparative study of ondansetron and metoclopramide in the prevention of nausea and vomiting following high-dose upper abdominal irradiation. *Clin Oncol* 1990; **2**: 71–5.

78. Collis CH, Priestman TJ, Priestman S et al, The final assessment of a randomized double blind comparative study of ondansetron vs metoclopramide in the prevention of nausea and vomiting following high dose upper abdominal irradiation. *Clin Oncol* 1991; **3**: 241–3.

79. Fitzpatrick PJ, Rider WD, Half-body radiotherapy. *Int J Radiat Oncol Biol Phys* 1976; **1**: 197–209.

80. Salazar OM, Rubin P, Keller B, Scarantino CW, Systemic (half-body) radiation therapy: response and toxicity. *Int J Radiat Oncol Biol Phys* 1978; **4**: 937–50.

81. Scarantino CW, Greven KM, Buss OH, Single dose large irradiation in drug resistant non Hodgkin lymphoma. *Int J Radiol Oncol Biol Phys* 1988; **14**: 1001–5.

82. Logue JP, Magee B, Hunter RD, Murdoch RD, The antimetic effect of granisetron in lower hemibody radiotherapy. *Clin Oncol R Coll Radiol* 1991; **3**: 247–9.

83. Prentice GH, Cunningham S, Gandhi L et al, Granisetron in the prevention of irradiation-induced emesis. *Bone Marrow Transplant* 1995; **15**: 445–8.

84. Belkacémi Y, Ozsahin M, Pène F et al, Total body irradiation prior to bone marrow transplantation: efficacy and safety of granisetron in the prophylaxis and control of radiation-induced emesis. *Int J Radiat Oncol Biol Phys* 1996; **36**: 77–82.

85. Gibbs SJ, Cassoni AM, A pilot study to evaluate the cost effectiveness of ondansetron and granisetron in fractionated total body irradiation. *Clin Oncol* 1996; **8**: 182–4.

86. Croockewit S, The efficacy of ondansetron in emesis induced by total body irradiation. Abstract, ESMO, Satellite Symposium, Zofran, Copenhagen, 1990.

87. Kaasa S, Kvaløy S, Lauvvang G, The role of ondansetron in patients receiving total body irradiation. Abstract, 7th ECCO: Progress in the Management of Emesis, Jerusalem, 1993.

88. Spitzer TR, Deeg HJ, Torrisi J, Total body irradiation induced emesis is universal after small dose fractions (120 cGy) and is not cumulative dose related. *Proc Am Soc Clin Oncol* 1990; **9**: 14.

89. Spitzer TR, Bryson JC, Cirenza E, Randomized double-blind, placebo-controlled evaluation of oral ondansetron in the prevention of nausea and vomiting associated with fractionated total body irradiation. *J Clin Oncol* 1994; **12**: 2432–5.

90. Walden ThL, Pritchard F, Bryson JC et al, Effect of ondansetron on serotonin levels in patients receiving total body irradiation. *Proc Am Soc Clin Oncol* 1994; **13**: 440.

91. Hewitt M, Cornish J, Pamphilon D, Oakhill A, Effective emetic control during conditioning of children for bone marrow transplantation using ondansetron, a 5-HT$_3$ antagonist. *Bone Marrow Transplant* 1991; **7**: 431–3.

92. Jürgens H, McQuade B, Ondansetron as prophylaxis for chemotherapy and radiotherapy induced emesis in children. *Oncology* 1992; **49**: 279–85.

93. Schwella N, König V, Schwerdtfeger R et al, Ondansetron for efficient emesis control during total body irradiation. *Bone Marrow Transplant* 1994; **13**: 169–71.

94. Priestman TJ, Roberts JT, Upadhyaya BK, Randomised double-blind trial of ondansetron and prochlorperazine in the prevention of fractionated radiotherapy induced emesis. *Proc Am Soc Clin Oncol* 1992; **9**: 1370.

95. Priestman TJ, Roberts JT, Upadhyaya BK, A prospective randomized double-blind trial comparing ondansetron versus prochlorperazine for the prevention of nausea and vomiting in patients undergoing fractionated radiotherapy. *Clin Oncol* 1993; **5**: 358–63.

96. Mirabell R, Coucke P, Behrouz F et al, Nausea and vomiting in fractionated radiotherapy: a prospective on-demand trial of tropisetron rescue for non-responders to metoclopramide. *Eur J Cancer* 1995; **31A**: 1461–4.

97. Rosenthal SA, Marquez CM, Hourigan HP, Ryu JK, Ondanstron for patients given abdominal radiotherapy. *Lancet* 1992; **339**: 490.

98. Spitzer TR, Clinical evidence for 5-HT$_3$ receptor antagonist efficacy in radiation induced emesis. In: *Serotonin and the Scientific Basis of Antiemetic Therapy* (Reynolds DJM, Andrews PLR, Davis CJ, eds) pp. 134–41. Oxford: Oxford Clinical Communications, 1995.

99. The Italian Group for Antiemetic Research, Dexamethasone, granisetron, or both for the prevention of nausea and vomiting during chemotherapy for cancer. *N Engl J Med* 1995; 332: 1–5.

100. Langham WH, *Radiobiological Factors in Manned Space Flight*. Washington, DC: National Academy of Sciences, National Research Council Publications, 1967: 1487.

101. Lushbaugh CC, Reflections on some recent progress in human radiobiology. *Adv Radiat Biol* 1969; 3: 277–315.

102. Lushbaugh CC, Human radiation tolerance. In: *Bioastronautics Data Book* (Parker Jr J, West VR, eds). Washington, DC: National Aeronautics and Space Administration, NASA-S-30006, 1973: 421–522.

103. Keitel-Wittig C, Riess H, Mechanism and therapy of cytotoxic induced emesis. *Sandorama* 1992; 4: 27–38.

9

Prevention of nausea and vomiting in repeat courses

Razvan A Popescu, David Cunningham

INTRODUCTION

The last four decades have seen a rapid rise in the use of highly emetogenic cytotoxic drugs and the development of more aggressive chemotherapy regimens in the treatment of malignancy.[1] The introduction of cisplatin, one of the most effective but also most emetogenic chemotherapy agents currently available, has spurned an exponential increase in studies of nausea and emesis control since the early 1980s.

Prior to the recognition of the efficacy of high-dose metoclopramide[2] and corticosteroids in relieving cisplatin-induced vomiting, patients treated with this agent had an average of 12 vomiting episodes per cycle.[3] Emesis was widely regarded as the worst side-effect of treatment.[4] The discovery in 1986 that 5-HT$_3$ receptor antagonists had antiemetic properties[5] led to rapid studies in patients unresponsive to standard antiemetic treatments. Leinbundgut and Lancranjan reported that tropisetron given to 11 patients receiving highly emetogenic chemotherapy totally controlled acute emesis in 31 of 47 courses, and major control was achieved in 43 of 47 chemotherapy courses.[6] Cunningham et al[7] showed that 14 of 15 patients receiving non-cisplatin chemotherapy

regimens received total protection from 16 mg ondansetron i.v. followed by three 4 mg oral doses. These initial observations have been confirmed in a multitude of clinical trials, showing 5-HT$_3$ receptor antagonists to be safe and effective in patients receiving highly emetogenic chemotherapy.[8,9] However, it has recently been estimated that between 10% and 15% of patients still choose to delay or curtail potentially curative treatment such as adjuvant chemotherapy because of problems with severe nausea and vomiting.[10]

Clinical studies of antiemetics have traditionally been performed in chemotherapy-naive patients who were studied during their first cycle of chemotherapy only.[11] More relevant for patients and oncologists alike, however, is the ability of an antiemetic drug or regimen to maintain efficacy during repeat cycles of chemotherapy administered over a period of several months. Such trials are more difficult and expensive to perform, and in their interpretation a variety of considerations must be drawn into account.

Firstly, three distinct types of emetic problems have been described in cancer patients receiving chemotherapy.[12] Acute chemotherapy-induced emesis occurs mostly within the first 1–4 hours following cytotoxic drug administration, with the important exception of carboplatin and cyclophosphamide,[13] which can cause a late onset of emesis. It usually resolves within 24 hours. Delayed chemotherapy-induced emesis has been reported following cisplatin treatment,[14,15] and is characterized by complete control of emesis in the first 24 hours, followed by development of nausea and vomiting in up to 93% of patients in whom antiemetic treatment is not continued over the next 4–5 days.[14] The severity of nausea and vomiting, both acute and delayed, depends on a number of factors, the most important of which is the type of cytotoxic drug that is used. Other important factors include the dose and number of cytotoxic drugs and the premorbid personality of the patient (for further discussion see Chapter 4). In patients with poor emesis control, anticipatory nausea and vomiting may develop. These begin before the administration of a repeat cycle of chemotherapy, and are conditioned responses, occurring mostly in young patients with poor control of emesis in prior chemotherapy cycles.[16,17] Receiving more than three chemotherapy cycles was shown to be an independent significant variable in predicting occurrence of anticipatory nausea.[16] When established, anticipatory nausea and vomiting are difficult to treat effectively, and this emphasizes the importance of good initial emesis control. All these three types of emesis may influence the response to antiemetic treatment in repeat cycles of chemotherapy, and may confound accurate reporting of acute emesis in multiple cycles.

Secondly, with repeat cycles of chemotherapy, patient numbers tend to decrease. Multiple reasons may contribute to this, including disease progression, lack of response, and various cytotoxic drug side-effects, but also poor emesis control. Good studies must list the causes of dropouts, and comparison of different reports must consider these in addition to patient characteristics at study onset. Large studies have shown that after three or four courses, over half the original number of patients are lost,[18,19] and after eight or ten courses, less than 10% remain evaluable. Especially in comparisons where the

additional benefit is modest, large patient numbers need to be enrolled for significant results to be attained.

STANDARD ANTIEMETIC REGIMENS WITH HIGH-DOSE METOCLOPRAMIDE OVER REPEAT CYCLES

Metoclopramide was the first antiemetic agent to demonstrate relevant antiemetic activity in patients treated with highly emetogenic chemotherapy. Substantial experience with this drug and various combinations with other antiemetics was gained,[2,20] and the combination of metoclopramide with dexamethasone and lorazepam or diphenhydramine was regarded as the optimal antiemetic treatment for both acute and delayed emesis in patients receiving high-dose cisplatin chemotherapy prior to the introduction of selective 5-HT$_3$ receptor antagonists.[21]

Efficacy of high-dose metoclopramide-containing antiemetic regimens is not maintained

Early uncontrolled observations of continued metoclopramide treatment during repeat courses of cisplatin suggested preservation of antiemetic efficacy (for a review see reference 2). This has been refuted by a number of clinical studies.

A multicentre double-blind randomized trial studied protection from nausea and vomiting by standard antiemetic regimens in 367 consecutive patients treated with various cisplatin-containing chemotherapy regimens.[22] Patients randomized to receive metoclopramide 3 mg/kg × 2 combined with dexamethasone and diphenhydramine experienced complete protection from nausea and vomiting in 72.5%/79.5%, compared with 55.8% and 65.1% in patients receiving metoclopramide 1 mg/kg × 4 and methylprednisolone. In subsequent cycles protection from emesis decreased significantly in both treatments.

Similarly, in a study of patients receiving

cisplatin doses of over $50 \, mg/m^2$ in repeat cycles, Roila[23] reported that 59% of patients given metoclopramide (3 mg/kg i.v. × 2) plus dexamethasone (20 mg i.v.) and diphenhydramine (50 mg i.v.) experienced no retching and vomiting and 50% had complete protection from nausea, but on subsequent cycles only 47% had no vomiting episodes.

A reduction in efficacy of a standard antiemetic combination over repeat cycles was also demonstrated in patients receiving moderately emetogenic chemotherapy. 107 female breast cancer patients receiving six consecutive cycles of adjuvant FAC chemotherapy (5-fluorouracil, doxorubicin, cyclophosphamide) received i.v. methylprednisolone, oral thiethilperazine and oral amitriptyline as antiemetic prophylaxis.[24] The complete protection rate (no vomiting) decreased continuously from 62.6% in the first course to 48.6% in the sixth, with a similar drop in major protection rate (0–2 vomiting episodes, 76.6% and 58% respectively).

Why does antiemetic efficacy decrease over repeat cycles?

These studies demonstrate that standard combinations of metoclopramide, corticosteroid and diphenhydramine are prone to lose their antiemetic efficacy when used in repeat cycles of highly or moderately emetogenic chemotherapy. A potential explanation for this phenomenon is the fact that emesis control and, more importantly, control of nausea are often unsatisfactory even during the initial course of chemotherapy in these patients, especially those receiving high-dose cisplatin chemotherapy (see Chapter 5). A larger proportion of patients thus treated are prone to develop anticipatory nausea than patients initially treated with more efficient antiemetic regimens containing 5-HT$_3$ antagonists.[25]

Work by Cubeddu and Hoffmann[26] may also contribute to our understanding of progressive loss of antiemetic efficiency. They investigated the urinary excretion of 5-hydroxyindoleacetic acid (5-HIAA), a serotonin metabolite, follow-

ing high-dose cisplatin chemotherapy. Increases in 5-HIAA excretion to 2.5–2.9 times baseline values were observed 4–8 hours following high-dose cisplatin administration, but daily 5-HIAA excretion was not different from pre-cisplatin levels on days 2–5. Together with the efficacy data for 5-HT$_3$ antagonists, this fits the current view that serotonin is an important contributor to acute high-dose cisplatin-induced nausea and vomiting. Interestingly, compared with the first cycle, higher and more sustained 5-HIAA levels were determined on subsequent courses of high-dose cisplatin. Thus the increased emetogenicity and poorer nausea and vomiting control attained on repeat courses may be also due to greater serotonin release. Metoclopramide (a mainly D2 antagonist with weak 5-HT$_3$ binding ability) may compete less efficiently for 5-HT$_3$ receptors with serotonin as the latter's concentration increases in repeat courses of highly emetogenic chemotherapy. Further increases in the metoclopramide dose to enhance its efficacy would, however, lead to an unacceptably high incidence of side-effects, the main one being extrapyramidal symptoms and leading currently in up to 15–20% of patients to change in antiemetic treatment.

5-HT$_3$ RECEPTOR ANTAGONISTS

5-HT$_3$ receptor antagonists have been shown to be superior to metoclopramide-containing standard antiemetic regimens in controlling acute cisplatin-induced nausea and vomiting. Initially used to rescue patients failing standard antiemetic treatment,[6,7,27] they were soon shown to be effective in controlling acute nausea and vomiting,[28,29] and have a favourable side-effect profile (for further discussion see Chapter 16). A huge expansion has occurred in the 5-HT$_3$ field, with currently more than 30 5-HT$_3$ antagonists under development for chemotherapy-induced nausea and vomiting.[30] Overall, these drugs are similar to the established 5-HT$_3$ antagonists, but long-term studies are not yet available. The following discussion will limit itself to data regarding ondansetron, granisetron and tropisetron used alone or in combination over repeat courses.

Ondansetron

Synergism of ondansetron and corticosteroids in highly emetogenic chemotherapy

The efficacy of ondansetron in highly emetogenic chemotherapy was proven in early studies against placebo[31] and against metoclopramide.[32] In the latter study ondansetron alone controlled acute vomiting induced by cisplatin 80–100 mg/m^2 in 29% of patients vs high-dose metoclopramide alone in 16%. While emesis control by ondansetron was significantly better, the question whether the addition of a corticosteroid has a synergistic activity with ondansetron was soon addressed, since the two drugs work in different ways.[33] Roila and colleagues published an elegant double-blind randomized crossover study comparing ondansetron and ondansetron plus dexamethasone[34] in chemotherapy-naive patients scheduled to receive at least two courses of a high-dose cisplatin-containing chemotherapy regimen. Out of 102 patients, 89 completed both cycles. Complete protection from emesis/nausea was achieved in 64%/66.3% of patients with ondansetron and 91%/88.8% with ondansetron plus dexamethasone. Of the patients expressing a treatment preference, 74% chose ondansetron and dexamethasone, compared with 26% preferring ondansetron alone.

A recent study confirmed the improved antiemetic efficiency of ondansetron when a corticosteroid was added, and studied the safety and efficiency of the combination over three cycles.[35] 102 patients receiving high-dose cisplatin-containing chemotherapy (50–120 mg/m^2, mean first dose 90 mg/m^2) were randomized to (A) 8 mg ondansetron i.v. and 120 mg methylprednisolone i.v. prior to chemotherapy followed by 12-hourly oral ondansetron 8 mg and methylprednisolone 16 mg for 3–5 days or (B) 8 mg ondansetron i.v. and placebo i.v. prior to chemotherapy, followed by 12-hourly oral ondansetron 8 mg and a placebo tablet for 3–5 days. Endpoints of the study were number of emetic episodes (defined as vomits or retches) during the first day, grade of nausea assessed by VAS and delayed emesis. Complete control of acute emetic episodes (0 episodes/day) was consistently and significantly better in the combination antiemetic schedule than in the ondansetron-plus-placebo group. For courses 1–3 these were 84.6% vs 65.3%, 83.3% vs 42.5% and 74.3% vs 54.3% respectively. Nausea on the first day of chemotherapy was significantly less in ondansetron plus methylprednisolone-treated patients than in controls for cycles 2 and 3, and the same applied for delayed emesis. Finally, overall control of emetic episodes over the whole course was better for patients also receiving methylprednisolone (54.2% vs 38.6% in the first cycle, 59% vs 29.2% in the third for complete emesis control, 75% vs 59.1% and 74.4% vs 38.2% respectively for complete or major control defined as 0–2 emesis episodes/day). Safety was excellent, with headaches as the most common adverse effect. Overall the ondansetron-plus-methylprednisolone group had fewer adverse effects than the ondansetron alone group. These results show that corticosteroids improve the antiemetic efficacy of ondansetron, and that the ondansetron-plus-methylprednisolone combination remains superior to ondansetron alone over repeat cycles.

Ondansetron and corticosteroids vs standard metoclopramide-containing regimens in repeat courses

Three pivotal studies have compared the combination of ondansetron and dexamethasone with best standard antiemetic treatment consisting of metoclopramide, dexamethasone and diphenhydramine or lorazepam in a minimum of three cycles of high-dose cisplatin chemotherapy.[23,36,37]

The Italian Group for Antiemetic Research randomized 289 patients receiving chemotherapy containing cisplatin (at least 50 mg/m^2) to (A) ondansetron 0.15 mg/kg before and after cisplatin and dexamethasone 20 mg before cisplatin or (B) metoclopramide 3 mg/kg before and after cisplatin + dexamethasone 20 mg + diphenhydramine 50 mg prior to cisplatin.[23] After the first cycle, 267 patients were evaluable for efficacy. Complete protection from vomiting was achieved in 78.7% of patients obtaining treatment A vs 59.5% of those obtaining treatment B during the first cycle. On subsequent cycles, ondansetron-plus-dexamethasone treatment retained its emesis-protective effect (74%), but the incidence of acute vomiting rose to 53% in those patients treated with the metoclopramide regimen. A reported benefit of ondansetron plus dexamethasone in controlling acute nausea has on reanalysis[38] been found to be due to a confounding effect.

In another study[37] the Italian Group for Antiemetic Research randomized 63 female patients with ovarian cancer undergoing cisplatin treatment to the same antiemetic regimens as detailed above (A = ondansetron plus dexamethasone, B = metoclopramide plus dexamethasone plus diphenhydramine). Ondansetron plus dexamethasone was more efficient than the standard conventional antiemetic regimen on days 1 and 2 of all three cycles. The efficiency in complete protection from acute vomiting decreased, however, from over 90% in the first course to over 70% in subsequent courses. Overall, ondansetron-plus-dexamethasone treatment was superior to metoclopramide, dexamethasone and diphenhydramine in controlling nausea and vomiting during the entire observation period (days 1–4) for all three studied courses.

Cunningham et al[36] recently reported on an international, multicentre, double-blind, double-dummy, parallel-group study comparing the efficacy and tolerability of ondansetron plus dexamethasone with metoclopramide plus dexamethasone plus lorazepam over three consecutive cycles of cisplatin chemotherapy. 237 chemotherapy-naive patients with a variety of primary tumour sites, scheduled to receive cisplatin 50–100 mg/m^2 as a single i.v. infusion over a period of up to four hours on day 1 and having no other aetiologies for emesis were included. The median cisplatin dose for the first course was 70.2 mg/m^2 for both antiemetic treatment arms. 117 patients were randomized to the O + D group and received ondansetron

8 mg i.v. plus dexamethasone 20 mg i.v. prior to cisplatin. On days 2–5 they were treated with ondansetron 8 mg bd orally and dexamethasone 4 mg bd orally. 120 patients were randomized to the M + D + L control antiemetic arm consisting of metoclopramide 3 mg/kg i.v., dexamethasone 20 mg i.v. and lorazepam 1.5 mg/m^2 i.v., maximum 3 mg, prior to chemotherapy followed by metoclopramide 3 mg/kg i.v. two hours post-chemotherapy then 40 mg tds orally and dexamethasone 4 mg bd orally on days 2–5. Intervention therapy with ondansetron 8 mg i.v. was available to patients who experienced three or more emetic episodes in the 24 hours following cisplatin infusion. Emetic episodes were defined as single vomits or retches separated from one another by at least one minute. Nausea was graded by patients as none, mild (did not interfere with normal life), moderate (interfered with normal daily life) and severe (bedridden due to nausea). 137 patients (61 in the O + D group and 76 in the M + D + L group) did not complete three courses of treatment. Withdrawal reasons were lack of response, adverse events, and disease progression leading to withdrawal from chemotherapy treatment. In addition, 17 patients (14%) withdrew from the M + D + L group because of extrapyramidal symptoms. During the first course of chemotherapy, patients receiving O + D had a significantly better control of nausea and vomiting for both day 1 and the five-day study period. In an intention-to-treat analysis, complete control of emesis was achieved in 73% vs 56% of patients treated with O + D vs M + D + L on day 1 ($p = 0.008$) and 54% vs 37% respectively for days 1–5 ($p = 0.014$). Similarly, none or mild nausea only was experienced by 64% vs 48% of patients ($p = 0.034$). Over the three courses of chemotherapy, 53% of patients in the O + D group vs 33% of M + D + L patients were completely free of emesis on day 1 of all their courses ($p = 0.002$), and the respective figures for days 1–5 were 41% and 24% ($p = 0.009$). Life tables shown in Figure 9.1 show the proportion of patients maintaining complete emesis and no/mild nausea control over courses 1–3. Side-effects

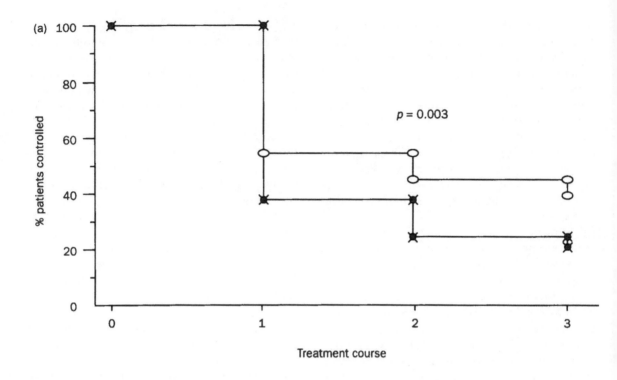

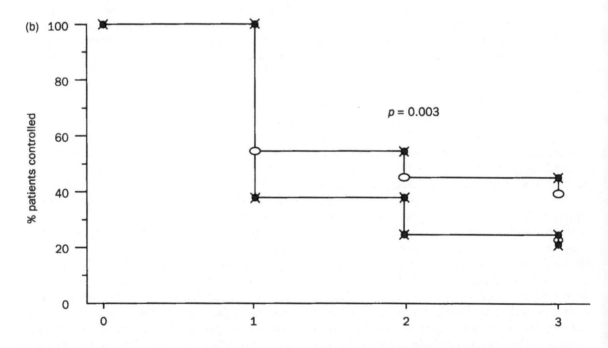

Figure 9.1 Maintenance of (a) complete emetic response and (b) nausea control (none or mild nausea) over courses 1–3, days 1–5 (intent-to-treat population): ○———○ , ondansetron regimen; ✷———✷ , metoclopramide regimen, with kind permission from Kluwer Academic Publishers.[36]

reported during all courses of antiemetic treatment were more frequent in the M + D + L group (78% vs 57%). The main adverse effects in the O + D group were constipation (25%) and headaches (19%); in the M + D + L group they were drowsiness (38%), extrapyramidal symptoms (20%), malaise/fatigue (16%), anxiety (11%) and dizziness (10%).

These studies demonstrated that ondansetron plus dexamethasone is more effective and better tolerated than standard antiemetic regimens (metoclopramide, dexamethasone plus lorazepam or diphenhydramine) in controlling high-dose cisplatin-induced emesis, and that the difference in antiemetic response is maintained over repeat cycles. However the life-table data of the study by Cunningham et al suggest that there is a decrease in overall emesis control as patients receive more chemotherapy courses even in the ondansetron-plus-dexamethasone regimen. The superiority of a 5-HT$_3$ antagonist plus corticosteroids over standard metoclopramide-based regimens argues convincingly that the former should be considered the new gold-standard antiemetic combination for prevention of high-dose cisplatin-induced nausea and vomiting over repeat courses.

Ondansetron and corticosteroids in moderately emetogenic chemotherapy

Ondansetron was shown to be good antiemetic prophylaxis in patients receiving a first course of non-cisplatin chemotherapy.[39] Its continued efficacy over repeat cycles in this setting and the potential benefit of dexamethasone maintenance has been examined by the NCI of Canada Clinical Trials Group.[40] The study population were 302 patients due to receive moderately emetogenic chemotherapy (defined as doxorubicin ≥40 mg/m^2 as a single agent or ≥25 mg/m^2 when administered in combination with other chemotherapy agents; epirubicin ≥74 mg/m^2 as a single agent or ≥50 mg/m^2 when administered in combination; cisplatin ≥20 mg/m^2 and <50 mg/m^2; carboplatin ≥300 mg/m^2 or cyclophosphamide ≥600 mg/m^2 when administered in combination). Three

antiemetic regimens were compared in a double-blind fashion in order to investigate the potential merits of splitting the day-1 ondansetron dose and of giving oral ondansetron on days 2–5 as antiemetic prophylaxis. There was no difference in antiemetic efficacy in patients given split dose ondansetron vs a single dose prior to chemotherapy for complete, complete plus major emesis response or severity of nausea in the first 24 hours. The overall response rate for five days determined in a subset of 189 patients receiving single-day chemotherapy was significantly superior in patients receiving ondansetron maintenance than patients in the placebo arm (59.6% vs 42.1% for complete response and 80.9% vs 66.3% complete plus major response respectively). This advantage was maintained in the 128 patients treated for a second and 103 patients treated for a third cycle on the same antiemetic protocol ($p = 0.004$, complete plus major response rates for five days for patients on maintenance ondansetron vs placebo 90.6% vs 79.2% for cycle 2 and 84.4% vs 76.5% for cycle 3). Patients who were receiving maintenance ondansetron and achieved a complete response in cycle 1 had a 90% probability of complete responses for both cycles 2 and 3. Patients given ondansetron on day 1 only had a similar preservation of antiemetic efficiency over the three studied courses, although the overall response was less favourable. This study established that ondansetron remains an efficient antiemetic in patients receiving moderately emetogenic chemotherapy over three treatment cycles, and that maintenance ondansetron decreases the probability and severity of delayed emesis. However, Jones et al[41] showed in a double-blind, crossover randomized study of patients receiving moderately emetogenic chemotherapy that dexamethasone was as effective as ondansetron in controlling delayed vomiting, but superior in control of nausea and more economical. Further comparisons between maintenance antiemetic treatment with ondansetron and corticosteroids in repeat courses of chemotherapy should be awaited.

Two studies showed ondansetron plus

dexamethasone to be better than a standard antiemetic regimen in controlling emesis in repeat cycles of chemotherapy containing cyclophosphamide $\geq 500 \, mg/m^2$ in women treated for breast cancer.[42,43] Soukop et al[42] treated patients with 16 mg dexamethasone i.v. followed by either 8 mg ondansetron (93 patients) or 60 mg metoclopramide (94 patients) prior to chemotherapy, followed by either 8 mg ondansetron or 20 mg metoclopramide orally tds for 5 days. 91% and 60% of patients in the ondansetron and metoclopramide groups respectively were free of emesis on day 1 and 81% vs 48% on days 1–5 of the first cycle. Over six courses, 67% of patients receiving ondansetron vs 28% of patients receiving meto-clopramide had a maximum of two emetic episodes on their worst day. Nausea and qual-ity-of-life data obtained using the Rotterdam Symptom Checklist were significantly better for patients treated with ondansetron over all cycles. Side-effects observed during treatment were minor, except for extrapyramidal symp-toms occurring in 19% of patients treated with metoclopramide and necessitating withdrawal of 15% of patients from their randomized antiemetic schedule. This carefully executed study showed ondansetron to be significantly superior to metoclopramide ($p < 0.001$) in all studied aspects over six cycles of treatment. A further study[43] randomized 64 chemotherapy-naive breast-cancer patients to ondansetron plus dexamethasone vs metoclopramide, dexa-methasone and orphenadrine, with ondan-setron or metoclopramide and dexamethasone as maintenance treatment, and followed them during six cycles of FEC/FAC chemotherapy. Complete and major control of acute emesis and major control of delayed emesis was supe-rior in the ondansetron-plus-dexamethasone treated patients through all cycles.

Granisetron

Granisetron is a potent and selective $5\text{-}HT_3$ receptor antagonist, shown to be efficient in control of chemotherapy-induced emesis by

high-dose cisplatin[44] or moderately emetogenic cytostatic chemotherapy.[45] Since the definition of antiemetic response in all granisetron trials is different and more stringent than for ondansetron or tropisetron, it shall be briefly enunciated here. By definition, complete control was attained in patients who experienced no vomiting and had no or only mild nausea. Partial control describes patients who experi-enced only one episode of vomiting, or, if no vomiting, recorded moderate to severe nausea in the studied time period. Patients having more than two episodes of vomiting regardless of nausea rating were described as having no control.

Open-label studies

Two reports[18,46] on safety and efficacy of repeated administration of granisetron in repeated cycles of chemotherapy will be dis-cussed here. Both were open-label studies per-formed in patients who had a good antiemetic response to granisetron during their first course of chemotherapy. 91 patients receiving 438 fur-ther cycles of chemotherapy were included in the first study.[46] Patients received either granisetron 40 µg/kg or a 3 mg total dose, with no other antiemetics allowed, over a median of four cycles. The recorded toxicity included mild headaches in 3.2% of the cycles and constipa-tion in 1.8% of cycles. The incidence of headache and constipation did not increase with multiple cycles of granisetron, and occur-rence of a side-effect did not predict recurrence in further cycles. Complete and partial antiemetic response was observed in 88–90% of all cycles, and was not significantly influenced by gender or age. Patients who had 'no control' were excluded from further treatment on repeat cycles. A total of 12 patients dropped out of the study – 4 after the first and after the second cycle, 2 after the third and 1 after the fourth and seventh cycles respectively. The patients remaining in the long-term study consistently had complete control rates of over 70%. Blijham summarized on behalf of the Granisetron Study Group the open-label granisetron results obtained in nine countries in 828 patients receiving a total of 2751 chemotherapy cycles.[18]

In the initial study, 574 patients were treated for 1966 cycles with a dose of granisetron of 40 µg/kg. From July 1989 onwards, the dosage regimen was simplified to a standard 3 mg dose, and 335 patients (including 81 transferred from study 1) were treated for 785 cycles. All patients included had had a favourable response to previous treatment with granisetron. A descriptive review of data only up to the eighth course of treatment was presented. With either regimen, approximately 60% of patients had complete control of acute emesis over eight cycles, and for the subgroup of patients receiving moderately emetogenic regimens complete control of acute emesis approached 70% in all treatment cycles. Emesis control in a subset of patients treated with high-dose cisplatin decreased from 59% in the first to 33.3% in the fifth cycle. This was attributed to a confounding effect: the percentage of complete responders was almost double in men than women, and the male:female ratio reversed during the course of the study from 1:0.6 at cycle one to 1:1.6 at cycle 5. Analysis of antiemetic response to high-dose cisplatin chemotherapy according to gender suggested that efficacy of granisetron is maintained over five additional cycles. Withdrawal from the long-term granisetron study was largely due to completion of chemotherapy treatment. However, 14.9% of patients discontinued treatment for reasons possibly related to poor emetic control, and 9.9% for unspecified reasons. Side-effects were headache and constipation, and they did not increase with repeat cycles. Granisetron appears to be thus an effective and safe agent in controlling nausea and vomiting in repeat chemotherapy courses. In estimating efficacy data from the above studies, it must be recalled that the Granisetron Study Group defines 'no control' as more than two emetic episodes over 24 hours, which is a very stringent standard. Exclusion of patients who experienced treatment failure, albeit stringently defined, may lead, however, to an overestimation of granisetron efficacy. It also precludes commenting on the ability of granisetron to maintain the same level of antiemetic control over consecutive cycles.

Granisetron with or without corticosteroids in controlled studies

A comparison of antiemetic efficacy of granisetron, dexamethasone and their combination over three courses of moderately emetogenic therapy has been published.[47] In a multicentre, randomized, double-blind study, 428 consecutive patients starting their first course of chemotherapy (including cyclophosphamide 600–1000 mg/m^2, doxorubicin ≥50 mg/m^2, epirubicin ≥75 mg/m^2 or carboplatin ≥300 mg/m^2 alone or in combination) were randomized to one of three antiemetic treatment arms. The first treatment consisted of 8 mg dexamethasone i.v. prior to chemotherapy and four doses of oral dexamethasone given six-hourly, starting immediately before administration of chemotherapy. In the second treatment patients received 3 mg of granisetron i.v. prior to chemotherapy administration and four placebo tablets taken six-hourly as in treatment arm 1. In the third regimen patients were given granisetron and dexamethasone (both i.v. and orally as in treatment arm 1). Patients' characteristics were similar in all three treatment groups. 398 patients were assessable at the end of the first cycle of chemotherapy, 354 after the second and 322 after the third cycle. The results of antiemetic efficacy over the three consecutive cycles of chemotherapy are presented in Table 9.1. A greater percentage of patients treated with the combination of granisetron and dexamethasone had complete protection from vomiting, nausea, and nausea and vomiting than patients treated with granisetron alone for all three courses of chemotherapy. Granisetron and dexamethasone in combination were superior to dexamethasone alone in complete protection from vomiting in the first two cycles only, and against nausea or nausea and vomiting only in the first cycle. Reasons for patient withdrawal during subsequent cycles of chemotherapy included interruption or change in chemotherapy, death or loss to follow-up in 34 patients, deviation from protocol in 19 patients, toxicity due to antiemetic treatment (1 patient in the granisetron group and 3 in the combination group) and lack of antiemetic efficiency (15 patients in the dexamethasone

Table 9.1 Antiemetic efficacy In all three consecutive cycles of chemotherapy,[47] reproduced by permission of WB Saunders Company

Efficacy	Cycle	Number of patients — DEX	GRAN	DEX Plus GRAN	DEX Mean	DEX ±SD	GRAN Mean	GRAN ±SD	DEX Plus GRAN Mean	DEX Plus GRAN ±SD	p
Percentage of complete protection from vomiting	1	132	134	132	70.5		72.4		92.4		0.0001
	2	113	116	125	77.0		75.0		91.2		0.0001
	3	101	107	114	83.2		68.2		90.4		0.0001
Percentage of complete protection from nausea	1	132	134	132	54.5		47.8		71.2		0.0005
	2	113	116	125	61.1		48.3		67.2		0.0005
	3	101	107	114	64.7		47.7		65.8		0.0005
Percentage of complete protection from both nausea and vomiting	1	132	134	132	49.2		42.5		69.7		0.0001
	2	113	116	125	55.7		44.0		66.4		0.0001
	3	101	107	114	61.8		42.1		63.2		0.0001
Number of emetic episodes[b]	1	39	37	10	4.80	3.9	4.08	3.0	2.70	2.2	NS
	2	26	29	11	3.31	3.4	3.59	2.5	2.18	0.9	NS
	3	17	34	11	3.53	4.0	3.09	2.1	2.36	1.7	NS
Maximal intensity of nausea[c]	1	60	70	38	1.63	0.8	1.64	0.8	1.55	0.8	NS
	2	44	56	41	1.57	0.8	1.72	0.8	1.88	1.8	NS
	3	35	56	39	1.46	0.7	1.80	0.8	1.51	0.6	NS
Time to start of vomiting (minutes)[d]	1	37	35	9	619	63	449	53	474	123	0.0036
	2	23	25	8	542	64	502	58	722	147	NS
	3	14	31	9	561	106	498	53	620	157	NS

Abbreviations: NS = not significant; DEX = dexamethasone; GRAN = granisetron. [a] Refers to G test. [b] Considering only the patients who vomited. [c] Considering only the patients who had nausea. [d] In 5 patients at the first, in 10 at the second, and in 8 at the third cycle of chemotherapy starting time of vomiting was not reported.

group, 10 patients in the granisetron group and only 2 patients in the combination group). The analysis of persistence of antiemetic efficacy was performed in the subgroup of 322 patients who completed all three cycles of chemotherapy. Complete protection from vomiting remained stable over the three cycles in the dexamethasone alone group (79.2%, 81.2% and 83.2% for courses 1–3 respectively) and the granisetron-plus-dexamethasone group (93.9%, 93.9% and 90.4% for courses 1–3), but decreased in the granisetron-alone group (77.6%, 75.5% and 68.2% for courses 1–3 respectively). A multifactorial analysis of the main prognostic factors of vomiting was performed. Variables predicting poor control in the first cycle were younger age, low alcohol intake and type of chemotherapy. For the second cycle the only significant effect was poor protection from vomiting in the first cycle. Complete protection from vomiting was obtained in 36.7% of patients who vomited in the first cycle compared to 90.5% in those who did not vomit. Antiemetic responses in the first and second courses of chemotherapy were by far the most powerful independent predictors of emesis in the third cycle. Prognostic factors for nausea were similar, but female sex was an additional independent predictor for nausea in all three courses. This careful investigation in a large number of patients receiving three moderately emetogenic chemotherapy treatments suggests that corticosteroids alone may be as or more effective in emesis control than granisetron alone, and preserve their antiemetic efficacy better over repeat cycles. The combination of the 5-HT₃ antagonist and dexamethasone, however, was superior to either single agent and was well tolerated, and should represent the standard against which antiemetic efficacy in cyclical chemotherapy should be investigated in further trials. The strong degree in which the response to the antiemetic treatment in the first course influenced the response to antiemetics in the subsequent courses of chemotherapy must caution our interpretation of the open-label granisetron studies detailed above. In those studies only patients having had a good response to granisetron in a prior cycle of

chemotherapy and requesting granisetron for further cycles were entered. Finally, the power of the initial level of emesis protection to predict nausea and vomiting in later courses should help rational antiemetic study design based on results obtained in the first treatment of chemotherapy-naive patients and strengthen the aim to achieve optimal emesis control from the onset of chemotherapy treatment.

Tropisetron

Leinbundgut and Lancranjan[6] published the first report demonstrating 5-HT₃ antagonist efficacy in humans on 11 patients treated with tropisetron during 47 cycles of cisplatin-containing chemotherapy. Patients had no acute retching or vomiting in 31 of 47 courses, 1 episode in 7 courses and 2 episodes in 5 courses. The effect was sustained, comparing favourably with metoclopramide. Many studies have since been published showing this selective 5-HT₃ receptor antagonist to be efficient in patients receiving their first course of high-dose cisplatin-containing chemotherapy.[48–50] 476 patients refractory to standard antiemetic treatment received 5 mg or 10 mg of tropisetron prior to their next course of chemotherapy,[51] with 62% achieving complete control of nausea and vomiting, and 91% complete or partial control (1–4 vomiting episodes or mild-to-moderate nausea). The authors also showed that 80% of patients with a complete response on cycle 1 also had a complete response on cycle 2.

Open-label studies

Sorbe[19,30,49,52] summarized the experience of safety and efficacy of tropisetron as antiemetic agent in patients treated for a variety of cancers recruited in 15 centres. 630 patients were included, 338 of whom had had previous exposure to chemotherapy. Cytotoxic agents used in treatment regimens included cisplatin (41%), carboplatin (23%), doxorubicin (27%) and epirubicin (24%). With single-agent tropisetron, 64% of patients had complete protection from acute nausea and vomiting, and delayed nausea and vomiting was prevented in 45–73% on days

2–6 during the first chemotherapy cycles. High-dose cisplatin-treated patients had lower response rates for acute nausea and vomiting than patients receiving non-cisplatin therapy (52% vs 72%). Treatment efficacy was reported as stable over 10 cycles, with 43 patients remaining evaluable at the end of the study. Patients not responding to antiemetic treatment were given rescue treatment with corticosteroids ± lorazepam and included in the analysis. Adverse effects were noted in 19–36% of cases during follow-up over repeat cycles, and consisted mostly of mild headache (16%) and constipation (5%).

Tropisetron with or without corticosteroids in controlled studies

Four studies were performed to investigate the benefit of addition of dexamethasone to tropisetron.[19,53–55] Addition of a corticosteroid significantly increased the efficacy of tropisetron[19] in patients who had insufficient emesis control on their first chemotherapy cycle on treatment with tropisetron alone, and in 126 patients scheduled to receive two cycles of moderately emetogenic chemotherapy the group randomized to receive dexamethasone on days 1–5 in addition to tropisetron orally had a greater control of acute and delayed vomiting and nausea than patients receiving the tropisetron–placebo treatment.[53] The magnitude of benefit of adding dexamethasone to tropisetron is illustrated in a multicentre study[54] in 160 chemotherapy-naive women with ovarian or endometrial carcinomas. 39% of the patients had a partial response in the first chemotherapy course to tropisetron 5 mg given i.v. on day 1 and orally on days 2–5, and were randomized to receive dexamethasone or placebo in course 2. Tropisetron plus dexamethasone prevented vomiting in 75% of patients vs 40% of patients receiving tropisetron plus placebo in the first 24 hours, and in 54% vs 20% of patients on days 1–6. 64% of the patients experienced no nausea on days 1–6 of the second course when receiving the tropisetron-and-dexamethasone combination vs 3% of patients receiving only tropisetron. While these data are encouraging, there are no studies investigating the persistence of this improved antiemetic effect of the tropisetron-and-dexamethasone combination over multiple cycles.

Tropisetron compared with standard metoclopramide-containing antiemetic treatment

A randomized crossover study comparing efficacy, toxicity and patient preference over three cycles of cisplatin-containing chemotherapy[56] compared tropisetron alone with a standard antiemetic regimen consisting of metoclopramide, dexamethasone, diphenhydramine and lorazepam. 62 chemotherapy-naive women were randomized. Complete protection from acute emesis was obtained in 48% of tropisetron-treated patients vs 29% of those treated with the conventional regimen. The superiority of tropisetron was most apparent in the first 12 hours following chemotherapy administration. The metoclopramide combination controlled delayed emesis better. However, a larger number of patients treated with the standard metoclopramide-containing regimen experienced side-effects, of which extrapyramidal symptoms were the most severe. Patients preferred the tropisetron regimen, and those receiving tropisetron for the first cycles had no drop in antiemetic efficacy in their three courses, but the patients treated first with the metoclopramide combination did. These results confirmed previous experience that proved tropisetron easier to administer, better tolerated and more efficacious than metoclopramide-based antiemetic regimens, and suggested that this advantage is maintained over three courses of chemotherapy. It is likely that, in analogy to ondansetron, the combination of tropisetron with dexamethasone, shown to be superior to tropisetron alone in patients starting highly emetogenic chemotherapy, will prove even more effective in comparison with standard regimens, and trials testing this hypothesis may be forthcoming.

Comparisons of 5-HT₃ antagonists

Various differences between ondansetron, granisetron and tropisetron have been described.[57]

Granisetron and tropisetron showed greater specificity and potency of binding to 5-HT$_3$ receptors, longer duration of action and terminal half-lives than ondansetron, and their pharmacokinetics were linear while ondansetron has a more complex dose–response pattern. Comparisons of reported efficacies of the different 5-HT$_3$ antagonists in highly or moderately emetogenic chemotherapy are difficult because of different study design and definitions of endpoints. Comparative studies that have been reported recently failed to identify significant differences in the three 5-HT$_3$ antagonists, both regarding efficacy and side-effects (for recent reviews see Chapter 7 and references 8 and 30). All studies have been of patients during their first course of chemotherapy only, with the exception of one study, which will be discussed here.[58] In this single-institution, prospective, randomized, open controlled trial, 117 chemotherapy-naive patients beginning chemotherapy containing cisplatin 80–100 mg/m^2 were randomized to receive ondansetron 24 mg i.v., granisetron 3 mg i.v. or tropisetron 5 mg i.v. and treated for a total of 463 cycles. Median cisplatin doses for the three groups were not indicated. The study endpoint was control of acute nausea and vomiting, defined as complete response (CR), major response (MR), minor response (MiR) and failure (F).[45,59] Over all cycles of treatment, ondansetron-treated patients achieved CR in 73.3%, MR in 20.7%, MiR in 1.3% and failure in 4.7%. For patients treated with granisetron, the corresponding figures were 72.1% CR, 19.4% MR, 3% MiR and 5.5% F, while patients receiving tropisetron achieved CR in 67.6%, MR in 17.6%, MiR in 10.1% and F in 4.7%. The differences in MR between ondansetron and tropisetron and in MiR between ondansetron, granisetron and tropisetron were significant. However, at study entry, tropisetron-treated patients may have had more advanced disease (Stage IV in 75% of patients in the tropisetron group vs 61.5 in the ondansetron group and 65.8% in the granisetron group). Control of emesis by the three 5-HT$_3$ antagonists for individual courses of chemotherapy is detailed in Table 9.2; there was no statistically significant difference

between the first and subsequent cycles in all treatment groups. Nineteen patients failing one antiemetic agent were crossed over to another drug. Of these, eight subsequently achieved MR and seven MiR, but four failed to achieve emesis control. The two major disadvantages of this study are the relatively small number of patients studied and its limitation to investigating only acute nausea and vomiting, while in the context of patients receiving cyclical chemotherapy control over the entire period is desired. Further larger studies are needed, addressing also the issue of delayed emesis control over repeat cycles, and possibly using the most efficacious antiemetic regimen against high-dose cisplatin-induced nausea, which includes corticosteroids.

Is the efficacy of 5-HT$_3$ antagonist prophylaxis maintained in patients receiving repeat courses of chemotherapy?

Few studies have been specifically designed to test the hypothesis that 5-HT$_3$ antagonist antiemetic activity does not decrease over repeat courses of chemotherapy. While open-label studies indicated that the efficacy of granisetron[18] or tropisetron[19] remained stable, patients failing antiemetic treatment were excluded from further cycles, tending to bias the results as detailed previously. The Italian Group for Antiemetic Research reported that efficacy of the ondansetron plus dexamethasone combination was preserved over three cycles of cisplatin chemotherapy,[23] but only patients who completed three cycles were included in the study. Cunningham et al,[36] reporting on the same drug combination, presented life tables suggesting a decrease of efficacy for patients achieving complete control. A study by deWit and colleagues[60] applied two different statistical analyses to data on emesis obtained during six cycles of treatment in patients given tropisetron prophylaxis. 83 patients receiving weekly cisplatin-containing chemotherapy at a dose of 70 mg/m^2 (when combined with etoposide) or 80 mg/m^2 as single agent were treated with tropisetron 5 mg

Table 9.2 Response rates to three antiemetics at the start of the first chemotherapy cycle compared with the second, third and subsequent cycles,[58] reprinted by permission of Wiley-Liss Inc, a subsidary of John Wiley and Sons Inc.

GRANISETRON

Response	1st cycle		2nd cycle		3rd cycle		Subsequent cycles	
	No.	%	No.	%	No.	%	No.	%
Complete response (CR)	32	84.2	22	66.7	20	74.1	45	67.2ª
Major response (MR)	4	10.5	9	27.3	6	22.2	13	19.4
Major efficacy (CR + MR)	36	94.7	31	93.9	26	96.3	58	86.6
Minor response (MiR)	1	2.6	—	—	—	—	4	6.0
Failures (F)	1	2.6	2	6.1	1	3.7	5	7.4
Total	38		33		27		67	

ONDANSETRON

Response	1st cycle		2nd cycle		3rd cycle		Subsequent cycles	
	No.	%	No.	%	No.	%	No.	%
Complete response (CR)	32	82.1	28	80.0	19	61.3	31	68.9ª
Major response (MR)	7	17.9	7	20.0	8	25.8	9	20.0
Major efficacy (CR + MR)	39	100.0	35	100.0	27	87.1	40	88.9
Minor responses (MiR)	—	—	—	—	1	32	1	2.2
Failures (F)	—	—	—	—	3	9.7	4	8.9
Total	39		35		31		45	

TROPISETRON

Response	1st cycle		2nd cycle		3rd cycle		Subsequent cycles	
	No.	%	No.	%	No.	%	No.	%
Complete response (CR)	29	72.5	24	66.7	19	65.5	28	65.1ª
Major response (MR)	6	15.0	7	19.4	5	17.2	8	18.6
Major efficacy (CR + MR)	35	87.5	31	86.1	24	82.8	36	83.7
Minor response (MiR)	3	7.5	4	11.1	4	13.8	4	9.3
Failures (F)	2	5.0	1	2.8	1	3.4	3	7.0
Total	40		36		29		43	

ª Chi-square test.
There were no statistically significant differences in response rates to antiemetic treatment in comparisons between the first and subsequent chemotherapy cycles.

i.v. on day 1, followed by oral tropisetron 5 mg daily on days 2–5. Over six consecutive cycles, complete protection rates against acute emesis decreased significantly from 71% in the first to 43% in the last cycle. Overall protection rates and protection against delayed emesis also decreased, from 95% to 72% and from 31% to 6% respectively. This decrease became only evident when cumulative protection rates, corresponding to a Kaplan–Meier analysis, were calculated. Calculation of conditional rates (including only those patients who were protected in previous cycles) failed to show the decrease in efficacy. The difference in response determined by the two methods is illustrated in Figure 9.2. These two reports[36,60] indicate that both ondansetron and tropisetron lose some of their efficacy when used in repeat courses of highly emetogenic chemotherapy, and it is possible that this represents a class effect. While antiemetic control has improved greatly over even a few years, this observation should encourage efforts to develop more efficient antiemetic schedules.

CONCLUSIONS

Much of the progress in controlling nausea and vomiting following cytotoxic chemotherapy made in recent years has been the result of understanding the mechanisms of emesis and the wide import into clinical practice of antiemetic regimens including high-dose metoclopramide, steroids and the group of 5-HT$_3$ receptor antagonists. The reports on which this experience is based have most often been studies of chemotherapy-naive patients undergoing their first cytotoxic treatment. While these have helped define endpoints and measures of response, and generated much data on safety, efficacy and potential synergism of different antiemetic drugs, the clinical setting in which these drugs are most frequently used is prevention of nausea and vomiting in patients receiving repeated cycles of chemotherapy. Studies designed to test optimal antiemetic treatment for these patients are scarce. They are more difficult to perform and interpret, and require a larger number of patients.

The best long-term studies currently available suggest that in patients treated with highly emetogenic chemotherapy schedules, 5-HT$_3$ receptor antagonists alone and in combination with corticosteroids maintain over repeated courses their superiority over antiemetic cocktails containing high-dose metoclopramide, corticosteroids and benzodiazepines. They are more efficient, easier to administer and better tolerated than previously used regimens, and

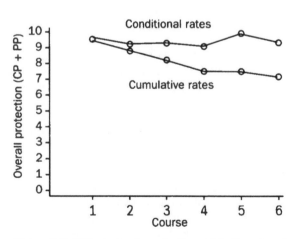
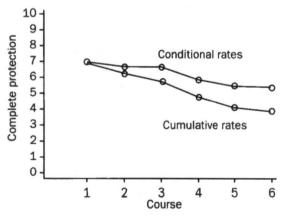

Figure 9.2 Differences in protection against acute emesis related or the conditional vs cumulative calculation method,[60] reproduced with permission of WB Saunders Company.

the combination of 5-HT$_3$ receptor antagonists and corticosteroids should be considered the gold antiemetic therapy standard in patients receiving repeat courses of highly emetogenic chemotherapy. For less emetogenic chemotherapy, the combination of 5-HT$_3$ receptor antagonists and corticosteroids remains the most efficient. Optimal dose and schedule for individual situations need careful consideration, however, since overtreatment is expensive but insufficient prophylaxis may create a resistance to antiemetic therapy that is difficult to over-

come. Indeed, level of control of nausea and vomiting in previous cycles has been shown to be the most powerful independent predictor of response in the following cycles.

With the best antiemetic prophylaxis, the majority of patients now experience no vomiting and only mild nausea following the administration of very emetogenic cytotoxics. Further research is needed to compare the efficacy of the different 5-HT$_3$ receptor antagonists and to establish the best and most economical antiemetic schedules for repeat courses of chemotherapy.

REFERENCES

1. O'Brien MER, Cunningham D, Anti-emetic therapy. In: *Treatment of Cancer* ed. P Price, K Sikora, pp. 975–84. London: Chapman & Hall, 1995.
2. Gralla RJ, Metoclopramide. A review of antiemetic trials. *Drugs* 1983; 25(Suppl 1): 63–73.
3. Grunberg SM, Hesketh PJ, Control of chemotherapy-induced emesis. *N Engl J Med* 1993; 329: 1790–6.
4. Morrow GR, The assessment of nausea and vomiting: past problems, current issues, and suggestions for future research. *Cancer* 1984; 53: 2267–78.
5. Miner WD, Sanger GJ, Inhibition of cisplatin-induced vomiting by selective 5-hydroxytryptamine M-receptor antagonism. *Br J Pharmacol* 1986; 88: 497–9.
6. Leinbundgut U, Lancranjan J, First results with ICS 205-930 (5-HT receptor antagonist) in prevention of chemotherapy-induced emesis. *Lancet* 1987; i: 1198.
7. Cunningham D, Pople A, Fort HT et al, Prevention of emesis in patients receiving cytotoxic drugs by GR38032F, a selective 5-HT$_3$ receptor antagonist. *Lancet* 1987; i: 1461–3.
8. Morrow GR, Hickok JT, Rosenthal SN, Comparisons of ondansetron (Zofran), granisetron (Kytril), and tropisetron (Navoban). *Cancer* 1995; 76: 343–57.
9. Jones AL, Cunningham D, The clinical care of patients receiving chemotherapy. In: *Emesis in Anti-Cancer Therapy* ed. PLR Andrews, GJ Sanger, pp. 229–46. London: Chapman & Hall, 1993.
10. Hickok JT, Morrow GR, A biobehavioral model of patient reported nausea: implications for clinical practice. *Adv Med Psychother* 1993; 6: 227–40.
11. Gralla RJ, Adverse effects of treatment. In: *Cancer: Principles and Practice of Oncology* ed. VT de Vita, S Hellman, SA Rosenberg, pp. 2338–48. Philadelphia: JB Lippincott, 1993.
12. Fiore JJ, Gralla RJ, Pharmacologic treatment of chemotherapy-induced nausea and vomiting. *Cancer Invest* 1984; 2: 351–61.
13. Fetting JH, Grochow LB, Folstein MF et al, The course of nausea and vomiting after high-dose cyclophosphamide. *Cancer Treat Rep* 1982; 66: 1487–93.
14. Kris MG, Gralla RJ, Clark RA et al, Incidence, course, and severity of delayed nausea and vomiting following the administration of high-dose cisplatin. *J Clin Oncol* 1985; 3: 1379–84.
15. Kris MG, Gralla RJ, Tyson LB et al, Controlling delayed vomiting: double-blind, randomized trial comparing placebo, dexamethasone alone, and metoclopramide plus dexamethasone in patients receiving cisplatin. *J Clin Oncol* 1989; 7: 108–14.
16. Alba E, Bastus R, de Andres L et al, Anticipatory nausea and vomiting: prevalence and predictors in chemotherapy patients. *Oncology* 1989; 46: 26–30.
17. Wilcox PM, Fetting JH, Nettesheim KM, Abeloff MD, Anticipatory vomiting in women receiving cyclophosphamide, methotrexate, and 5-FU (CMF) adjuvant chemotherapy for breast carcinoma. *Cancer Treat Rep* 1982; 66: 1601–4.
18. Blijham GH, Does granisetron remain effective over multiple cycles? The Granisetron Study Group. *Eur J Cancer* 1992; 28A(Suppl 1): S17–21.
19. Sorbe BG, Hogberg T, Glimelius B et al, Navoban (tropisetron) alone and in combination with dexamethasone in the prevention of

chemotherapy-induced nausea and vomiting: the Nordic experience. The Nordic Antiemetic Trial Group. *Anticancer Drugs* 1995; 6(Suppl 1): 31–6.

20. Cunningham D, Evans C, Gazet JC et al, Comparison of antiemetic efficacy of domperidone, metoclopramide and dexamethasone in patients receiving outpatient chemotherapy regimens. *Br Med J* 1987; **295**: 250.

21. Gralla R, The management of chemotherapy induced nausea and vomiting. *Med Clin N Am* 1987; **71**: 289–301.

22. Roila F, Tonato M, Basurto C et al, Protection from nausea and vomiting in cisplatin-treated patients: high-dose metoclopramide combined with methylprednisolone versus metoclopramide combined with dexamethasone and diphenhydramine: a study of the Italian Oncology Group for Clinical Research. *J Clin Oncol* 1989; **7**: 1693–700.

23. Roila F, Ondansetron plus dexamethasone compared to the 'standard' metoclopramide combination. *Oncology* 1993; **50**: 163–7.

24. Martin M, Diaz Rubio E, Casado A et al, Progressive loss of antiemetic efficacy during subsequent courses of chemotherapy. *Eur J Cancer* 1992; **28**: 430–2.

25. The Italian Group for Antiemetic Research, Cisplatin-induced delayed emesis: pattern and prognostic factors during three subsequent cycles. *Ann Oncol* 1994; **5**: 585–9.

26. Cubeddu LX, Hoffmann IS, Participation of serotonin on early and delayed emesis induced by initial and subsequent cycles of cisplatinum-based chemotherapy: effects of antiemetics. *J Clin Pharmacol* 1993; **33**: 691–7.

27. Cassidy J, Raina V, Lewis C et al, Pharmacokinetics and anti-emetic efficacy of BRL 43694, a new selective 5-HT$_3$ antagonist. *Br J Cancer* 1988; **58**: 651–3.

28. De Mulder PHM, Seynaeve C, Vermorken JB et al, Ondansetron compared with high-dose metoclopramide in prophylaxis of acute and delayed cisplatin-induced nausea and vomiting. *Ann Int Med* 1990; **113**: 834–40.

29. Chevallier B, Efficacy and safety of granisetron compared with high-dose metoclopramide plus dexamethasone in patients receiving high-dose cisplatin in a single-blind study. *Eur J Cancer* 1990; **26**(Suppl 1): S33–6.

30. Sorbe B, 5-HT$_3$ receptor antagonists as antiemetic agents in cancer chemotherapy. *Exp Opin Invest Drugs* 1996; **5**: 389–407.

31. Cubeddu LX, Hoffman IS, Fuenmayor NT et al, Efficacy of ondansetron (GR 38032F) and the role of serotonin in cisplatin-induced nausea and vomiting. *N Engl J Med* 1990; **322**: 810–16.

32. Marty M, Pouillart P, Scholl S et al, Comparison of the 5-hydroxytryptamine$_3$ (serotonin) antagonist ondansetron (GR 38032F) with high-dose metoclopramide in the control of cisplatin-induced emesis. *N Engl J Med* 1991; **322**: 816–21.

33. Cunningham D, Turner A, Hawthorn J et al, Ondansetron with or without dexamethasone to treat chemotherapy induced emesis. *Lancet* 1989; i: 1323.

34. Roila F, Tonato M, Cognetti F et al, Prevention of cisplatin-induced emesis: a double-blind multicenter randomized crossover study comparing ondansetron and ondansetron plus dexamethasone. *J Clin Oncol* 1991; **9**: 675–8.

35. Chevallier B, Marty M, Paillarse JM, Methylprednisolone enhances the efficacy of ondansetron in acute and delayed cisplatin-induced emesis over at least three cycles. Ondansetron Study Group. *Br J Cancer* 1994; **70**: 1171–5.

36. Cunningham D, Dicato M, Verweij J et al, Optimum anti-emetic therapy for cisplatin induced emesis over repeat courses: ondansetron plus dexamethasone compared with metoclopramide, dexamethasone plus lorazepam. *Ann Oncol* 1996; **7**: 277–82.

37. Italian Group for Antiemetic Research, Ondansetron plus dexamethasone versus metoclopramide plus dexamethasone plus diphenhydramine in cisplatin-treated patients with ovarian cancer. *Support Care Cancer* 1994; **2**: 167–70.

38. Italian Group for Antiemetic Research, On the relationship between nausea and vomiting in patients undergoing chemotherapy. *Support Care Cancer* 1994; **2**: 171–6.

39. Frashini G, Antiemetic activity of ondansetron in cancer patients receiving non-cisplatin chemotherapy. *Semin Oncol* 1992; **19**(Suppl 10): 41–7.

40. Kaizer L, Warr D, Hoskins P et al, Effect of schedule and maintenance on the antiemetic efficacy of ondansetron combined with dexamethasone in acute and delayed nausea and emesis in patients receiving moderately emetogenic chemotherapy: a phase III trial by the National Cancer Institute of Canada Clinical Trials Group. *J Clin Oncol* 1994; **12**: 1050–7.

41. Jones AL, Hill AS, Soukop M et al, Comparison of dexamethasone and ondansetron in the prophylaxis of emesis induced by moderately emetogenic chemotherapy. *Lancet* 1991; **338:** 483–7.

42. Soukop M, McQuade B, Hunter E et al, Ondansetron compared with metoclopramide in the control of emesis and quality of life during repeated chemotherapy for breast cancer. *Oncology* 1992; **49:** 295–304.

43. Campora E, Giudici S, Merlini L et al, Ondansetron and dexamethasone versus standard combination antiemetic therapy. A randomized trial for the prevention of acute and delayed emesis induced by cyclophosphamide-doxorubicin chemotherapy and maintenance of antiemetic effect at subsequent courses. *Am J Clin Oncol* 1994; **17:** 522–6.

44. Cupissol DR, Serrou B, Caubel M, The efficacy of granisetron as a prophylactic anti-emetic and intervention agent in high dose cisplatin induced emesis. *Eur J Cancer Clin Oncol* 1990; **26**(Suppl 1): S23–7.

45. Smith IE, on behalf of the Granisetron Study Group. A comparison of two dose levels of granisetron in patients receiving moderately emetogenic cytostatic chemotherapy. *Eur J Cancer Clin Oncol* 1990; **26**(Suppl): S19–23.

46. de Wet M, Falkson G, Rapoport BL, Repeated use of granisetron in patients receiving cytostatic agents. *Cancer* 1993; **71:** 4043–9.

47. The Italian Group for Antiemetic Research, Persistence of efficacy of three antiemetic regimens and prognostic factors in patients undergoing moderately emetogenic chemotherapy. *J Clin Oncol* 1995; **13:** 2417–26.

48. Dogliotti L, Antonacci RA, Paze E et al, Three years' experience with tropisetron in the control of nausea and vomiting in cisplatin-treated patients. *Drugs* 1992; **43**(Suppl 3): S6–10.

49. Sorbe B, Tropisetron in the prevention of chemotherapy induced nausea and vomiting: the Nordic experience. *Ann Oncol* 1993; **4**(Suppl 3): S39–42.

50. de Bruijn KM, Tropisetron: a review of the clinical experience. *Drugs* 1992; **43**(Suppl 3): 11–22.

51. Bleiberg H, Van Belle S, Paridaens R et al, Compassionate use of a 5-HT$_3$ receptor antagonist, tropisetron, in patients refractory to standard antiemetic treatment. *Drugs* 1992; **43** (Suppl 3): 27–32.

52. Sorbe B, Andersson H, Schmidt M et al, Tropisetron (Navoban) in the prevention of chemotherapy-induced nausea and vomiting – the Nordic experience. *Support Care Cancer* 1994; **2:** 393–9.

53. Adams M, Soukop M, Barley V. Tropisetron alone or in combination with dexamethasone for the prevention and treatment of emesis induced by non-cisplatin chemotherapy: a randomized trial. *Anticancer Drugs* 1995; **6:** 514–21.

54. Schmidt M, Sorbe B, Hogberg T et al, Efficacy and tolerability of tropisetron and dexamethasone in the control of nausea and vomiting induced by cisplatin. *Ann Oncol* 1993; **4**(Suppl 3): 31–4.

55. Van Belle SJ, Cocquyt VF, Bleiberg H et al, Optimal combination therapy with Navoban (tropisetron) in patients with incomplete control of chemotherapy-induced nausea and vomiting. The Belgian Navoban Group. *Anticancer Drugs* 1995; **6**(Suppl 1): 22–30.

56. Chang TC, Hsieh F, Lai-CH et al, Comparison of the efficacy of tropisetron versus a metoclopramide cocktail based on the intensity of cisplatin-induced emesis. *Cancer Chemother Pharmacol* 1996; **37:** 279–85.

57. Andrews PLR, Bhandari P, Davey PT et al, Are all 5-HT$_3$ receptor antagonists the same? *Eur J Cancer Clin Oncol* 1992; **28A**(Suppl 1): S2–6.

58. Mantovani G, Maccio A, Bianchi A et al, Comparison of granisetron, ondansetron, and tropisetron in the prophylaxis of acute nausea and vomiting induced by cisplatin for the treatment of head and neck cancer: a randomised controlled trial. *Cancer* 1996; **77:** 941–8.

59. Kamanabrou D, on behalf of the Granisetron Study Group. Intravenous granisetron – establishing the optimal dose. *Eur J Cancer Clin Oncol* 1992; **28A**(Suppl 1): S6–11.

60. deWit R, Schmitz PIM, Verveij J et al, Analysis of cumulative probabilities shows that the efficacy of 5-HT$_3$ antagonist prophylaxis is not maintained. *J Clin Oncol* 1996; **14:** 644–51.

10

Anticipatory nausea and vomiting: models, mechanisms and management

Gary R Morrow, Joseph A Roscoe

CONTENTS • Introduction • Prevalence of anticipatory nausea and vomiting • Aetiology of anticipatory nausea and vomiting • Treatment of ANV • Summary

INTRODUCTION

Patients have reported nausea and vomiting following the administration of chemotherapy ever since drugs were first used to treat cancer. Fortunately, since that time, pharmacological control of chemotherapy-induced nausea and emesis has improved. However, even now, cancer patients may develop as much apprehension and dread about treatment and the side-effects of treatment as they do about their disease. If not adequately controlled, these side-effects can lead to further complications such as anorexia and metabolite imbalance, along with contributing to a general deterioration of the cancer patient's psychological and physical condition. Many cancer patients treated with chemotherapy request dosage reductions or even stop potentially curative treatment prematurely owing to inadequately controlled nausea and vomiting.[1-4] The impact of inadequately controlled nausea/vomiting on patient quality of life is also substantial.

Investigators also recognized that nausea and vomiting could arise in anticipation of a chemotherapy treatment. Approximately 15 years ago, we noted that some patients reported nausea and emesis prior to a second or subsequent course of chemotherapy.[5,6] We have labelled this phenomenon anticipatory nausea and vomiting (ANV). Many patients have not reported ANV spontaneously, because they believe it to be clearly psychological in origin. As one of our early patients explained, 'I must have lost my mind; now I become sick even thinking about the treatment. Please don't tell my doctor.'

ANV, which develops in approximately 30% of patients by the fourth treatment cycle, appears to link psychological, neurological and physiological systems.[2] Once they develop, ANV cannot be controlled by pharmacological means, including the new 5-HT$_3$ receptor antagonists. Fortunately, behavioural interventions have been effective in mitigating these side-effects. This chapter will examine these interventions as well as the prevalence and aetiology of ANV.

PREVALENCE OF ANTICIPATORY NAUSEA AND VOMITING

The prevalence of anticipatory nausea and vomiting in adult and paediatric cancer chemotherapy patients has been reported in a

Table 10.1 Prevalence of anticipatory side-effects in cancer chemotherapy patients

Authors	Number studied	Anticipatory nausea	Anticipatory vomiting[a]
Alba et al[30]	175	26%	12%
Andrykowski and Redd[46]	78	33%	—
Andrykowski et al[20]	71	37%	—
Andrykowski and Redd[46]	77	57%	—
Cella et al[8]	60	63%	—
Challis and Stam[52]	70	30%	14%
Chin et al[43]	40	40%	22%
Cohen[31]	149	42%	27%
Dobkin and Morrow[16]	125	32%	12%
Dolgin et al[39]	80	29%	20%
Fdez-Arguelles et al[88]	72	31%	—
Fetting et al[32]	123	31%	17%
Hursti et al[89]	39	67%	0%
Ingle et al[33]	60	25%	—
Kvale et al[53]	31	39%	—
Love et al[34]	126	38%	—
Morrow and Dobkin[13]	736	26%	8%
Morrow[14]	1985	33%	8%
Nesse et al[22]	18	44%	—
Nerenz et al[42]	61	24%	—
Nicholas[7]	71	18%	—
Nicholas[90]	50	42%	—
Olafsdottir et al[91]	50	40%	14%
Palmer et al[92]	24	22%	9%
Razavi et al[23]	47	26%	2%
Schultz[45]	68	31%	—
Scogna and Smalley[93]	41	37%	—
Stefanek et al[38]	121	33%	18%
Stockhorst et al[94]	55	18%	0%
van Komen and Redd[35]	100	33%	11%
Watson et al[36]	95	23%	4%
Weddington et al[41]	17	53%	12%
Weddington et al[40]	50	38%	—
Wilcox et al[15]	52	33%	33%
Wilson et al[37]	66	20%	8%
TOTAL	4370	29%	11%
Median		35%	13%
Range	17–1985	18–63%	0–27%

[a] — indicates that the factor was not investigated independently.

number of studies (summarized in Table 10.1). On the lower end of estimates, 18% of 71 patients examined by Nicholas[7] reported anticipatory side-effects, while Cella et al[8] reported that over half of 60 patients previously treated for Hodgkin's disease developed ANV.

Several factors have been proposed to account for variation in prevalence rates.[2,6,9–12] The following are among the most commonly expressed explanations for differences in prevalence rates of anticipatory nausea.

- Nausea and vomiting side-effects can occur *during* chemotherapy with some drugs. While some investigators have considered this an anticipatory phenomenon and recorded it as such, it is more likely a physiological response.
- Some researchers have studied anticipatory nausea and vomiting symptoms independently of each other, whereas other researchers have combined them and viewed the symptoms as one phenomenon.
- Prevalence rates may be influenced by the type of chemotherapeutic drugs administered to cancer patients, since post-treatment side-effects vary across different treatment regimens.
- The time frame in which ANV symptoms were studied has differed across studies. For example, Morrow et al[13,14] assessed patients prior to their fourth chemotherapy cycle, whereas Wilcox et al[15] did so prior to the tenth chemotherapy cycle.
- A portion of the variation in prevalence rates may be due to different measurement methodology. A variety of self-reporting measures have been used to assess ANV across studies.[11] Some studies involved interviewing patients by asking retrospective questions,[16] whereas others used patient-completed logs during and following treatment.[17]
- Because ANV is not consistent within individuals across chemotherapy trials, prevalence rates will also vary, depending on whether the data is interpreted cross-sectionally or longitudinally. For example, data from a series of 1985 consecutive

patients of ours[14] taken before each of his or her first four chemotherapy treatments showed that 33% experienced ANV at least once prior to a treatment, but only half of this group actually experienced these symptoms at the fourth treatment.

Perhaps the best way to avoid some of the methodological and definitional issues associated with this field of research is to look primarily at the University of Rochester Cancer Center study. We collected data on 2877 patients assessed with the same scale (Morrow Assessment of Nausea and Emesis[18]), at a standard time (prior to the fourth chemotherapy cycle). It appears that the cross-sectional prevalence rate is around 20%, with approximately one third of all patients experiencing ANV at least once by the fourth treatment.

AETIOLOGY OF ANTICIPATORY NAUSEA AND VOMITING

Several potential correlates of anticipatory nausea and vomiting have been studied. This section begins with a detailed examination of how available data support a model of ANV development based on learning principles. The relationship between anxiety and ANV will then be discussed. Studies exploring associations among demographic, clinical and psychological variables of ANV are then presented and reviewed.

Conditioning mechanism of ANV

Several characteristics of ANV suggested that its mechanisms might fit within a learning model. Subsequent studies by our group and several others in the United States and Europe confirmed that the development of ANV involves elements of classical conditioning.[2,19–21]

Classical conditioning is also known as *Pavlovian conditioning* after the Russian scientist who was able to induce dogs to salivate at the sound of a bell that had been repeatedly paired with the ingestion of food. In this paradigm, an

The first few chemotherapy treatments

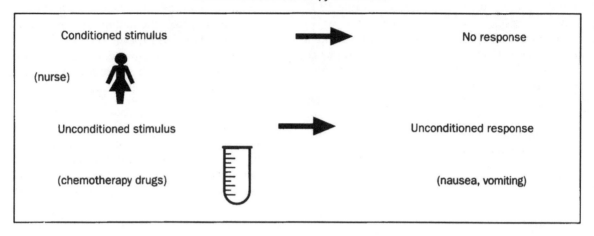

After several chemotherapy treatments

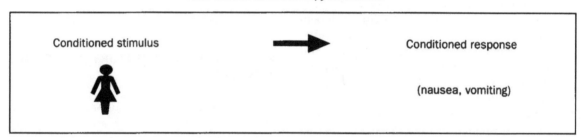

Figure 10.1 Learning model of ANV (adapted from Morrow[95], with permission).

unconditioned response (such as salivation) that typically results from an unconditioned stimulus (the presentation of food) can be elicited by a conditioned stimulus (such as the ringing of a bell) that is present at the same time as the unconditioned stimulus.

How might this paradigm apply to chemotherapy? Figure 10.1 shows how a learning model might account for the development of anticipatory side-effects. Potential conditioned stimuli (such as the sight of the nurse, or other sights, sounds or smells of the clinic) are present while the chemotherapeutic agents (unconditioned stimulus) that produce the unconditioned response (nausea and emesis) are administered. Over several trials (chemotherapy cycles), the conditioned response stimuli (sights, sounds and even thoughts of the clinic) can be learned; they then produce what is now the conditioned response of ANV. No data convincingly contradict the conclusion that ANV is learned. Among the supporting lines of evidence are the following.

- Anticipatory side-effects rarely develop unless post-treatment side-effects have

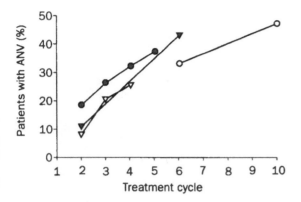

Figure 10.2 Incidence of ANV (at least one occurrence): O, Andrykowski et al[20], n = 71; ●, Morrow[14], n = 1119; Δ, Razavi et al[23], n = 47; ▲, Love et al[3], n = 147. Adapted from Morrow[95], wtih permission.

occurred. Very few patients in our series of over 4000 developed anticipatory nausea without having experienced post-treatment nausea at least once.

- Conditioning is more successful with a greater number of learning trials. The frequency of ANV increases almost linearly with the number of chemotherapy cycles given. We and others have found that by the fourth treatment cycle, approximately 30% of patients experience ANV. Figure 10.2 summarizes four studies[3,14,20,23] that report the incidence of ANV measured at least twice during the course of chemotherapy. The studies differ in oncological diagnoses, chemotherapeutic agents, antiemetic agents and number of patients. Nonetheless, despite these differences, all the studies show an increase in the incidence of ANV with repeated chemotherapy cycles. The trend in all four studies appears to be linear and increasing. Each of the studies reports that by the fourth treatment cycle, approximately 20–35% of patients experience anticipatory side-effects.

- The development of ANV is significantly correlated with the occurrence of post-treatment side-effects. The more severe the post-treatment nausea and emesis produced, the more frequent the development of ANV.[14]

Anxiety as contributor and consequence

Several investigators have speculated that anxiety may be involved in the development of anticipatory side-effects. Houts et al[24] have proposed four potential ways in which anxiety might relate to anticipatory side effects:

1. anticipatory nausea causes pretreatment anxiety;
2. pretreatment anxiety causes anticipatory nausea;
3. anticipatory nausea and pretreatment anxiety are both caused by post-treatment nausea;
4. pretreatment anxiety facilitates the conditioning process of anticipatory side-effects.

These are some data that lend partial support to each of the four potential explanations.

However, in order to examine separately each of the potentially competing hypotheses, experiments would have to be designed that would isolate a particular portion of the chemotherapy treatment. This, unfortunately, is not possible in a clinical setting, since chemotherapy is given in repeated cycles. Andrykowski et al[20] and Andrykowski[25] provided evidence that elevated levels of state anxiety may precede the initial occurrence of anticipatory symptoms. These authors caution, however, that the relationship between anxiety and anticipatory side-effects may not be a strictly causal one. Their data also support a view that anxiety may be heightened following a particular chemotherapy treatment and that, in turn, the increased anxiety may increase post-treatment nausea/vomiting, which in turn may increase susceptibility to conditioning on the next chemotherapy cycle. This circular process may facilitate and promote a conditioning process rather than serve as a direct cause itself. Thus the explanation that anxiety is involved in some form in the conditioning of side-effects is the most plausible of the four. It is likely that some degree of anxiety facilitates the conditioning process by alerting or sensitizing the patient in much the same way that somebody who is mildly anxious may be quite prone to suddenly notice and become concerned over a physical sensation such as irregular heartbeats that had probably been present for a period of time.

A further complication to fully understanding the relationship between anxiety and ANV is that chemotherapy-related nausea and vomiting can produce anxiety,[26] and anxiety can itself become a conditioned response.[27,28] This may lead to a situation in which both ANV and anticipated anxiety develop as a consequence of repeated nausea-producing chemotherapy treatments,[2,6,29] with each possibly contributing to the magnitude of the other.

Table 10.2 Demographic variables associated with anticipatory nausea and vomiting

Authors	n	Gender	Age	Race
Alba et al[30]	175	×	Younger	—
Andrykowski et al[20]	71	—	×	—
Challis and Stam[52]	70	×	×	—
Cohen[31]	149	×	Younger	—
Dolgin et al[39]	80	×	×	×
Fetting et al[32]	123	Female	Younger	×
Ingle et al[33]	60	×	Younger	×
Love et al[34]	126	—	Younger	×
Morrow[6]	225	×	Younger	×
Morrow[14]	1985	Female	Younger (nausea)	×
			× (vomiting)	
Nesse et al[22]	18	×	×	—
Schultz[45]	68	×	×	—
Stefanek et al[38]	121	Female	×	—
van Komen and Redd[35]	100	×	Younger	—
Watson et al[36]	95	×	Younger	—
Weddington et al[41]	17	×	×	—
Weddington et al[40]	50	×	×	×
Wilson et al[37]	66	Female	Younger	×
Association found:	—	4/16	10/18	0/8

Key: × indicates that the factor was investigated and was not found to correlate with ANV.
— indicates that the factor was not investigated.

Univariate correlates of anticipatory nausea and vomiting

A number of characteristics have been examined for their possible role in how anticipatory side-effects develop. They fit loosely in categories of demographic, clinical, psychological and physiological characteristics.

Demographic variables

Table 10.2 summarizes the types of demographic variables examined for a correlation with anticipatory side-effects. Every investigator who has included[6,14,30-37] has found an association between age (that is, being younger than 50 years old) and experiencing ANV. Only four of the sixteen studies investigating gender[14,32,37,38] found it to be associated with ANV symptomatology. None of seven studies including data on ethnicity.[6,32-34,37,39,40] have reported a relationship between race and anticipatory side-effects. Education level and socioeconomic and marital status do not appear to be critical factors for the development of ANV symptoms.[6,32,41] Overall, with the exception of age and gender, there appears to be little association between patient demographic characteristics and the development of anticipatory side-effects. The effect of age has been found to be independent of other factors such as amount and type of chemotherapeutic drug given. Younger patients have also been found to experience greater nausea/vomiting as a result of anaesthesia. Whether or not some common mechanism is responsible for both findings is a topic for further research.

Clinical variables

Table 10.3 summarizes results of clinical variables examined for their association to ANV. A significant positive correlation between the number of treatments received and development of ANV was found in ten of the fifteen studies looking at this variable. Seven of eight studies that examined a potential relationship between how much nausea and vomiting a chemotherapy drug typically caused after treatment (its emetic potential) and ANV reported a significant relationship. It was, however, the largest of these studies[14] with 1985 patients that found a non-significant relationship. Virtually all researchers reported a significant relationship between post-chemotherapy nausea and vomiting respectively and ANV symptoms. Other clinical variables found to be associated with increased ANV in at least one study include being treated in the presence of other patients,[35] the presence of strong taste sensations during chemotherapy,[6,42] and greater post-treatment dizziness or light-headedness, and delayed onset of PCNV.[6,43]

Psychological variables

Consistent with a view that emotions and cognitions may contribute to the development of ANV,[35,44,45] anxiety, depression, hostility and coping styles in cancer chemotherapy patients have been studied.

As shown in Table 10.4, all fourteen of the investigations that examined state anxiety levels found that they were significantly elevated in patients with ANV compared with patients without ANV. The cause-and-effect relationship of these two variables, if any, is not clear. Two out of three investigations found trait anxiety related to ANV. Love et al,[34] using a prospective research design, studied 126 cancer patients being treated with chemotherapy for breast cancer ($n = 94$) and malignant lymphoma ($n = 32$). Patients were interviewed repeatedly during their initial six months of chemotherapy. 38% of the patients developed ANV, with patients who experienced anxiety during injections significantly more likely to develop anticipatory nausea than non-anxious patients. Interestingly, the association between anxiety and anticipatory nausea was not statistically significant during the first two chemotherapy cycles, but became significant by the sixth cycle. Andrykowski and Redd[46] also reported that the relationship between anxiety and ANV should be qualified according to the treatment time frame. To determine if there were different patterns of infusion-related state anxiety and post-treatment nausea prior to AN onset, AN patients were divided into early (i.e. prior to chemotherapy cycle number 7) and late (i.e. following chemotherapy cycle number 7) onset groups. According to this distinction,

Table 10.3 Clinical variables associated with anticipatory nausea and vomiting

Authors	n	Number of Rx	Emetic potential	Post-Rx nausea		Post-Rx vomiting	
				S	D	S	D
Alba et al[30]	175	*	*	*	*	*	×
Andrykowski et al[20]	71	a	—	*	—	*	—
Andrykowski and Redd[46]	77	*	—	*	—	—	—
Challis and Stam[52]	70	*	*	*	*	*	*
Chin et al[43]	40	—	—	*	×	*	×
Cohen[31]	149	×	—	—	—	—	b*
Dobkin and Morrow[16]	125	—	—	—	b*	—	b*
Dolgin et al[39]	80	×	*	*	—	*	×
Fetting et al[32]	123	—	—	—	*	—	*
Ingle et al[33]	58	×	—	*	—	—	—
Morrow[6]	225	—	*	*	*	*	*
Morrow[58]	176	—	—	*	—	*	—
Morrow[14]	1985	*	×	*	*	*	×
Nerenz et al[42]	61	—	—	—	×	—	×
Nesse et al[22]	18	*	—	*	*	*	*
Nicholas[90]	71	*	—	—	*	—	*
Stefanek et al[38]	121	×	—	×	*	×	×
Stockhorst et al[94]	55		*	—	b*	—	b*
van Komen and Redd[35]	100	*	—	*	—	*	—
Watson et al[36]	95	×	*	—	—	—	—
Weddington et al[41]	17	*	—	—	—	—	—
Weddington et al[40]	50	*	—	—	b×	—	b×
Wilcox et al[15]	52	—	*	*	—	*	—
Associations found:		10/15 (67%)	7/8 (87%)	13/14 (93%)	10/13 (77%)	11/12 (92%)	8/15 (53%)

Key: × indicates that the factor was studied and was not found to correlate with ANV.
— indicates that the factor was not studied.
* indicates that the factor was found to correlate significantly with ANV.
Rx = chemotherapy regimen; S = severity; D = duration.
a indicates length of infusion.
b indicates frequency (rather than duration).

anxiety appeared to contribute to the development of AN only for patients who were in the late-onset group. A clear, direct relationship between anxiety and ANV development has not been found.

Depression and hostility were found to be significantly elevated in ANV patients in three out of six studies and in two out of four respectively. Coping styles were not found to be consistently different in ANV patients. Altmaier et

Table 10.4 Psychological variables associated with anticipatory nausea and vomiting

Authors	n	Anxiety	Depression	Hostility	Coping
Ahles et al[44]	9	* (state)	—	—	—
Altmaier et al[47]	9	* (state)	—	×	O
Andrykowski et al[20]	71	* (state)	—	—	—
Andrykowski and Redd[46]	77	++ (state)	—	—	—
Chin et al[43]	40	* (state)	—	—	—
Challis and Stam[52]	70	* (state)	×	—	—
Cohen[31]	31	* (state)	*	—	—
		× (trait)			
Houts et al[24]	90	* (state)	—	—	—
Ingle et al[33]	58	* (state)	×	*	*
Morrow[14]	1985	* (state)	*	*	—
		* (trait)			
Nerenz et al[42]	18	* (state)	—	—	**
Razavi et al[23]	47	* (state)	—	—	—
Shultz[45]	68	* (state/trait)	—	—	—
van Komen and Redd[35]	100	* (trait)	*	—	—
Watson et al[36]	95	* (state)	×	—	—
Wilson et al[37]	66	+	+	×	—
Associations found:	2234	14/14 (state)	3/6	2/4	1/3
		2/3 (trait)			

Key: × indicates that there was no difference between ANV and non-ANV patients.
    — indicates that the factor was not investigated.
    * indicates that the measure was significantly elevated in ANV patients.
    O indicates that the measure was depressed in ANV patients.
    ** indicates that 'more attempts to cope' were made.
    + indicates that conflicting results were found between measures.
    ++ indicates that anxiety was significantly elevated only in late onset of ANV patients.

al[47] reported that patients with ANV exhibited a coping style that was 'inhibitive rather than facilitative in nature'. In contrast, Ingle et al,[33] found a greater number of 'attempts to cope' with chemotherapy and a higher level of hostility in patients with ANV compared with patients without ANV. Coping styles are, however, difficult hypothetical constructs to operationalize; it is therefore possible that these divergent findings reflect measurement variance rather than actual differences in responses.

Physiological variables

The neural pathway between the vomiting centre (an area in the dorsolateral reticular formation of the medulla) and the vestibular system has been implicated in motion-induced nausea and vomiting as well as vomiting from poisons given to animals.[48] Thus, a possible relationship between susceptibility to motion sickness and chemotherapy nausea/vomiting has been studied. Using a case control methodology, we showed that cancer patients who self-report a susceptibility to motion sickness (compared with patients without susceptibility) had (a) significantly more side-effects from chemotherapy drugs;[49] (b) significantly more post-treatment nausea and vomiting;[50] and (c) significantly more anticipatory nausea and vomiting.[51] Later studies[30,36,52] did not find this relationship.

It is known that autonomic, particularly sympathetic, reactivity correlates with the development of conditioned responses. Kvale[53,54] has demonstrated a connection between autonomic reactivity and subsequent development of ANV. Patients in both studies that experienced ANV showed significantly increased sympathetic reactivity as compared with patients who did not experience ANV. Similarly, Challis and Stam[52] found that patients who experienced ANV showed significantly higher levels of awareness concerning their autonomic activity as compared with patients who did not experience ANV. Another group of investigators found increased parasympathetic autonomic conditionability, measured by the development of conditioned heart-rate deceleration, in patients with a history of conditioned nausea in response to chemotherapy; patients without conditioned nausea did not develop the conditioned heart-rate deceleration.[55] These findings are suggestive of a meditational role for autonomic reactivity in ANV development.

Multivariate correlates of anticipatory side-effects

Several studies have built on some of the earlier promising univariate findings, and have used multivariate procedures to examine potential joint or interactive relationships among variables that might be associated with the development of anticipatory side-effects.

Morrow[6] reported results from a two-group discriminate analysis on 225 cancer patients. Overall, an 80% accurate classification was achieved, with 42% of patients experiencing ANV and 91% of patients not experiencing ANV correctly classified based on a combination of age, severity and duration of post-

chemotherapy nausea and vomiting. Cohen[31] reported that the frequency of vomiting during/after chemotherapy sessions and age (younger than 50 years old) accounted for 32% of the variance in the occurrence of anticipatory nausea.

Andrykowski, Redd, and Hatfield[20] studied 26 patients who displayed anticipatory side-effects and 45 who did not. While seven variables entered into a hierarchical regression analysis accounted for about half (47%) of the variance in group membership, post-treatment nausea alone accounted for about a quarter (24%). State anxiety and length of time it took to give the chemotherapeutic drug were the only two other variables giving a significant increment in explained variance.

Ingle et al[33] used a three-group ('conditioned, may be conditioned, and not conditioned') discriminant analysis involving seven variables from 58 adult cancer patients in order to determine the best set of 'predictors' for patients with ANV. These authors reported an overall assignment rate (by regression) of 71% to the three groups based on age (younger than 50 years old), post-chemotherapy nausea and vomiting, anxiety, and 'coping effort'.

Van Komen and Redd[35] administered the Millon Behavioral Health Inventory[56] and the Spielberger State-Trait Anxiety Inventory[57] to 59 cancer patients in order to examine potential personality factors hypothesized to be associated with ANV symptomatology. The most important discriminator variables found were social alienation, future despair (depression) and gastrointestinal susceptibility. Trait anxiety was also shown to be higher in patients with ANV compared with patients without ANV. Interestingly, patients who received chemotherapy in a group setting were more likely to experience ANV than patients who were treated on an individual basis.

A study was made of 176 consecutive ambulatory patients with histologically confirmed cancer who were being treated at three geographically separate hospitals at the University of Rochester Cancer Center; the study was carried out at the time of their fourth chemotherapy treatment.[58] Patients found to experience anticipatory nausea and vomiting were significantly more likely to have four or more of the following characteristics compared with patients who did not report anticipatory side-effects (Table 10.5):

1. age (less than 50 years);
2. the experience of nausea and/or vomiting after their last chemotherapy treatment;
3. describing nausea after the last treatment as 'moderate, severe, or intolerable';
4. describing vomiting after the last treatment as 'moderate, severe, or intolerable';
5. reporting the side-effect 'warm or hot all over' after their last treatment;
6. susceptibility to motion sickness;
7. experiencing 'sweating after their last treatment';
8. experiencing 'generalized weakness after their last chemotherapy treatment'.

These results were replicated in a prospective study.[19] Following their first chemotherapy treatment, 530 consecutive cancer patients were asked the previously reported eight questions. The outcome measure was whether or not they had developed anticipatory nausea/vomiting by the time of their fourth chemotherapy treatment. Those patients who had four or more of the eight characteristics were predicted to develop anticipatory side-effects. Those with three or fewer were predicted not to. While a significant association was found between these characteristics and subsequent development of anticipatory side-effects for 345 patients entered into the study and followed through their fourth chemotherapy treatment, the prediction was much more accurate in identifying patients who did not develop subsequent ANV than those who did.

These characteristics may help to screen patients following their first chemotherapy treatment to determine their potential to develop anticipatory side-effects. Enhanced efforts at emetic control along with early intervention with behavioural techniques may be warranted for patients considered to be particularly at risk.[6,59–62]

Table 10.5 Patient characteristics associated with the development of anticipatory nausea and vomiting[63]

- Age less than 50
- Nausea/vomiting after last chemotherapy session
- Post-treatment nausea described as 'moderate, severe or intolerable'
- Post-treatment vomiting described as 'moderate, severe or intolerable'
- Feeling warm or hot all over after last chemotherapy session
- Susceptibility to motion sickness
- Sweating after last chemotherapy session
- Generalized weakness after last chemotherapy session

Patients with fewer than three of the above eight characteristics have been found unlikely to develop ANV.[51,58,95]

TREATMENT OF ANV

Antiemetics do not control ANV once it has developed, and indeed have been found by some investigators to paradoxically increase symptoms,[21,58,63–65] perhaps by acting as conditioned stimuli themselves.[65] Once developed, ANV does not appear to improve spontaneously.[64,65]

Pharmacological treatment

A preliminary study by Razavi et al[23] does suggest, however, that a potentially useful pharmacological preventive intervention may be low-dose alprazolam (0.5–2 mg) taken daily. This double-blind, placebo-controlled study of 57 women with breast cancer in a psychological support programme that included progressive muscle relaxation training (discussed below) found a significantly higher occurrence of anticipatory nausea (18% vs 0%) in the placebo arm as compared with the alprazolam arm of the study. This significant difference between groups was found prior to the third treatment, but not at later treatments.

The mechanisms by which anticipatory side-effects develop suggest a further therapeutic approach: the degree to which *post-treatment* side-effects can be controlled is the degree to which *anticipatory* side-effects will fail to develop. Simply stated, without an unconditioned response (post-treatment nausea and vomiting), the conditioned response (anticipatory nausea and vomiting) will not develop. Some evidence indicates that this approach may succeed for anticipatory vomiting, but not for anticipatory nausea.

Behavioural treatment

As a learned phenomenon, ANV is treatable by means of behavioural approaches based on learning principles. Research on the behavioural treatment of conditioned adverse effects of chemotherapy has centred on four principal approaches: progressive muscle relaxation training, systematic desensitization, hypnosis and cognitive distraction.

Progressive muscle relaxation training

Progressive muscle relaxation training (PMRT) enables individuals to achieve a state of muscle relaxation in anticipation of, or in response to, a variety of specific situations that may produce tension or anxiety, such as receipt of chemotherapy. A series of randomized clinical trials has demonstrated the efficacy of relaxation-based behavioural treatments.[61,64] The technique involves learning to relax by actively tensing and then relaxing specific muscle groups in a progressive manner. It is often combined with guided imagery in which the individual visualizes pleasant, soothing images or scenes while relaxed. PMRT is generally taught to individual patients by a trained therapist, following which the subject is requested to practise the technique at home using either an audiotape made during the training session or a set of written instructions.

The ability of patients to relax themselves after one or at most a few therapist-directed sessions can enhance the cost-effectiveness of the procedure by limiting therapist involvement, and also facilitate its continued effectiveness over time.[59,66-69] In one randomized study, use of an audiotape alone was not effective in teaching patients with anticipatory nausea and vomiting to relax prior to being exposed to a systematic desensitization procedure.[11]

PMRT appears to exert its greatest effects against adverse events that develop after administration of chemotherapy, including post-chemotherapy nausea and vomiting, anxiety and physiological (autonomic) arousal; it has been less effective against anticipatory symptoms.[59,68-71] PMRT plus guided imagery also results in less nausea during chemotherapy, can prevent the development of conditioned side-effects, and can also decrease the frequency and severity of conditioned side-effects that have already developed.[70,72] It may act to prevent the development of ANV by decreasing anticipatory anxiety, thought to be a factor in the production of conditioned side-effects, especially in patients using a blunting coping style.[73]

Systematic desensitization

The technique of systematic desensitization (SD), commonly used to treat learning-based difficulties such as fears and phobias, is particularly effective for ANV. One way in which phobias may develop is by means of the classical conditioning mechanism described previously. In many respects, anticipatory side-effects display characteristics of phobic behaviours, although the match is far from perfect. Nonetheless, a learning-based treatment approach definitely reduces ANV.

SD involves the counterconditioning of a response incompatible with those stimuli that typically elicit a maladaptive reaction. In terms of ANV, the theory predicts that these symptoms would be reduced if patients could be taught an incompatible response (such as muscle relaxation), rather than the conditioned response of nausea and vomiting, in response to the conditioned stimuli (the clinic, the nurse).

Patients are taught an active behavioural intervention called *Jacobsonian progressive muscle relaxation*. They then construct a hierarchy of stimuli that appear to elicit the ANV. This hierarchy typically involves moving progressively closer to the location where the chemotherapy is administered. For example, patients often begin to experience ANV a day or two prior to chemotherapy as they think about it. The intensity of ANV often increases on the morning of the chemotherapy visit and increases again as the patient travels to the clinic. Further increases occur as patients walk towards the hospital, approach the door of the treatment centre, enter the room where treatment is administered, and see the drug-administration apparatus. SD operates by encouraging patients to imagine going through this sequence while they are deeply relaxed. Rather than learning feelings of nausea as a response to the chemotherapy experience, relaxation is counter-conditioned as a response. We and others have found that this treatment is successful in over half the patients to whom it is administered.[61,71,74-76]

Additional clinical trials have shown that these behavioural techniques can be taught to oncologists and oncology nurses. We have reported teaching this treatment approach to oncologists, nurses and other behavioural psychologists.[64] The results of this study showed that medical oncologists and nurses were as effective in using this treatment as were experienced behavioural psychologists. Therefore, with proper instruction, this treatment approach can be learned and used successfully by clinic personnel. It does, however, require time and effort that may not be available in all treatment situations.

Hypnosis
Hypnosis, also known as suggestive therapy and trance therapy, is a self-control technique in which patients learn to invoke a physiological state incompatible with nausea and vomiting.[60] In the method usually used to produce the altered state of consciousness, induction of total body relaxation is followed by presentation of restful psychic imagery. Suggestions for

specific treatment objectives, such as increasing food intake, can then be made,[77,78] and patients can undergo chemotherapy while hypnotized.[60] Furthermore, while in the trance, subjects can be taken through a series of events (for example, those associated with anticipatory nausea and vomiting), a technique similar to SD.[60]

Thus hypnosis involves a passive type of muscle relaxation and possibly also distraction.[60,77-79] Although the initial sessions are usually therapist-directed, some patients can learn to induce the state themselves, and thus no therapist need be present during chemotherapy.[77] Although hypnosis was the first psychological technique used to control ANV, few controlled studies have been done. It has been most often used with children and adolescents.[21,77,78,80] This may be also because children often experience undesirable side-effects from antiemetic drugs, and so some antiemetics are not used with children.[78] Children are also more readily hypnotized than adults.[81]

In a controlled experiment, Cotanch and colleagues[78] randomly assigned 12 young people aged 10–18 years to receive either a relaxation/self-hypnosis intervention or standard treatment. The intervention significantly reduced the frequency, severity and duration of chemotherapy-related emesis, and the intensity and duration of nausea. Oral intake was also significantly enhanced, and the patients reported feeling less bothered by the chemotherapy experience.

Zeltzer, LeBaron and Zeltzer[80] compared hypnotherapy with supportive counselling, and suggested that non-specific therapy effects such as demand characteristics and/or attention may contribute to treatment changes found. In their study, 19 children, aged 6–17 years, were randomly assigned to a hypnotherapy or a supportive counselling group. Children in both groups reported reductions in nausea and vomiting, and rated chemotherapy as 'less noxious' following intervention. There were, however, no statistically or clinically significant differences in outcome found between the two approaches, whereas a later study by Zeltzer et al[82] with 54 paediatric cancer patients showed a significant reduction group as compared with those in either the non-hypnotic distraction/ relaxation group or the attention placebo (control) group.

Overall, it appears that studies using hypnosis for ANV control have shown that this intervention may be beneficial for children. Less evidence is available demonstrating its usefulness for adults. In order to establish the effectiveness of hypnotherapy for cancer chemotherapy patients, studies with larger sample sizes in which patients are randomly assigned to treatment or appropriate control groups are needed.

Hypnosis has certain advantages. There are no undesirable side-effects. Little training is needed to learn the induction techniques. No special equipment is needed. Hypnosis requires little physical effort on the patient's part. However, misconceptions about the procedure may lead some patients to refuse to try it;[21] cultural factors may play a role in patient acceptance of hypnosis.[83]

In summary, hypnosis can reduce anticipatory as well as post-chemotherapy nausea and vomiting, and improve negative affect and quality of life. However, alternative procedures may be just as effective.[21,80]

Cognitive distraction

It has been suggested that cognitive distraction (CD) is the common element responsible for the success of both relaxation training and hypnosis in decreasing conditioned nausea in adult patients receiving chemotherapy for cancer.[79,84] CD is presumed to act by focusing patients' attention away from nausea and vomiting or the stimuli associated with these phenomena.[84]

Redd and colleagues[84] investigated this hypothesis in two experiments in paediatric patients with documented ANV from cancer chemotherapy using commercially available video games to distract patients. In the first, 26 children were randomly assigned to the video game intervention or a control group, and in the second, 15 of the 26 children were studied using a multiple-baseline design in which the nausea was assessed with and without video game playing in the same group of children. In both experiments, patients had significant

reductions in conditioned nausea after video games. The changes in nausea could not be attributed to either antiemetic medication or physical relaxation (which did not take place).

In the first controlled study of CD in adults, 60 patients, stratified by level of anxiety, were randomly assigned to receive CD (video games), PMRT with guided imagery, or no intervention, and were followed through five consecutive chemotherapy sessions during which antiemetic medication was kept relatively constant. Patients receiving either intervention had significantly less nausea prior to chemotherapy than those in the control condition; there were no significant differences for the two treatment groups on nausea or other outcome measures. Anxiety level did not influence the effectiveness of either treatment modality.[85] These investigators and others[60,84] have concluded that CD is responsible for at least some of the effects of PMRT on reducing ANV by interfering with the development or expression of this conditioned side-effect.

CD may be especially attractive for paediatric patients, who sometimes have difficulty mastering relaxation and hypnosis.[84] Furthermore, it may be cost-effective, since it does not need to be administered by a trained therapist.[84,85] Video games in particular are inexpensive, effective distracters that can be individualized, require no training or professional assistance, and can result in sustained distraction over time.[79] However, the effects have been noted to decrease over successive chemotherapy sessions.[85]

SUMMARY

Since it is likely that multiple emetic mechanisms operate at different points in time to cause emesis following chemotherapy, and currently available pharmacological agents are unable to provide complete protection from either anticipatory or post-treatment nausea and emesis associated with this form of cancer treatment, a multidisciplinary approach has been advocated that includes the best possible pharmacological control of post-chemotherapy nausea and vomiting, providing adequate information to patients in order to modify their expectations, drugs as needed to decrease anxiety, and adjunctive behavioural treatment, ideally given prophylactically.[58,63,77,86,87] Furthermore, if ANV are caused by a behavioural process (i.e. a classical conditioning process),

behavioural methods of treatment may be particularly appropriate.[6,60,61,69] In addition, behavioural interventions that prevent the development, or decrease the severity, of post-treatment nausea and vomiting may prevent the occurrence of ANV.[61]

REFERENCES

1. Hoagland AC, Morrow GR, Bennett JM, Carnrike CL Jr, Oncologists' views of cancer patient noncompliance. *Am J Clin Oncol* 1983; **6**: 239–44.
2. Burish TG, Carey MP, Conditioned aversive responses in cancer chemotherapy patients: theoretical and developmental analysis. *J Consult Clin Psychol* 1986; **54**: 593–600.
3. Love RR, Leventhal H, Easterling DV, Nerenz DR, Side effects and emotional distress during cancer chemotherapy. *Cancer* 1989; **63**: 604–12.
4. Holland J, Psychological aspects of oncology. *Med Clin North Am* 1977; **61**: 737–48.
5. Morrow GR, Behavioral treatment of anticipatory nausea and vomiting during chemotherapy. *Proc Annu Meet Am Soc Clin Oncol* 1981; **22**: 396.
6. Morrow GR, Prevalence and correlates of anticipatory nausea and vomiting in chemotherapy patients. *J Natl Cancer Inst* 1982; **68**: 585–8.
7. Nicholas DR, Prevalence of anticipatory nausea and emesis in cancer chemotherapy patients. *J Behav Med* 1982; **5**: 461–3.
8. Cella DF, Pratt A, Holland JC, Long-term conditioned nausea and anxiety persisting in cured Hodgkin's patients after chemotherapy. *Proc Annu Meet Am Soc Clin Oncol* 1984; **3**: 73.
9. Andrykowski MA, Definitional issues in the study of anticipatory nausea in cancer chemotherapy. *J Behav Med* 1986; **9**: 33–41.
10. Duigon A, Anticipatory nausea and vomiting associated with cancer chemotherapy. *Oncol Nurs Forum* 1986; **13**: 35–40.
11. Morrow GR, The assessment of nausea and vomiting: Past problems, current issues, and suggestions for future research. *Cancer* 1984; **53**: 2267–78.
12. Nicholas DR, Hollandsworth JG, Assessment of anticipatory nausea and vomiting in cancer patients undergoing chemotherapy: theoretical and methodological considerations. *J Psychosoc Oncol* 1986; **4**: 61.
13. Morrow GR, Dobkin PL, Behavioral approaches for the management of adverse side effects of cancer treatment. *Psychiatr Med* 1987; **5**: 299–314.
14. Morrow GR, Current data on an ongoing series of chemotherapy patients. Submitted for publication.
15. Wilcox PM, Fetting JH, Nettesheim KM, Abeloff MD, Anticipatory vomiting in women receiving cyclophosphamide, methotrexate, and 5-FU (CMF) adjuvant chemotherapy for breast carcinoma. *Cancer Treat Rep* 1982; **66**: 1601–4.
16. Dobkin PL, Morrow GR, Long-term side effect in patients who have been treated successfully for cancer. *J Psychosoc Oncol* 1985; **3**: 23–51.
17. Burish TG, Carey MP, Conditioned responses to cancer chemotherapy: Etiology and treatment. In: *Impact of Psychoendocrine Systems in Cancer and Immunity* (Fox BHN, ed.). Toronto: CJ Hogrefe, 1984.
18. Morrow GR, A patient report measure for the quantification of chemotherapy induced nausea and emesis: psychometric properties of the Morrow assessment of nausea and emesis (MANE). *Br J Cancer Suppl* 1992; **19**: S72–4.
19. Morrow GR, Lindke J, Black PM, Predicting development of anticipatory nausea in cancer patients: prospective examination of eight clinical characteristics. *J Pain Symptom Manage* 1991; **6**: 215–23.
20. Andrykowski MA, Redd WH, Hatfield AK, Development of anticipatory nausea: a prospective analysis. *J Consult Clin Psychol* 1985; **53**: 447–54.
21. Carey MP, Burish TG, Etiology and treatment of the psychological side effects associated with cancer chemotherapy: a critical review and discussion. *Psychol Bull* 1988; **104**: 307–25.
22. Nesse RN, Carli T, Curtis GC, Kleinman PD, Pretreatment nausea in cancer chemotherapy: a conditioned response. *Psychosom Med* 1980; **42**: 33–6.

23. Razavi D, Delvaux N, Farvacques C et al, Prevention of adjustment disorders and anticipatory nausea secondary to adjuvant chemotherapy: a double-blind, placebo-controlled study assessing the usefulness of alprazolam. *J Clin Oncol* 1993; **11**: 1384–90.

24. Houts P, Morrow GR, Lipton A et al, The role of pretreatment anxiety in anticipatory nausea among cancer patients receiving chemotherapy. Unpublished manuscript, University of Pennsylvania, 1984.

25. Andrykowski MA, The role of anxiety in the development of anticipatory nausea in cancer chemotherapy: a review and synthesis. *Psychosom Med* 1990; **52**: 458–75.

26. Jacobsen PB, Bovbjerg DH, Redd WH, Anticipatory anxiety in women receiving chemotherapy for breast cancer. *Health Psychol* 1993; **12**: 469–75.

27. Hall JF, The conditional emotional response as a model of Pavlovian conditioning. *Pavlovian J Biol Sci* 1986; **21**: 1–11.

28. Rachman S, Neo-conditioning and the classical theory of fear acquisition. *Clin Psychol Rev* 1991; **11**: 155–73.

29. Sabbioni ME, Bovbjerg DH, Jacobsen PB et al, Treatment related psychological distress during adjuvant chemotherapy as a conditioned response. *Ann Oncol* 1992; **3**: 393–8.

30. Alba E, Bastus R, de Andres L et al, Anticipatory nausea and vomiting: prevalence and predictors in chemotherapy patients. *Oncology (Huntingt)* 1989; **46**: 26–30.

31. Cohen RE, Distress associated with anti-neoplastic chemotherapy: prediction, assessment, and treatment. State University of New York, Albany, 1982 (doctoral dissertation).

32. Fetting JH, Wilcox PM, Iwata BA et al, Anticipatory nausea and vomiting in an ambulatory medical oncology population. *Cancer Treat Rep* 1983; **67**: 1093–8.

33. Ingle RJ, Burish TG, Wallston KA, Conditionability of cancer chemotherapy patients. *Oncol Nurs Forum* 1984; **11**: 97–102.

34. Love RR, Nerenz DR, Leventhal H, Anticipatory nausea with cancer chemotherapy: Development through two mechanisms. *Proc Annu Meet Am Soc Clin Oncol* 1982; **2**: 242.

35. van Komen RW, Redd WH, Personality factors associated with anticipatory nausea/vomiting in patients receiving cancer chemotherapy. *Health Psychol* 1985; **4**: 189–202.

36. Watson M, McCarron J, Law M, Anticipatory nausea and emesis, and psychological morbidity: assessment of prevalence among out-patients on mild to moderate chemotherapy regimens. *Br J Cancer* 1992; **66**: 862–6.

37. Wilson JP, Rahdert ER, Black CD et al, Identifying anxiety and/or depression in emesis-prone cancer chemotherapy patients. *Proc Annu Meet Am Soc Clin Oncol* 1986; **5**: 239.

38. Stefanek ME, Sheidler VR, Fetting JH, Anticipatory nausea and vomiting: does it remain a significant clinical problem? *Cancer* 1988; **62**: 2654–7.

39. Dolgin MJ, Katz ER, McGinty K, Siegel SE, Anticipatory nausea and vomiting in pediatric cancer patients. *Pediatrics* 1985; **75**: 547–52.

40. Weddington WW, Miller NJ, Sweet DL, Anticipatory nausea and vomiting associated with cancer chemotherapy. *J Psychosom Res* 1984; **28**: 73–7.

41. Weddington WW Jr, Miller NJ, Sweet DL, Anticipatory nausea and vomiting associated with cancer chemotherapy. *N Engl J Med* 1982; **307**: 825–6.

42. Nerenz DR, Leventhal H, Easterling DV, Love RR, Anxiety and drug taste as predictors of anticipatory nausea in cancer chemotherapy. *J Clin Oncol* 1986; **4**: 224–33.

43. Chin SB, Kucuk O, Peterson R, Ezdinli EZ, Variables contributing to anticipatory nausea and vomiting in cancer chemotherapy *Am J Clin Oncol* 1992; **15**: 262–7.

44. Ahles TA, Cohen RE, Little D et al, Toward a behavioral assessment of anticipatory symptoms associated with cancer chemotherapy. *J Behav Ther Exp Psychiatry* 1984; **15**: 141–5.

45. Schultz LS, Classical (Pavlovian) conditioning of nausea and vomiting in cancer chemotherapy. *Proc Annu Meet Am Soc Clin Oncol* 1980; **21**: 244.

46. Andrykowski MA, Redd WH, Longitudinal analysis of the development of anticipatory nausea. *J Consult Clin Psychol* 1987; **55**: 36–41.

47. Altmaier EM, Ross WE, Moore K, A pilot investigation of the psychologic functioning of patients with anticipatory vomiting. *Cancer* 1982; **49**: 201–4.

48. Money KE, Cheung BS, Another function of the inner ear: facilitation of the emetic response to poisons. *Aviation, Space Environ Med* 1983; **54**: 208–11.

49. Morrow GR, The effect of a susceptibility to motion sickness on the side effects of cancer chemotherapy. *Cancer* 1985; **55**: 2766–70.

50. Morrow GR, Susceptibility to motion sickness

and chemotherapy-induced side-effects. *Lancet* 1984; i: 390–1.

51. Morrow GR, Susceptibility to motion sickness and the development of anticipatory nausea and vomiting in cancer patients undergoing chemotherapy. *Cancer Treat Rep* 1984; **68**: 1177–8.

52. Challis GB, Stam HJ, A longitudinal study of the development of anticipatory nausea and vomiting in cancer chemotherapy patients: the role of absorption and autonomic perception. *Health Psychol* 1992; **11**: 181–9.

53. Kvale G, Hugdahl K, Asbjornsen A et al, Anticipatory nausea and vomiting in cancer patients. *J Consult Clin Psychol* 1991; **59**: 894–8.

54. Kvale G, Psychol C, Hugdahl K, Cardiovascular conditioning and anticipatory nausea and vomiting in cancer patients. *Behav Med* 1994; **20**: 78–83.

55. Fredrikson M, Hursti T, Salmi P et al, Conditioned nausea after cancer chemotherapy and autonomic nervous system conditionability. *Scand J Psychol* 1993; **34**: 318–27.

56. Millon J, Green CJ, Meagher RB, The MBHI: a new inventory for the psychodiagnostician in medical settings. *Prof Psychol* 1979; **10**: 529.

57. Spielberger CD, Gorsuch RL, Lushene R, *The State-Trait Anxiety Inventory (STAI)*. Palo Alto: Consulting Psychologists Press, 1968.

58. Morrow GR, Clinical characteristics associated with the development of anticipatory nausea and vomiting in cancer patients undergoing chemotherapy treatment. *J Clin Oncol* 1984; **2**: 1170–6.

59. Morrow GR, Dobkin PL, Anticipatory nausea and vomiting in cancer patients undergoing chemotherapy treatment: prevalence, etiology, and behavioral interventions. *Clin Psychol Rev* 1988; **8**: 517–56.

60. Redd WH, Andrykowski MA, Behavioral intervention in cancer treatment: controlling aversion reactions to chemotherapy. *J Consult Clin Psychol* 1982; **50**: 1018–29.

61. Morrow GR, Morrell C, Behavioral treatment for the anticipatory nausea and vomiting induced by cancer chemotherapy. *N Engl J Med* 1982; **307**: 1476–80.

62. Morrow GR, Behavioral management of chemotherapy-induced nausea and vomiting in the cancer patient. *The Clinical Oncologist* 1986; **1**: 11–14.

63. Morrow GR, Chemotherapy-related nausea and vomiting: etiology and management. *CA Cancer J Clin* 1989; **39**: 89–104.

64. Morrow GR, Asbury R, Hammon S et al, Comparing the effectiveness of behavioral treatment for chemotherapy-induced nausea and vomiting when administered by oncologists, oncology nurses, and clinical psychologists. *Health Psychol* 1992; **11**: 250–6.

65. Morrow GR, Arseneau JC, Asbury RF et al, Anticipatory nausea and vomiting with chemotherapy. *N Engl J Med* 1982; **306**: 431–2.

66. Burish TG, Lyles JN, Effectiveness of relaxation training in reducing the aversiveness of chemotherapy in the treatment of cancer. *J Behav Ther Exp Psychiatry* 1979; **10**: 357–61.

67. Spiegel D, Spiegel H, Hypnosis in psychosomatic medicine. *Psychosomatics* 1980; **21**: 35–41.

68. Lyles JN, Burish TG, Krozely MG, Oldham RK, Efficacy of relaxation training and guided imagery in reducing the aversiveness of cancer chemotherapy. *J Consult Clin Psychol* 1982; **50**: 509–24.

69. Burish TG, Carey MP, Krozely MG, Greco FA, Conditioned side effects induced by cancer chemotherapy: prevention through behavioral treatment. *J Consult Clin Psychol* 1987; **55**: 42–8.

70. Burish TG, Jenkins RA, Effectiveness of biofeedback and relaxation training in reducing the side effects of cancer chemotherapy. *Health Psychol* 1992; **11**: 17–23.

71. Morrow GR, Effect of the cognitive hierarchy in the systematic desensitization treatment of anticipatory nausea in cancer patients: a component comparison with relaxation only, counseling, and no treatment. *Cognit Ther Res* 1986; **10**: 421–46.

72. Burish TG, Vasterling JJ, Carey MP et al, Posttreatment use of relaxation training by cancer patients. *Hosp J* 1988; **4**: 1–8.

73. Lerman C, Rimer B, Blumberg B et al, Effects of coping style and relaxation on cancer chemotherapy side-effects and emotional responses. *Cancer Nurs* 1990; **13**: 308–15.

74. Elam CL, Andrykowski MA, Admission interview ratings: relationship to applicant academic and demographic variables and interviewer characteristics. *Acad Med* 1991; **66**: S13–15.

75. Hailey BJ, White JG, Systematic desensitization for anticipatory nausea associated with chemotherapy. *Psychosomatics* 1983; **24**: 287–91.

76. Hoffman ML, Hypnotic desensitization for the management of anticipatory emesis in chemotherapy. *Am J Clin Hypn* 1982; **2–3**: 173–6.

77. LaBaw W, Holton C, Tewell K, Eccles D, The use of self-hypnosis by children with cancer. *Am J Clin Hypn* 1975; **17**: 233–8.

78. Cotanch P, Hockenberry M, Herman S, Self-hyp-

nosis as antiemetic therapy in children receiving chemotherapy. *Oncol Nurs Forum* 1985; **12**: 41–6.

79. Kolko DJ, Rickard-Figueroa JL, Effects of video games on the adverse corollaries of chemotherapy in pediatric oncology patients: a single-case analysis. *J Consult Clin Psychol* 1985; **53**: 223–8.

80. Zeltzer L, LeBaron S, Zeltzer PM, The effectiveness of behavioral intervention for reduction of nausea and vomiting in children and adolescents receiving chemotherapy. *J Clin Oncol* 1984; **2**: 683–90.

81. Olness K, Imagery (self-hypnosis) as adjunct therapy in childhood cancer: clinical experience with 25 patients. *Am J Pediatr Hematol/Oncol* 1981; **3**: 313–21.

82. Zeltzer LK, Dolgin MJ, LeBaron S, LeBaron C, A randomized, controlled study of behavioral intervention for chemotherapy distress in children with cancer. *Pediatrics* 1991; **88**: 34–42.

83. Zeltzer L, Kellerman J, Ellenberg L, Dash J, Hypnosis for reduction of vomiting with chemotherapy and disease in adolescents with cancer. *J Adolesc Health Care* 1983; **4**: 77–84.

84. Redd WH, Jacobsen PB, Die-Trill M et al, Cognitive/attentional distraction in the control of conditioned nausea in pediatric cancer patients receiving chemotherapy. *J Consult Clin Psychol* 1987; **55**: 391–5.

85. Vasterling J, Jenkins RA, Tope DM, Burish TG, Cognitive distraction and relaxation training for the control of side effects due to cancer chemotherapy. *J Behav Med* 1993; **16**: 65–80.

86. Fallowfield LJ, Behavioural interventions and psychological aspects of care during chemotherapy. *Eur J Can* 1992; **28A**(Suppl 1): S39–41.

87. Andrews PLR, Sanger GJ (eds), *Emesis in Anti-Cancer Therapy. Mechanisms and Treatment.* London: Chapman & Hall.

88. Fdez-Arguelles P, Guerrero J, Duque A et al, Nauseas y vomitos anticipatorios en pacientes cancerosos sometidos a tratamiento de quimioterapia. Paper presented at the 6th Eupsyca Symposium, Zaragoza, Spain, 1985.

89. Hursti T, Fredrikson M, Furst LJ et al, Poster presented at the Joint ESPO–BPOG Conference, London, Royal College of Physicians, 1989.

90. Nicholas DR, Anticipatory nausea in cancer chemotherapy: cognitive, motoric, and physiological components. University of Southern Mississippi, 1983 (Masters thesis).

91. Olafsdottir M, Sjoden P, Westling B, Prevalence and prediction of chemotherapy-related anxiety, nausea and vomiting in cancer patients. *Behav Res Ther* 1986; **24**: 59–66.

92. Palmer BV, Walsh GA, McKinna JA, Greening WP, Adjuvant chemotherapy for breast cancer: side effects and quality of life. *Br Med J* 1980; **281**: 1594–7.

93. Scogna DM, Smalley RV, Chemotherapy-induced nausea and vomiting. *Am J Nurs* 1979; **79**: 1562–4.

94. Stockhorst U, Klosterhalfen S, Klosterhalfen W et al, Anticipatory nausea in cancer patients receiving chemotherapy: classical conditioning etiology and therapeutical implications. *Integr Physiol Behav Sci* 1993; **28**: 177–81.

95. Morrow GR, Behavioural factors influencing the development and expression of chemotherapy induced side effects. *Br J Cancer Suppl* 1992; **19**: S54–60; discussion S60–3.

11

Are there differences between 5-HT$_3$ receptor antagonists?

Jørn Herrstedt

INTRODUCTION

Since the first clinical studies investigating the effect of 5-hydroxytryptamine$_3$ (5-HT$_3$) receptor antagonists were published in 1987,[1,2] investigators – and the involved pharmaceutical companies – have discussed whether there are any differences within this group of important antiemetics. The question is not difficult to answer, because differences do obviously exist! A more interesting question is, however, whether these differences have any clinical significance. As an attempt to answer the latter question, this chapter will briefly review preclinical and clinical studies of the different 5-HT$_3$ antagonists, but will mainly focus on comparative studies of the clinical available agents ondansetron, granisetron, tropisetron and dolasetron.

DEVELOPMENT OF 5-HT$_3$ ANTAGONISTS

The 5-HT$_3$ receptor was identified 40 years ago, but initially referred to as the 'M' receptor.[3] In 1986, Bradley et al[4] reclassified 5-HT receptors, and the 'M' receptor was then classified as the 5-HT$_3$ receptor. Today seven classes (and several subgroups) of 5-HT receptors are recognized (5-HT$_1$, . . . , 5-HT$_7$),[5] but although 5-HT$_{1A}$, 5-HT$_{2A/2C}$ and 5-HT$_4$ receptors seem to be involved in the induction of emesis,[6–8] 5-HT$_3$ antagonists are, so far, the only clinically useful antiemetics among the 5-HT agonists/antagonists.

The recognition that metoclopramide in high doses blocks not only dopamine D$_2$ but also 5-HT$_3$ receptors,[9] and probably exerts its antiemetic effect by antagonism of the 5-HT$_3$ receptors,[10,11] soon led to the development of more potent and selective 5-HT$_3$ antagonists, as shown in Table 11.1.

Ondansetron, granisetron and tropisetron are already established antiemetics, and others will soon follow (dolasetron), whereas the development of some of the other 5-HT$_3$ antagonists has been stopped for unknown reasons (bemesetron and eusetron) or because of adverse events (batanopride and RS-42358-197).[12,13]

PRECLINICAL DIFFERENCES

Besides differences in structure, the 5-HT$_3$ receptor antagonists differ in potency, selectivity and duration of action in animal models.

Table 11.1 Serotonin (5-HT₃) antagonists as antiemetics	
Azasetron	Y-25130
Batanopride	BMY-25801
Bemesetron	MDL 72222
Dazopride	AHR-5531
Dolasetron	MDL 73,147EF
Eusetron	RG 12915
Granisetron	BRL 43694
Itasetron	DAU 6215
Ondansetron	GR 38032
Pancopride	LAS 30451
Renzapride	BRL 24924
Tropisetron	ICS 205-930
Zacopride	AHR-111906
Zatosetron	LY 277359

Structure–potency relationships

The development of the 5-HT₃ antagonists occurred through different pathways, as has previously been described in detail,[14,15] and is addressed in Chapters 1 and 3. Realizing the weak 5-HT₃ antagonist activity of metoclopramide, a natural approach was the development of different substituted benzamides such as dazopride, batanopride, zacopride and renzapride. Although most of these drugs are very potent at the 5-HT₃ receptor, the antiemetic effect is not always optimal. For example, the antiemetic efficacy of renzapride is less than that of MDL 72222, in spite of the fact that renzapride is approximately 10 times more potent than MDL 72222 as a 5-HT₃ receptor antagonist. It has been hypothesized that this is due to the ability of renzapride to stimulate gastric motility, possibly by agonism at 5-HT₄ receptors.[16] MDL 72222 was the first selective 5-HT₃ antagonist and the predecessor of dolasetron (MDL 73147EF). Other approaches to the development of selective 5-HT₃ antagonists concentrated on compounds containing an indole or tropane

nucleus (tropisetron, granisetron, ondansetron).

The potency and 5-HT₃ receptor affinity of ondansetron,[17,18] granisetron,[17,19] tropisetron[17,20,21] and dolasetron[22,23] have been investigated in different animal models, such as rats (Bezold–Jarisch effect), guinea pigs (isolated ileum) and rabbits (isolated heart and isolated muscle). Differences in potency appeared in these models, but seem to be of little, if any, clinical relevance, because of the favourable safety profile of the 5-HT₃ antagonists.

Selectivity of receptor binding

The importance of selectivity for the 5-HT₃ receptor has been a major topic of discussion.[24] Most, but not all, of the drugs in Table 11.1, are highly selective. In fact, zacopride[16,25] and azasetron[26] are capable of inducing emesis in ferrets and dogs respectively. Two explanations for this phenomena have been hypothesized.[27] Zacopride is a racemic mixture of an S-enantiomer with agonist effect and an R-enantiomer with antagonist activity at the 5-HT₃ receptor.[28] In addition, the 5-HT₄ receptor agonist activity of zacopride is thought to contribute to the induction of emesis,[29] although this has recently been called into question.[6] It should be emphasized that ondansetron, granisetron, tropisetron and dolasetron all have an affinity 250–1000 times greater for the 5-HT₃ receptor than for any other receptor. Ondansetron has minimal affinity for 5-HT₁ᵦ, 5-HT₂c (previously named 5-HT₁c), α₁-adrenergic and μ opioid receptors,[17] granisetron for 5-HT₁ₐ receptors,[30] tropisetron for 5-HT uptake[17] and 5-HT₄ receptors (antagonist),[31] and dolasetron for benzodiazepine receptors.[22] Also, batanopride has a favourable receptor binding profile, but causes hypotension when given in effective doses.[12]

Other preclinical differences

It has been stressed that the dose–response curves of granisetron and tropisetron are linear (in ferrets), whereas the curve for ondansetron is nonlinear.[24] Tropisetron and granisetron also seemed to be longer-acting than ondansetron. In two studies of vagal 5-HT$_3$ receptors in the rat[32] and in the rabbit,[33] the 5-HT$_3$ antagonist effect of ondansetron, but not of granisetron and tropisetron, was surmounted by increasing the concentration of 5-HT. This is in accordance with a recent study in which ondansetron was demonstrated to act as a competitive inhibitor of rat 5-HT$_3$ receptors.[34] Such experimental differences are, however, only of interest if they result in clinically meaningful differences.

CLINICAL PHARMACOKINETICS

The importance of the differences in elimination half-life $T_{1/2}$ between the 5-HT$_3$ antagonists has been debated. A number of factors, such as age, systemic clearance, co-administration of antineoplastic drugs, changes in protein binding, involvement of the hepatic cytochrome P450 enzyme system in the metabolism, and disease of the patients, could influence the plasma half-life.[35] $T_{1/2}$ of granisetron[35] and ondansetron[36] is shorter in healthy volunteers than in cancer patients (ondansetron 3 versus 5 hours, granisetron 3–4 versus 9–12 hours). This could of course be due to the fact that healthy volunteers are usually younger than cancer patients. Dolasetron is rapidly metabolized to hydrodolasetron ($T_{1/2}$ = 10 minutes), which is considered to cause most of the antiemetic effect, and has a higher receptor binding affinity and a longer $T_{1/2}$ (7–9 hours) than the parent compound.[37] The cytochrome P450 enzyme system participates in the metabolism of ondansetron,[38] granisetron,[39] dolasetron[38] and tropisetron,[40] but is of major significance for the metabolism of tropisetron only. Tropisetron undergoes metabolism by the cytochrome P450 2D6 isoenzyme system, which shows phenotypic populations of poor and extensive metabolizers. This means that the $T_{1/2}$ of tropisetron is 7.3 hours in most patients, but is prolonged to 30 hours[40] in poor metabolizers (1 out of 12 in Caucasians). The clinical relevance of these observations is questionable, since the duration of antiemetic effect of the 5-HT$_3$ antagonists is probably better correlated with interactions at the receptor level than with plasma half-life.

The oral absorption of ondansetron, granisetron and dolasetron is almost complete, and is unaffected by co-administration with food. The bioavailability is, however, decreased to 60%, 60% and 75% respectively,[35–37] owing to hepatic first-pass metabolism. Also, tropisetron is well absorbed, with a bioavailability of approximately 60% for the recommended 5 mg dose.[41] The bioavailability of larger doses approaches 100%, because of saturation kinetics of the first-pass metabolism.

DOSE-FINDING STUDIES

The finding of the optimal dose and schedule for the 5-HT$_3$ antagonists has been a subject of major interest. There is persistent confusion regarding the dosage of granisetron and ondansetron, due to the lack of clear-cut conclusive dose-finding studies, resulting in differences in the official recommended doses in different countries. In Table 11.2 a summary of the recommended intravenous and oral doses (adults) is given.

Table 11.2 Intravenous and oral doses of 5-HT$_3$ antagonists

Antiemetic	Dose	
	Intravenous	Oral
Ondansetron	8–32 mg × 1	8 mg × 2
Granisetron	1–3 mg × 1	1 mg × 2[a]
Tropisetron	5 mg × 1	5 mg × 1[b]
Dolasetron	1.8 mg/kg × 1	200 mg × 1[c]

[a] Can also be prescribed as 2 mg × 1.
[b] Dose not verified in double-blind trials.
[c] Effect of doses >200 mg not investigated.

Ondansetron

Ondansetron was primarily investigated in intravenous doses of 8 mg × 3, 0.15 mg/kg × 3 or 8 mg as a bolus infusion followed by a 24-hour continuous infusion of 1 mg/hour. Subsequent studies demonstrated that the schedule could be simplified to a single dose given before chemotherapy without loss of antiemetic effect.[42-44] In two studies[43,45] there were no differences between single doses of 8 mg and 32 mg, whereas in a third study[44] the 32 mg dose was slightly superior to the 8 mg.

Initial studies of oral ondansetron used 8 mg × 3, but 8 mg × 2 offers the same degree of antiemetic protection.[46]

Granisetron

Granisetron was investigated as a single intravenous dose. Up to two rescue doses within the initial 24 hours after chemotherapy were allowed. However, no substantial data have supported the use of these rescue doses. A dose of 40 µg/kg (or 3 mg) was considered optimal, but recent studies have indicated that 10 µg/kg (or 1 mg) is just as efficacious.[47,48] This is supported by a study including 987 patients, in which no significant differences were obtained between granisetron 10 or 40 µg/kg (or ondansetron).[49] The oral dose of granisetron is 1 mg × 2 daily. A large study (697 patients) concluded that granisetron could be given as a single oral dose of 2 mg without loss of efficacy.[50]

Tropisetron

Tropisetron was investigated from the beginning in single intravenous and oral doses, but the quantity of dose-finding data is limited compared with that for ondansetron and granisetron. An intravenous dose of 5 mg administered before chemotherapy is as effective as 10, 20 or 40 mg, and superior to 2 mg.[51,52] The oral maintenance dose of tropisetron is 5 mg × 1.

Dolasetron

Single intravenous doses of 0.6, 1.2, 1.8, 2.4 and 3.0 mg/kg have been compared in patients receiving cisplatin.[53] The 1.8 mg/kg seems to produce optimal results, with no advantages with higher doses. This has been confirmed in comparative trials of different doses of dolasetron versus metoclopramide[54,55] or ondansetron[56] or granisetron.[57] Division of the 1.8 mg/kg into three doses of 0.6 mg/kg produced inferior results.[58]

Three studies compared the efficacy of single oral doses of 25, 50, 100 and 200 mg. Pooled data from these trials showed that the 100 and 200 mg doses were superior to lower doses, and indicated that the 200 mg dose was superior to 100 mg,[59] although a statistically significant difference was not obtained. It is not known if oral doses higher than 200 mg will increase the efficacy.

ANTIEMETIC EFFECT OF 5-HT$_3$ ANTAGONISTS

The clinical development of the 5-HT$_3$ antagonists also went through different pathways. Ondansetron was investigated using the best-known antiemetic, metoclopramide, as a comparator, whereas granisetron and tropisetron were compared with metoclopramide-based combinations. Dolasetron has, as described above, been compared with metoclopramide,[54,55] ondansetron[56] and granisetron.[57]

Several randomized, double-blind trials have shown that the antiemetic effect of both ondansetron, granisetron and tropisetron is improved by the addition of dexamethasone. In a recent trial, the antiemetic effect of dolasetron was also improved when used in combination with dexamethasone.[60]

Three randomized, double-blind studies, one including chemotherapy-naive patients[61] and two[62,63] including patients refractory to previous antiemetic therapy, showed that the combination of ondansetron plus the dopamine antagonist metopimazine is superior to ondansetron alone. Another dopamine antagonist, haloperidol, was able to improve the antiemetic effect of tropisetron in a trial using historical controls,[64] and the combination of granisetron and the antihistamine hydroxyzine hydrochloride decreased the severity of nausea (but not vomiting) in an open trial comparison with granisetron alone.[65]

The role of the 5-HT₃ antagonists in the treatment of acute and delayed nausea and vomiting is described in detail in Chapters 5 and 6.

COMPARATIVE STUDIES OF 5-HT₃ ANTAGONISTS

Owing to differences in doses, comparator arms and trial methodology,[66] early clinical studies were unsuitable for exposing possible differences between 5-HT₃ antagonists. This led several investigators to initiate comparative studies including two or more 5-HT₃ antagonists. Today approximately 30 comparative studies have been completed. A summary of these, in patients receiving cisplatin-based chemotherapy,[45,49,56,57,67-72] is given in Table 11.3, while Table 11.4 summarizes studies in patients undergoing treatment with moderately emetogenic chemotherapy.[60,67,73-81] Another eight studies,[82-89] which all used an open trial design, and so far have been published as abstracts only, will not be discussed further. Although the quantity of comparative data is substantial, a number of the studies quoted are of limited value, owing to methodological pitfalls. A crucial factor is the sample size, which determines the minimal realistic difference that a study has the power to detect (MIREDIF). The MIREDIF, however, depends not only on the sample size, but also on the level of significance (Type I error) and the power of the study (1-Type II error) chosen. It is therefore important that a precalculation of the necessary sample size is done, using clinically relevant Type I and II errors. Other important factors are the use of a double-blind design and of relevant dose schedules of the 5-HT₃ antagonists.

Taking note of the above comments about methodology, it is obvious that the overall qual-ity of comparative studies in patients receiving cisplatin-based chemotherapy (Table 11.3) is greater than that of studies in patients exposed to moderately emetogenic chemotherapy (Table 11.4). The discussion below concerns comparative studies investigating the effect of 5-HT₃ antagonists on acute emesis. The number of patients given in the tables are those who were included in the analysis for efficacy. As can be seen, the evaluable parameters emphasized are complete control on day 1 and, in studies using a crossover design, also patient preference. Complete control is defined as absence of emetic episodes, independent of nausea. A better definition would have been absence of emetic episodes and of nausea. This information is, however, not available from all the studies. Other evaluable parameters will be included, in case they make a decisive contribution to the interpretation. Finally, a few comments on the sparse data on delayed emesis will be stated.

The safety of 5-HT₃ antagonists in comparative studies has recently been reviewed in detail.[90] Although side-effects were reported at different frequencies from one study to another, no major differences between the different agents were found.

Cisplatin-based chemotherapy

Ten studies compared two or more 5-HT₃ antagonists in patients receiving cisplatin-based chemotherapy (Table 11.3). Seven of these studies were double-blind.

Open studies

Three studies used an open design, and included 101,[70] 117[69] and 166[67] patients respectively. They all compared ondansetron given as a single intravenous (i.v.) dose of 24 mg,[67,69] or as three divided doses of 8 mg,[70] with granisetron 3 mg i.v. One of the studies[69] included a third arm in which patients received 5 mg of i.v. tropisetron. The studies by Gebbia et al[67] and Mantovani et al[69] included chemotherapy-naive patients, and used a parallel design and a MIREDIF of 20%. In both

Table 11.3 Comparative studies of 5-HT₃ antagonists in patients receiving cisplatin-based chemotherapy

Authors	Design[a]	Number of patients	Cisplatin (mg/m²)	Antiemetics day 1 (i.v.)[b]	MIREDIF[c]	Control, day 1, no EE[d] (%)	Preferences[d,e]
Audhuy et al[57]	DB, P	474	≥80	DOL 1.8 mg/kg DOL 2.4 mg/kg GRA 3 mg	15%	54 47 48	—
Gebbia et al[67]	O, P	166	≥70	OND 24 mg GRA 3 mg	20%	52 49	—
Hesketh et al[56]	DB, P	609	≥70	DOL 1.8 mg/kg DOL 2.4 mg/kg OND 32 mg	15%	44.4 40.0 42.7	—
IGAR[68]	DB, P	966	≥50	OND 8 mg + DEX 20 mg or GRA 3 mg + DEX 20 mg	10%	79.3 79.9	—
Mantovani et al[69]	O, P	117	80–100	OND 24 mg GRA 3 mg TRO 5 mg	20%	73.3 72.1 67.6	—
Martoni et al[70]	O, CO	101	50–70	OND 8 mg × 3 GRA 3 mg	15%	68 71	25% OND 45% GRA 30% NP
Marty et al[71]	DB, P	231	≥50	OND 32 mg TRO 5 mg	20%	65 54	—
Navari et al[49]	DB, P	987	≥60	OND 0.15 mg/kg × 3 GRA 10 µg/kg GRA 40 µg/kg	6 h in time to first EE[d]	51 47 48	—
Noble et al[72]	DB, CO	309	≥15/day or ifos[f] >1200/day	OND 8 mg × 3 GRA 3 mg	16% in 5-day control	39.8[g] 44.0	25.9% OND 34.4% GRA 39.7% NP
Ruff et al[45]	DB, P	496	≥50	OND 8 mg OND 32 mg GRA 3 mg	15%	59 51 56	—

[a] CO, crossover; DB, double-blind; O, open; P, parallel. [b] DOL, dolasetron; OND, ondansetron; GRA, granisetron; TRO, tropisetron; DEX, dexamethasone. [c] MIREDIF, minimal relevant difference that the study had the power to detect. [d] EE, emetic episode. [e] NP, no preference. [f] ifos, ifosamide. [g] Control, day 1–5 (no EE).

Table 11.4 Comparative studies of 5-HT$_3$ antagonists in patients receiving moderately emetogenic chemotherapy

Authors	Design[a]	Number of patients	Chemotherapy (mg/m²)[b]	Antiemetics day 1[c]	MIREDIF[d]	Control, day 1, no EE[e] (%)	Preferences[f]
Bonneterre et al[73]	O, CO	150	FEC and other	OND 8 mg i.v. + 8 mg × 2 p.o. GRA 3 mg i.v.	20%	77 72	34% OND 27% NP 39% GRA
Campora et al[74]	O, P	40	FAC/FEC	OND 8 mg i.v. + 8 mg × 2 p.o. TRO 5 mg i.v.	?	65.4 75.5	—
Fauser et al[75]	DB, P	399	C, A, CP other	DOL 25 mg p.o. DOL 50 mg p.o. DOL 100 mg p.o. DOL 200 mg p.o. OND 8 mg × 3–4 p.o.	25%	45.0 49.4 60.5 76.3 72.3	—
Gebbia et al[67]	O, P	158	CMF, FAC, FEC, other	OND 16 mg i.v. GRA 3 mg i.v.	20%	69 67	—
Jantunen et al[76]	O, CO	39	CMF, CP other	OND 8 mg i.v. + 8 mg × 2 p.o. + DEX TRO 5 mg i.v. + DEX	?	97 82	33% OND 49% NP 18% TRO
Jantunen et al[77]	O, CO	130	FAC/FEC other	OND 8 mg i.v. GRA 3 mg i.v. TRO 5 mg i.v.	?	68.5 80.0 74.6	17% OND 42% GRA 15% TRO 26% NP
Lofters and Zee[60]	DB, P	696	Moderately emetogenic	OND 32 mg i.v. ± DEX DOL 2.4 mg/kg ± DEX	?	67.0 57.0	—
Massida et al[78]	O, P	122	E, DTIC, other	OND 16 mg i.v. GRA 3 mg i.v. TRO 5 mg i.v.	?	69 68 78	—
Perez et al[79]	DB, CO	623	FAC	OND 32 mg i.v. GRA 10 µg/kg	?	62 58	51% OND 49% GRA[g]
Pion et al[80]	DB, CO	188	Moderately emetogenic	OND 8 mg × 2 p.o. GRA 1 mg × 2 p.o.	?	68.5 73.3	No difference[h]
Stewart et al[81]	DB, P	488	CMF	OND 8 mg i.v. + 8 mg p.o. OND 8 mg × 2 p.o. GRA 3 mg i.v.	15%	78 78 81	—

[a] CO, crossover; DB, double-blind; O, open; P, parallel. [b] C, cyclophosphamide; A, Adriamycin; E, epirubicin; F, 5-fluorouracil; DTIC, dacarbazine; CP, carboplatin; M, methotrexate. [c] DOL, dolasetron; OND, ondansetron; GRA, granisetron; TRO, tropisetron; DEX, dexamethasone. [d] MIREDIF, minimal relevant difference that the study had the power to detect. [e] EE, emetic episode. [f] NP, no preference. [g] Number of patients with no preference not specified. [h] Percentage not reported.

studies a precalculation of the sample size was done. Mantovani et al increased the power of the study to 90%, by following the patients during a total of 463 cycles. This means of course, that patients were chemotherapy-naive in one third of the cycles only. In the study by Gebbia et al the power was lower than the reported 80%, because only 166 patients were evaluable for efficacy, instead of 182 as estimated. None of the studies showed any statistically significant differences in complete protection from acute emesis (CR) between granisetron (49%) and ondansetron (52%)[67] or between granisetron (72.1%), ondansetron (73.3%) and tropisetron (67.6%)[69] (Table 11.3).

Martoni et al[70] compared granisetron and ondansetron in 101 chemotherapy-naive patients using a crossover design. No significant difference in CR was found (71% vs 68%, Table 11.3), but more patients preferred granisetron (45% vs 25%, $p = 0.003$). The fact that patients' preference also depended on the sequence of antiemetics in the crossover, and especially the use of an open study design, implies a significant deterioration in the quality of this information.

Double-blind studies

Only two comparative studies have so far included dolasetron – one in comparison with ondansetron[56] and one with granisetron.[57] Hesketh et al[56] compared single i.v. doses of dolasetron 1.8 mg/kg, dolasetron 2.4 mg/kg and ondansetron 32 mg in a parallel study in 609 patients naive to cisplatin-based chemotherapy. Patients were stratified according to dose of cisplatin (70–90 mg/m² or >90 mg/m²). The study had a power of 80% and a MIREDIF of 15%. No significant differences between ondansetron and dolasetron were seen, but less nausea was noted with dolasetron 1.8 mg/kg than with 2.4 mg/kg ($p = 0.044$). CR (whole patient population) was 44.4% and 40.0% with dolasetron 1.8 mg/kg and 2.4 mg/kg respectively, and 42.7% with ondansetron (Table 11.3). In another parallel study[57] the same two doses of dolasetron were compared with a single 3 mg i.v. dose of granisetron. The patient population consisted of 474 patients, and both chemotherapy-naive patients and patients who had previously received chemotherapy were included. Although the sample size was smaller than in the other study, the MIREDIF (15%) and the power (80%) of the study was the same, because the Type I error chosen was 10%, instead of the usual 5%. CR was achieved by 54, 47 and 48% of patients receiving 1.8 mg/kg dolasetron, 2.4 mg/kg dolasetron and granisetron respectively. The authors concluded that granisetron and dolasetron were equally effective in preventing nausea and vomiting from cisplatin-based chemotherapy, and that the 1.8 mg/kg dose of dolasetron was optimal for further clinical development.

Marty et al[71] compared ondansetron 32 mg with tropisetron 5 mg, both given as a single i.v. dose before chemotherapy. This parallel study included 231 chemotherapy-naive patients, of whom 65% obtained CR with ondansetron and 54% with tropisetron ($p = 0.052$). The total control of acute nausea was 62% with ondansetron and 66% with tropisetron. The authors emphasized that the control obtained with tropisetron is consistent with other trials. In contrast, the ondansetron complete response rate of 65% is, for unknown reasons, higher than in other trials investigating a 32 mg dose of ondansetron.

Four studies compared ondansetron and granisetron[45,49,68,72] in patients not previously exposed to treatment with cisplatin-containing chemotherapy; one study[72] used a crossover design, the others a parallel design. The crossover study by Noble and colleagues[72] compared a single dose of granisetron (3 mg i.v.) with divided doses of ondansetron (8 mg × 3 i.v.) in 309 patients receiving five-day fractionated chemotherapy with cisplatin or ifosfamide (Table 11.3). There were no differences in complete protection from vomiting on day 1 (94.5% vs 90.7% in course 1) or during days 1–5 (ondansetron 39.5% vs granisetron 44.0%, both courses combined). Significantly more patients preferred granisetron (34.4% vs 25.9%, $p = 0.048$), but as many as 39.7% did not express a preference for either of the two treatments (Table 11.3). Ruff et al[45] compared two doses of ondansetron (8 mg and 32 mg × 1 i.v.) with granisetron 3 mg in 496 patients. Complete control of emesis was reported in 59% of patients in the 8 mg ondansetron group compared with 51% in the 32 mg ondansetron group and 56% in patients receiving granisetron. No significant differences were found in this study, which had a power of 80% to detect differences of 15% or more. Besides emphasizing the similar efficacy of ondansetron and granisetron, the study found no differences between the 8 and 32 mg doses of ondansetron. Navari et al[49] compared single doses of 10 and 40 µg/kg granisetron with three divided doses of ondansetron (0.15 mg/kg) in 987 patients. The number of patients included provided 90% power to detect a six-hour difference in time to event (first emetic episode). As can be seen from Table 11.3, no significant difference in CR was obtained between patients receiving ondansetron (51%) and granisetron 10 and 40 µg/kg (47% and 48%) respectively. Furthermore, no differences in time to first emesis or nausea were seen.

As previously described, the antiemetic effect of 5-HT₃ antagonists is improved by the addition of dexamethasone, and the combination of a 5-HT₃ antagonist plus dexamethasone is often considered as the antiemetic regimen of choice for the prevention of acute cisplatin-induced emesis.[91] So far, only one study of patients receiving cisplatin has investigated possible differences between 5-HT₃ antagonists in combination with dexamethasone. In a large parallel study,[68] 966 patients were randomized to antiemetic therapy with ondansetron 8 mg i.v. plus dexamethasone 20 mg i.v. or granisetron 3 mg i.v. plus dexamethasone 20 mg i.v. The study was designed to detect differences of 10% or more with a power of 90–96%. The complete protection rates from acute vomiting were almost identical, since 79.3% of patients receiving ondansetron plus dexamethasone, compared with 79.9% of patients receiving granisetron plus dexamethasone, had no emesis. There was no difference in the protection rates from acute nausea either (72.0% vs 71.8%).

Moderately emetogenic chemotherapy

Eleven studies have addressed possible differences between 5-HT₃ antagonists in patients exposed to moderately emetogenic chemotherapy (Table 11.4). Five of these studies are double-blind, but so far three of these have been published as abstracts only. Only half of the studies seem to have speculated on the necessary size of the patient population.

Open studies

Ondansetron was compared with granisetron in two studies, both designed to detect differences of at least 20%. Bonneterre et al[73] compared ondansetron 8 mg i.v. followed by two oral doses of 8 mg with a single i.v. dose of granisetron 3 mg, in 175 chemotherapy-naive patients. 150 patients were evaluable for crossover analysis. Complete protection from acute emesis was obtained in 77% of patients receiving ondansetron and in 72% receiving granisetron. Ondansetron was the treatment preferred by 34% of the patients, and granisetron was preferred by 39%. None of these differences were statistically significant. Gebbia et al[67] compared single doses of ondansetron 16 mg and granisetron 3 mg in a parallel study. A total of 158 chemotherapy-naive patients were evaluable for efficacy. No differences were seen, with complete response rates of 69% (ondansetron) and 67% respectively.

Four studies compared the antiemetic effect of tropisetron and ondansetron; two of these also included a comparison with granisetron. Campora et al[74] followed 40 women during three cycles of adjuvant FAC/FEC chemotherapy. They found no differences in antiemetic effect between a single dose of tropisetron 5 mg and multiple doses of ondansetron. Massida et al[78] compared tropisetron 5 mg, ondansetron 16 mg and granisetron 3 mg (single i.v. doses) in a parallel study including 122 patients, primarily women. No data on previous chemotherapy were available. A numerically higher response rate was obtained with tropisetron (78%), but this was not significantly different from response rates obtained in patients randomized to treatment with ondansetron (68%) or granisetron (67%). Jantunen et al have performed two studies in patients receiving moderately emetogenic chemotherapy. Both studies used a crossover design, and included a mixture of chemotherapy-naive patients and patients who had previously received chemotherapy. The first study[76] compared a single dose of tropisetron with divided doses of ondansetron, both combined with dexamethasone, in 39 evaluable patients. A significantly higher response rate was seen with ondansetron (97% vs 82%, $p = 0.026$), but, as the authors emphasized themselves, this could be due to differences in the dose schedules and the open trial design. In the second study[77] 166 patients were randomized to tropisetron 5 mg, ondansetron 8 mg or granisetron 3 mg given as single i.v. doses. Patients were followed during three cycles of chemotherapy, and 130 patients were evaluable for crossover analysis. As can be seen in Table 11.4, more patients preferred treatment with granisetron (42%) than with tropisetron (15%) or ondansetron (17%), and granisetron was also superior to ondansetron in terms of complete control of vomiting ($p = 0.034$). Again, one should be cautious not to attach too much importance to these results, because of a number of methodological problems.

Double-blind studies

Two studies, using a parallel design, investigated ondansetron versus dolasetron.[60,75] In the study by Fauser et al[75] four different doses of dolasetron were compared with oral ondansetron. Dolasetron was given as a single dose of 25 mg, 50 mg, 100 mg or 200 mg and ondansetron as 8 mg × 3–4 (Table 11.4). Although 399 patients were included, the MIREDIF of the study was as high as 25%, because patients were randomized to one of five treatments. Patients were stratified by gender and by history of previous chemotherapy (naive/non-naive). The 200 mg dose of dolasetron was superior to lower doses, with complete response rates of 45% (25 mg), 49.4% (50 mg), 60.5% (100 mg) and 76.3% (200 mg) respectively (≤ 0.0188). The complete response

rate with ondansetron was 72.3%, which was not significantly different from the 200 mg dolasetron dose. A lower score on the 100 mm visual analogue scale for nausea was seen with the 200 mg dolasetron dose, than with ondansetron ($p = 0.0061$) and with lower doses of dolasetron (≤ 0.0019). It should, however, be noted that the nausea scores for ondansetron and for dolasetron 100 mg and 200 mg were all very low (3.0 mm, 3.5 mm and 0.0 mm respectively), compared with 25 mg and 50 mg of dolasetron (29.0 mm and 31.0 mm). The safety profile was identical between ondansetron and dolasetron, with no linear trend with dolasetron dose for overall adverse events. Lofters and Zee[60] randomized 709 patients, in a 2 × 2 factorial design, to antiemetic therapy with dolasetron 2.4 mg/kg or ondansetron 32 mg, both given as a single i.v. dose before chemotherapy. Half of the patients in each group were randomized to additional treatment with i.v. dexamethasone. A total of 696 patients were evaluable. Complete control from acute emesis was obtained in 67% receiving ondansetron and 57% receiving dolasetron (both ± dexamethasone, $p = 0.13$).

Three studies[79-81] (two[79,80] published so far as abstracts only) compared ondansetron with granisetron. Stewart et al[81] investigated the antiemetic effect of ondansetron 8 mg i.v. + 8 mg orally versus 8 mg × 2 orally versus granisetron 3 mg i.v. in a parallel study. A total of 540 patients (488 evaluable for effect) scheduled to receive their first course of cyclophosphamide-based chemotherapy were included. The study had a power of 80% to detect a MIREDIF of 15%. Both ondansetron regimens resulted in complete protection from acute emesis in 78% of the patients compared with 81% in patients who received granisetron. The study supports the lack of difference between ondansetron and granisetron, but also suggests that the i.v. bolus infusion of ondansetron could be replaced by an oral dose, although a little more patients in the oral than in the i.v. ondansetron group received antiemetic rescue (2 vs 8%). An interesting crossover study[79] compared granisetron 10 µg/kg with ondansetron 32 mg in 623 breast-cancer patients, receiving their first course of cyclophosphamide–doxorubicin-containing chemotherapy. No data are yet available on the power of the study, but a course 1 analysis in, for example, 600 evaluable patients will result in a power of 90% to detect a MIREDIF of approximately 13%. A crossover analysis will of course increase the power. A preliminary analysis showed equal protection from acute emesis (CR 58% with granisetron, 62% with ondansetron), whereas more ondansetron patients had no nausea at 24 hours (48% vs 39%, $p = 0.035$). There was no significant difference in patient preference. Another crossover study[80] compared oral granisetron (1 mg bid) and oral ondansetron (8 mg bid) in 188 chemotherapy-naive patients. Preliminary data indicated no difference in patients' preference, or in the complete protection from acute emesis in course 1 (73.3% with granisetron vs 68.5% with ondansetron). It was stated that a higher complete protection rate and less nausea was obtained in the granisetron arm in course 2, but further interpretation of this study will have to await full publication.

Delayed emesis

The role of 5-HT₃ antagonists in the treatment of delayed emesis is reviewed in Chapter 6. It is obvious that the antiemetic effect of 5-HT₃ antagonists is modest in the delayed phase, compared with the significant effect during the initial 24 hours after chemotherapy.

None of the comparative studies quoted above were designed with the specific purpose of evaluating delayed nausea and vomiting. A number of the studies did, nevertheless, include efficacy data of delayed emesis.

In patients receiving cisplatin (Table 11.3), six studies evaluated the first 24 hours after chemotherapy only,[45,49,56,57,69,70] and one included patients receiving fractionated chemotherapy.[72] One study did evaluate the delayed phase,[68] but, recognizing that 5-HT₃ antagonists are not first choice in the treatment of delayed emesis, patients received dexamethasone and metoclopramide. This means that only two of the studies evaluated the effect of 5-HT₃ antagonists in

delayed emesis. No differences between granisetron and ondansetron[67] or between ondansetron and tropisetron[71] were seen.

Eight of the studies in patients receiving moderately emetogenic chemotherapy assessed delayed emesis.[60,67,73,74,78–81] Only four of these[67,73,74,81] have been published as full papers. In two of these,[73,81] patients received granisetron 3 mg i.v. on day 1 and no further antiemetic therapy compared with ondansetron 8 mg i.v. (or orally) followed by ondansetron 8 mg × 2–3. The studies therefore do not contribute to disclosing possible differences between the 5-HT₃ antagonists in the delayed phase. The other two trials found no differences between ondansetron and granisetron[67] or ondansetron and tropisetron.[74]

CONCLUSIONS

The 5-HT₃ antagonists have improved the treatment of acute emesis and quality of life in patients receiving chemotherapy. Early studies demonstrated differences in receptor specificity and pharmacokinetics, but the clinical importance of these differences has been questioned.

It seems unlikely that the 5-HT₃ antagonists exhibit clinically relevant differences in patients exposed to cisplatin-based chemotherapy. Double-blind studies,[49,56,68] which included sufficient numbers of patients to unmask differences of 10–15%, are remarkably concordant. No such differences in antiemetic effect or tolerability were found.

Studies in patients receiving moderately emetogenic chemotherapy are less conclusive. Many of these included a limited number of patients, used an open design or possessed other methodological problems. It has previously been pointed out that more patients preferred granisetron to ondansetron in crossover studies, but it was also stressed that limitations in methodology prevent a final conclusion.[90] It is therefore of major interest that in a double-blind trial[79] including 623 patients, preliminary results did not differ as regards patients' preference for granisetron (49%) or ondansetron (51%).

There are specific subgroups of patients in which no substantial dose-finding or comparative data are available. These groups include patients receiving multiple-day or multiple cycles of chemotherapy and paediatric patients. In patients subjected to high-dose chemotherapy with stem-cell support, preliminary data suggest that higher than conventional doses of 5-HT$_3$ antagonists are necessary to obtain optimum antiemetic effect.

Today, the clinician should choose the least expensive of the 5-HT$_3$ antagonists available. Future studies may reveal differences between the agents in small subgroups of patients.

REFERENCES

1. Leibundgut U, Lancranjan I, First results with ICS 205-930 (5-HT$_3$ receptor antagonist) in prevention of chemotherapy induced emesis. *Lancet* 1987; i: 1198.
2. Cunningham D, Hawthorn J, Pople A et al, Prevention of emesis in patients receiving cytotoxic drugs by GR38032F, a selective 5-HT$_3$ receptor antagonist. *Lancet* 1987; i: 1461–2.
3. Gaddum JH, Picarelli ZP, Two kinds of tryptamine receptor. *Br J Pharmacol Chemother* 1957; **12**: 323–8.
4. Bradley PB, Engel G, Fenuik W et al, Proposals for the classification and nomenclature of functional receptors for 5-hydroxytryptamine. *Neuropharmacology* 1986; **25**: 563–76.
5. Hoyer D, Clarke DE, Fozard JR et al, International Union of Pharmacology classification of receptors for 5-hydroxytryptamine (serotonin). *Pharmacol Rev* 1994; **46**: 157–203.
6. Tonini M, 5-HT$_4$ receptor involvement in emesis. In: *Serotonin and the Scientific Basis of Anti-Emetic Therapy* (Reynolds DJM, Andrews PLR, Davis CJ, eds). Oxford: Oxford Clinical Communications, 1995: 192–9.
7. Okada F, Torii Y, Saito H, Matsuki N, Antiemetic effects of serotonergic 5-HT$_{1A}$ receptor agonists in *Suncus murinus*. *Jap J Pharmacol* 1994; **64**: 109–14.
8. Okada F, Saito H, Matsuki N, Blockade of motion- and cisplatin-induced emesis by a 5-HT$_2$ receptor agonist in *Suncus murinus*. *Br J Pharmacol* 1995; **114**: 931–4.
9. Fozard JR, Neuronal 5-HT receptors in the periphery. *Neuropharmacology* 1984; **23**: 1473–86.
10. Miner WD, Sanger GJ, Inhibition of cisplatin-induced vomiting by selective 5-hydroxytryptamine M-receptor antagonism. *Br J Pharmacol* 1986; **88**: 497–9.
11. Costall B, Domeney AM, Naylor RJ, Tattersall FD, 5-Hydroxytryptamine M-receptor antagonism to prevent cisplatin-induced emesis. *Neuropharmacology* 1986; **25**: 959–61.
12. Herrstedt J, Jeppesen BH, Dombernowsky P, Dose-limiting hypotension with the 5-HT$_3$ antagonist batanopride (BMY 25801). *Ann Oncol* 1991; **2**: 154–5.
13. Kowalczyk BA, Dvorak CA, Total synthesis of the 5-HT$_3$ receptor antagonist palonosetron. *Synthesis* 1996; **7**: 816–18.
14. King FD, Sanger GJ, 5-HT$_3$ receptor antagonists. *Drugs Future* 1989; **14**: 875–89.
15. Richardson BP, The discovery of selective 5-hydroxytryptamine-3 (5-HT$_3$) receptor antagonists. In: *Serotonin and the Scientific Basis of Anti-Emetic Therapy* (Reynolds DJM, Andrews PLR, Davis CJ, eds). Oxford: Oxford Clinical Communications, 1995: 50–9.
16. Sanger GJ, New antiemetic drugs. *Can J Physiol Pharmacol* 1990; **68**: 314–24.
17. Van Wijngaarden I, Tulp MTM, Soudijn W, The concept of selectivity in 5-HT receptor research. *Eur J Pharmacol* 1990; **188**: 301–12.
18. Butler A, Hill JM, Ireland SJ et al, Pharmacological properties of GR38032F, a novel antagonist at 5-HT$_3$ receptors. *Br J Pharmacol* 1988; **94**: 397–412.
19. Sanger GR, Nelson DR, Selective and functional 5-hydroxytryptamine$_3$ receptor antagonism by BRL 43694 (granisetron). *Eur J Pharmacol* 1989; **159**: 113–24.
20. Richardson BP, Engel G, Donatsch P, Stadler PA, Identification of serotonin M-receptor subtypes and their specific blockade by a new class of drugs. *Nature* 1985; **316**: 126–31.
21. Kutz K, Pharmacology, toxicology and human pharmacokinetics of tropisetron. *Ann Oncol* 1993; **4**(Suppl 3): S15–18.
22. Miller RC, Galvan M, Gittos MW et al, Pharmacological properties of dolasetron, a potent and selective antagonist at 5-HT$_3$ receptors. *Drug Dev Res* 1993; **28**: 87–93.

23. Boeijinga PH, Galvan M, Baron BM et al, Characterization of the novel 5-HT₃ antagonist MDL 73147EF (dolasetron mesilate) and MDL 74156 in NG108-15 neuroblastoma × glioma cell. *Eur J Pharmacol* 1992; **219**: 9–13.

24. Andrews PLR, Bhandari P, Davey PT et al, Are all 5-HT₃ receptor antagonists the same? *Eur J Cancer* 1992; **28A**(Suppl 1): 2–6.

25. King GL, Emesis and defecations induced by the 5-hydroxytryptamine₃ (5-HT₃) receptor antagonist zacopride in the ferret. *J Pharmacol Exp Ther* 1990; **253**: 1034–41.

26. Fukuda T, Setoguchi M, Inaba K et al, The antiemetic profile of Y-25130, a new selective 5-HT₃ receptor antagonist. *Eur J Pharmacol* 1991; **196**: 299–305.

27. Sanger GJ, The pharmacology of anti-emetic agents. In: *Emesis in Anti-Cancer Therapy: Mechanisms and Treatment* (Andrews PLR, Sanger GJ, eds). London: Chapman & Hall, 1993: 179–210.

28. Middlefell VC, Price TL, 5-HT₃ receptor agonism may be responsible for the emetic effects of zacopride in the ferret. *Br J Pharmacol* 1991; **103**: 1011–12.

29. Bhandari P, Andrews PLR, Preliminary evidence for the involvement of the putative 5-HT₄ receptor in zacopride- and copper-sulphate-induced vomiting in the ferret. *Eur J Pharmacol* 1991; **204**: 273–80.

30. Freeman AJ, Cunningham KT, Tyers MB, Selectivity of 5-HT₃ receptor antagonists and anti-emetic mechanisms of action. *Anti-Cancer Drugs* 1992; **3**: 79–85.

31. Clarke DE, Craig DA, Fozard JR, The 5-HT₄ receptor: naughty but nice. *Trends Pharmacol Sci* 1989; **10**: 385–6.

32. Newberry NR, Watkins CJ, Sprosen TS et al, BRL 46470 potently antagonizes neural responses activated by 5-HT₃ receptors. *Neuropharmacology* 1993; **32**: 729–35.

33. Elliot P, Seemungal BM, Wallis DJ, Antagonism of the effects of 5-hydroxytryptamine on the rabbit isolated vagus nerve by BRL 43694 and metoclopramide. *Naunyn-Schmiedeberg's Arch Pharmacol* 1990; **341**: 503–9.

34. Csillik-Perczel V, Bakonyi A, Yemane T et al, GYKI-46903, a non-competitive antagonist for 5-HT₃ receptors. *Pharmacol Toxicol* 1996; **79**: 32–9.

35. Yarker YE, McTavish D, Granisetron: an update of its therapeutic use in nausea and vomiting induced by antineoplastic therapy. *Drugs* 1994; **48**: 761–93.

36. Wilde MI, Markham A, Ondansetron: a review of its pharmacology and preliminary clinical findings in novel applications. *Drugs* 1996; **52**: 773–94.

37. Galvan M, Claverie N, Hahne W, Pharmacology and metabolism of dolasetron mesilate. *Eur Hosp Pharmacy* 1996; **2**(Suppl 1): S12–14.

38. Sanwald P, David M, Dow J, Characterization of the cytochrome P450 enzymes involved in the in vitro metabolism of dolasetron. Comparison with other indole-containing 5-HT₃ antagonists. *Drug Metab Dispos* 1996; **24**: 602–9.

39. Bloomer JC, Baldwin SJ, Smith GJ et al, Characterisation of the cytochrome P450 enzymes involved in the in vitro metabolism of granisetron. *Br J Clin Pharmacol* 1994; **38**: 557–66.

40. Lee CR, Plosker GL, McTavish D, Tropisetron: a review of its pharmacodynamic and pharmacokinetic properties, and therapeutic potential as an antiemetic. *Drugs* 1993; **46**: 925–43.

41. De Bruijn KM, Tropisetron: a review of the clinical experience. *Drugs* 1992; **43**(Suppl 3): 11–22.

42. Marty M, d'Allens H et le Groupe Multicentrique Francais, Etude randomisée en double-insu comparant l'efficacité de l'ondansetron selon deux modes d'administration: injection unique et perfusion continue. *Cahiers Cancer* 1990; **2**: 541–6.

43. Seynaeve C, Schuller J, Buser K et al, Comparison of the anti-emetic efficacy of different doses of ondansetron, given as either a continuous infusion or a single intravenous dose, in acute cisplatin-induced emesis. A multi-centre, double-blind, randomised, parallel group study. *Br J Cancer* 1992; **66**: 192–7.

44. Beck TM, Hesketh PJ, Madajewicz S et al, Stratified, randomized, double-blind comparison of intravenous ondansetron administered as a multiple-dose regimen versus two single-dose regimens in the prevention of cisplatin-induced nausea and vomiting. *J Clin Oncol* 1992; **10**: 1969–75.

45. Ruff P, Paska W, Goedhals L et al, on behalf of the Ondansetron and Granisetron Emesis Study Group, Ondansetron compared with granisetron in the prophylaxis of cisplatin-induced acute emesis: a multicentre double-blind, randomised, parallel group study. *Oncology* 1994; **51**: 113–18.

46. Dicato MA, Oral treatment with ondansetron in an outpatient setting. *Eur J Cancer* 1991; **27**(Suppl 1): S18–19.

47. Riviere A, on behalf of The Granisetron Study Group, Dose finding study of granisetron in

patients receiving high-dose cisplatin chemotherapy. *Br J Cancer* 1994; **69**: 967–71.

48. Navari RM, Kaplan HG, Gralla RJ et al, Efficacy and safety of granisetron, a selective 5-hydroxy-tryptamine-3 receptor antagonist, in the prevention of nausea and vomiting induced by high-dose cisplatin. *J Clin Oncol* 1994; **12**: 2204–10.

49. Navari R, Gandara P, Hesketh P et al, Comparative clinical trial of granisetron and ondansetron in the prophylaxis of cisplatin-induced emesis. *J Clin Oncol* 1995; **13**: 1242–8.

50. Ettinger DS, Eisenberg PD, Fitts D et al, A double-blind comparison of the efficacy of two dose regimens of oral granisetron in preventing acute emesis in patients receiving moderately emetogenic chemotherapy. *Cancer* 1996; **78**: 144–51.

51. Van Belle SJP, Stamatakis L, Bleiberg H et al, Dose-finding study of tropisetron in cisplatin-induced nausea and vomiting. *Ann Oncol* 1994; **5**: 821–5.

52. Dogliotti L, Antonacci RA, Pazè E et al, Three years' experience with tropisetron in the control of nausea and vomiting in cisplatin-treated patients. *Drugs* 1992; **43**(Suppl 3): 6–10.

53. Thant M, Pendergrass K, Harman G et al, Double-blind, randomized study of the dose-response relationship across five single doses of i.v. dolasetron mesylate (DM) for prevention of acute nausea and vomiting after cisplatin chemotherapy (CCT). *Proc Am Soc Clin Oncol* 1996; **15**: 533 (abst).

54. Chevallier B, Cappelaere P, Splinter T et al, A double-blind, multicentre comparison of intravenous dolasetron mesylate and metoclopramide in the prevention of nausea and vomiting in cancer patients receiving high-dose cisplatin chemotherapy. *Support Care Cancer* 1997; **5**: 22–30.

55. Fauser AA, Bleiberg H, Chevallier B et al, A double-blind randomized, parallel study of i.v. dolasetron mesilate versus i.v. metoclopramide in patients receiving moderately emetogenic chemotherapy. *Cancer J* 1996; **9**: 196–202.

56. Hesketh P, Navari R, Grote T et al, Double-blind, randomized comparison of the antiemetic efficacy of intravenous dolasetron mesylate and intravenous ondansetron in the prevention of acute cisplatin-induced emesis in patients with cancer. *J Clin Oncol* 1996; **14**: 2242–9.

57. Audhuy B, Cappelaere P, Martin M et al, A double-blind, randomised comparison of the anti-emetic efficacy of two intravenous doses of dolasetron mesilate and granisetron in patients receiving high dose cisplatin chemotherapy. *Eur J Cancer* 1996; **32A**: 807–13.

58. Harman GS, Omura GA, Ryan K et al, A randomized, double-blind comparison of single-dose and divided multiple-dose dolasetron for cisplatin-induced emesis. *Cancer Chemother Pharmacol* 1996; **38**: 323–8.

59. Rubinstein E, Fauser A, Grote T et al, Determination of optimal dolasetron mesylate (DM) dose in prevention of acute nausea and vomiting (ANV) after moderately emetogenic chemotherapy (MECT) using pooled data from three pivotal trials. *Proc Am Soc Clin Oncol* 1996; **15**: 532 (abst).

60. Lofters WS, Zee B, Dolasetron (DOL) vs ondansetron (OND) with and without dexamethasone (DEX) in the prevention of nausea (N) and vomiting (V) in patients (PTS) receiving moderately emetogenic chemotherapy. *Support Care Cancer* 1995; **3**: 338 (abst).

61. Herrstedt J, Sigsgaard T, Handberg J et al, Randomized, double-blind comparison of ondansetron versus ondansetron plus metopimazine as antiemetic prophylaxis during platinum-based chemotherapy in patients with cancer. *J Clin Oncol* 1997; **15**: 1690–6.

62. Herrstedt J, Sigsgaard T, Boesgaard M et al, Ondansetron plus metopimazine compared with ondansetron alone in patients receiving moderately emetogenic chemotherapy. *N Engl J Med* 1993; **328**: 1076–80.

63. Depierre A, Lebeau B, Chevallier B, Votan B, Efficacy of ondansetron (O), methylprednisolone (M) plus metopimazine (MPZ) in patients previously uncontrolled with dual therapy in cisplatin containing chemotherapy. *Ann Oncol* 1996; **7**(Suppl 5): 134 (abst).

64. Bregni M, Siena S, Di Nicola M et al, Tropisetron plus haloperidol to ameliorate nausea and vomiting associated with high-dose alkylating agent cancer chemotherapy. *Eur J Cancer* 1991; **27**: 561–5.

65. Tsukuda M, Furukawa S, Kokatsu T et al, Comparison of granisetron alone and granisetron plus hydroxyzine hydrochloride for prophylactic treatment of emesis induced by cisplatin chemotherapy. *Eur J Cancer* 1995; **31A**: 1647–9.

66. Herrstedt J, We still need common criteria for the assessment of nausea and vomiting. *Eur J Cancer* 1994; **30A**: 1217.

67. Gebbia V, Cannata G, Testa A et al, Ondansetron versus granisetron in the prevention of chemotherapy-induced nausea and vomiting. *Cancer* 1994; **74**: 1945–52.

68. Italian Group for Antiemetic Research, Ondansetron versus granisetron, both combined with dexamethasone, in the prevention of cisplatin-induced emesis. *Ann Oncol* 1995; **6**: 805–10.

69. Mantovani G, Macciò A, Bianchi A et al, Comparison of granisetron, ondansetron, and tropisetron in the prophylaxis of acute nausea and vomiting induced by cisplatin for the treatment of head and neck cancer: a randomized controlled trial. *Cancer* 1996; **77**: 941–8.

70. Martoni A, Angelelli B, Guaraldi M et al, An open randomised cross-over study on granisetron versus ondansetron in the prevention of acute emesis induced by moderate dose cisplatin-containing regimens. *Eur J Cancer* 1996; **32A**: 82–5.

71. Marty M, Kleisbauer J-P, Fournel P et al, Is Navoban® (tropisetron) as effective as Zofran® (ondansetron) in cisplatin-induced emesis? *Anti-Cancer Drugs* 1995; **6**(Suppl 1): 15–21.

72. Noble A, Bremer K, Goedhals L et al, on behalf of the Granisetron Study Group, A double-blind, randomised, crossover comparison of granisetron and ondansetron in 5-day fractionated chemotherapy: assessment of efficacy, safety and patient preference. *Eur J Cancer* 1994; **30A**: 1083–8.

73. Bonneterre J, Hecquet B, on behalf of The French Northern Oncology Group, Granisetron (IV) compared with ondansetron (iv plus oral) in the prevention of nausea and vomiting induced by moderately emetogenic chemotherapy. A cross-over study. *Bull Cancer* 1995; **82**: 1038–43.

74. Campora E, Simoni C, Rosso R, Tropisetron verso ondansetron nella prevenzione e controllo dell'emesi in pazienti sottoposte a chemioterapia con FAC/FEC per carcinoma mammario metastatico o operato. *Minerva Med* 1994; **85**: 25–31.

75. Fauser AA, Duclos B, Chemaissani A et al, Therapeutic equivalence of single oral doses of dolasetron mesilate and multiple doses of ondansetron for the prevention of emesis after moderately emetogenic chemotherapy. *Eur J Cancer* 1996; **32A**: 1523–9.

76. Jantunen IT, Kataja VV, Johansson RT, Ondansetron and tropisetron with dexamethasone in the prophylaxis of acute vomiting induced by non-cisplatin-containing chemotherapy. *Acta Oncol* 1992; **31**: 573–5.

77. Jantunen IT, Muhonen TT, Kataja VV et al, 5-HT₃ receptor antagonists in the prophylaxis of acute vomiting induced by moderately emetogenic chemotherapy – a randomised study. *Eur J Cancer* 1993; **29A**: 1669–72.

78. Massida B, Laconi S, Foddi MR et al, Prevention of non-cisplatin induced emesis: role of the antagonists of 5-HT₃ receptors. *Ann Oncol* 1994; **5**(Suppl 8): 204 (abst).

79. Perez EA, Lembersky B, Kaywin P et al, Intravenous (iv) granisetron vs ondansetron in the prevention of cyclophosphamide–doxorubicin-induced emesis in breast cancer patients: a double-blind crossover study. *Proc Am Soc Clin Oncol* 1996; **15**: 543 (abst).

80. Pion JM, Fournier C, Darloy F et al, Oral granisetron vs oral ondansetron, a comparative double-blind cross-over multicenter study of preventive anti-emetic in moderately emetogenic chemotherapy by The French Northern Oncology Group (FNOG). *Proc Am Soc Clin Oncol* 1996; **15**: 530 (abst).

81. Stewart A, McQuade B, Cronje JDE et al, Ondansetron compared with granisetron in the prophylaxis of cyclophosphamide-induced emesis in out-patients: a multicentre, double-blind, double-dummy, randomised, parallel-group study. *Oncology* 1995; **52**: 202–10.

82. Bianchi A, Macciò A, Curreli L et al, Comparison of granisetron vs ondansetron vs tropisetron in the prophylaxis of acute nausea and vomiting induced by high-dose cisplatin for treatment of primary head and neck cancer: an open randomized controlled trial. *Ann Oncol* 1996; **7**(Suppl 5): 135 (abst).

83. Cho JY, Park JO, Rha SY et al, A comparative study of granisetron i.v. versus ondansetron i.v./oral in the prevention of nausea and vomiting associated with moderately emetogenic chemotherapy. *Ann Oncol* 1996; **7**(Suppl 5): 142 (abst).

84. Massida B, Ionta MT, The 5-HT₃-receptor-antagonists in the prevention of acute and delayed emesis induced by standard or accelerated chemotherapy for breast cancer. *Support Care Cancer* 1996; **4**: 250 (abst).

85. Mylonakis N, Tsavaris N, Karabelis A et al, A randomized comparative study of antiemetic activity of ondansetron (Ond) vs tropisetron (Tr) in patients receiving moderately emetogenic chemotherapy. *Support Care Cancer* 1996; **4**: 252 (abst).

86. Tsavaris N, Kosmas C, Samarkos M et al, Randomized comparative study of antiemetic activity of metoclopramide (M) vs ondansetron (Od) vs tropisetron (T) vs granisetron (G) in patients receiving moderately emetogenic chemotherapy. *Support Care Cancer* 1996; **4**: 252 (abst).

87. Crenier L, Lemoine F, Bastin G et al, A comparative study on the efficacy of the different 5-HT$_3$ antagonists to control acute emesis in blood stem cells transplantation. *Support Care Cancer* 1996; **4**: 253 (abst).

88. Harris E, Hakimian D, Dempsey C, Clark C, Comparative outcomes of granisetron and ondansetron for prevention of chemotherapy induced nausea and vomiting. *Proc Am Soc Clin Oncol* 1996; **15**: 540 (abst).

89. Spina M, Valentini M, Fedele P et al, Randomized comparison of granisetron vs ondansetron in patients with HIV-related non-Hodgkin's lymphoma (HIV-NHL) receiving moderately emetogenic chemotherapy (CT) regimens. *Proc Am Soc Clin Oncol* 1995; **14**: 532 (abst).

90. Aapro MS, Are there any true clinical differences between 5-HT$_3$ receptor antagonists? In: *Serotonin and the Scientific Basis of Anti-Emetic Therapy* (Reynolds DJM, Andrews PLR, Davis CJ, eds). Oxford: Oxford Clinical Communications, 1995: 164–72.

91. Tonato M, Roila F, Principles of supportive care. Antiemetics. In: *Textbook of Medical Oncology* (Cavalli F, Hansen HH, Kaye SB, eds). London: Martin Dunitz, 1997: 363–72.

Quality of life

Stein Kaasa

INTRODUCTION

Most people have an intuitive understanding of the term 'quality of life' (QOL). It is related to an individual's experience of his or her life and living situation. It is a subjective individual issue, and is not directly observable or measurable. Therefore the concept has to be defined, operationalized and developed in order to be measurable in a scientific way.

In the social sciences QOL was introduced as an indicator of social progress in the late 1950s and early 1960s.[1,2] These subjective measures were introduced in addition to the more traditional indicators, such as economic welfare. A decade or two later, in health-care research, assessments of physical, emotional and social aspects of life were performed in patients with advanced breast cancer.[3] In contrast to previous measures, such as the Karnofsky Performance Status,[4] the method of Priestman and Baum[3] method was a patient rating scale. This study actually used the recommendations of Karnofsky from 1949. Furthermore, it showed that important information may be obtained by asking patients to complete questionnaires directly instead of the regular patriarcathic method 'through the doctor'. During the last few decades, a large number of measures of QOL have been developed and validated specifically for health care.

Anecdotal evidence suggests that nausea and vomiting may have major impact on patients' QOL. Patients have reported that nausea and vomiting are their first concern when receiving chemotherapy.[5] Unfortunately, the study in question was performed almost 15 years ago, before the new antiemetics were developed. Furthermore, the interpretation of the impact of chemotherapy may also have changed during these years, both from a health-care perspective and from a patient perspective. When considering this type of information, whether one is a patient or a doctor may dramatically influence the answer. For example, in studies assessing treatment intensity, side-effects and expected outcome, the discrepancies between nurses and doctors on one side and patients on the other are substantial.

The impact of acute and long-term toxicities on patients' QOL have been explored in some studies[6,7] with different designs, goals, outcome measures, antineoplastic treatment and antiemetic treatment. It seems, however, that patients may tolerate treatment-related toxicity better than was first expected.

The introduction of 5-hydroxytryptamine (5-HT$_3$) receptor antagonists has had a major impact on the control of chemotherapy- and radiotherapy-induced nausea and vomiting. The acute effect seems to be superior to the late effect. Between 55% and 75% of patients receiving 5-HT$_3$ antagonist and dexamethasone in a Canadian survey experienced vomiting or nausea during the first week after treatment.[8] Several factors associated with post-treatment nausea and vomiting have been described, such as type of chemotherapy, site of radiation, female gender, young age, pre-existing anxiety and nausea, low alcohol consumption, motion sickness and previous experience with emetogenic treatment.

QOL has been shown to be a major predictor of survival in patients with advanced cancer.[9,10] Correlations have been documented between QOL domains and emesis. Therefore it is reasonable to ask whether QOL can be used as a predictor, for example, for post-chemotherapy nausea and vomiting. Relationships between emesis and QOL have been assessed in some studies;[11,12] however, large prospective studies are rare.

In order to better understand patients' QOL, well-conducted studies with high compliance rate should be performed. Identical or similar outcome measures should be used in repeated studies in order to compare data. Furthermore, these measures should be tested for validity and reliability. The scoring methods and the ways in which the data are reported should also be standardized.

A better clinical understanding of the measure should be given high priority, including norms for non-cancer populations. This chapter will focus primarily on how to measure QOL in cancer patients, QOL and emesis, and finally QOL data from a normal Norwegian population. Further details on measurement of QOL in clinical trials, are given in references 13 and 14.

HEALTH-RELATED QOL

The WHO definition of health[15] and the Karnofsky Performance Status have, in a broad sense, coloured the definition of QOL in oncology and health care in general. Health-related QOL (HRQOL) is defined as a multidimensional concept consisting of physical, social and emotional (psychological) dimensions. These dimensions have been broken down further into subdimensions, such as physical concerns, functional ability, family well-being, emotional well-being, spirituality, treatment satisfaction, future orientation, sexuality/intimacy, social function and occupational function.

Measures

In selecting measures in clinical studies, the issues most likely to be affected by the cancer and/or the treatment should be included. Whenever possible, patients' self-reported data should be collected. Most researchers have therefore agreed upon the use of questionnaires. However, in some studies, diary cards may be used to collect details of single symptoms, such as emesis or pain. It may be a difficult task for clinicians to select the appropriate measure to use in a given trial. A series of methods have been developed and tested. Recommendations with regard to the use of measures have been given by several cooperative groups. These recommendations are partly based upon the content, the layout, the scoring procedure and the development process of the various instruments.

The different instruments can be divided into cancer-specific measures, general (generic) health measures, and more-specific measures, such as scales measuring anxiety/depression, coping, family support, spiritual well-being, emesis, etc. It is outside the scope of this chapter to give a detailed overview of all these measures. However, those used most frequently in oncology will be discussed.

There is no gold-standard instrument for measuring cancer-related QOL. However, it seems worthwhile to concentrate on as few measures as possible in cancer clinical trials in order to be able to compare data between studies. The methods should be multidimensional, having a standard format, and scoring procedures, and ideally being cross-culturally developed and validated. Furthermore, it may also be reasonable to choose measures used in earlier studies on similar populations.

Generic measures evaluate health and/or psychosocial related issues. Many of these have been used in a variety of studies; however, one limitation is that many of these methods, such as the Sickness Impact Profile,[16] are lengthy and not optimal for use in clinical trials. Some of the generic measures, such as the SF-36 Health Survey (SF-36),[17] the Nottingham Health Profile[18] and the Quality of Life Well Being Scale,[19] are shorter and may be used in clinical trials. The SF-36 has been translated and validated in the International Quality of Life Assessment (IQOLA) Project.[20] It has now been translated into 11 languages and has been cross-culturally validated. In addition, researchers from more than 25 other countries are translating and validating the SF-36 using IQOLA Project methods.

CANCER-SPECIFIC INSTRUMENTS

In recent years, efforts have been made to design and validate cancer-specific instruments. These include the Functional Living Index – Cancer (FLIC),[21] the Rotterdam Symptom Check List (RSLC),[22] the Cancer Rehabilitation Evaluating System (CARES),[23] the EORTC Core Quality of Life Questionnaire (EORTC QLQ-

Table 12.1 Content areas of the EORTC QLQ-C30

Quality of life domains	Number of items within scales/single items
Functioning scales/items	
Physical	5
Role	2
Emotional	4
Cognitive	2
Social	2
Global quality of life	2
Symptom scales/items	
Fatigue	3
Nausea and vomiting	2
Pain	2
Dyspnoea	1
Sleep disturbance	1
Appetite loss	1
Constipation	1
Diarrhoea	1
Financial impact	1
TOTAL	30

C30),[24] and Functional Assessment of Cancer Therapy – General (FACT-G).[25] All of these instruments have been used in various cancer clinical trials. The last two are the most recently developed, and are now widely used in Europe and in the USA.

EORTC QLQ-C30 and modules

The EORTC is one of the largest and oldest clinical trials groups in Europe. An early goal of the Study Group on Quality of Life within the EORTC was to achieve consensus on how to measure and to develop measures for QOL.[26] Because of the absence of other well-validated cancer-specific QOL instruments consisting of multidimensional subscales and not yielding a single measure, a long-term process of instrument development was started. The Core Quality of Life instrument consisting of 30 items was developed and tested. This instrument consists of six functioning scales, three symptom scales and six single items (Table 12.1). The reliability of the QLQ-C30 has been confirmed in several studies measuring its internal consistency,[24,27–33] and, in one study, measuring the test/retest reliability.[34] The validity has been assessed by examining the QLQ's ability to distinguish between subgroups of patients found on the basis of their clinical or treatment status (so-called known-group comparisons). Two studies[28,35] have tested the validity of the construct by correlating the QLQ-C30 with a general health questionnaire. On the basis of data from the reliability and validity studies, the QLQ-C30 has undergone minor modifications. The latest version of the QLQ-C30, Version 3.0 has a new role-functioning scale yielding highly satisfactory reliability. Furthermore, the physical and role-functioning scale in Version 3.0 has been changed to a Likert-type response set rather, as earlier, being dichotomized.

The QLQ-C30 has been translated into 27 languages (Table 12.2), and has been found to be cross-culturally reliable and valid. A scoring manual is produced by the Study Group on Quality of Life, which includes information about various versions of the instrument, modules, scoring procedures, handling of missing data, etc.[36]

Table 12.2 Overview of the translation of the EORTC QLQ-C30, Version 2.0 (April 1997)

Language	Status
African	In preparation
Bulgarian	Final
Chinese	Final
Croatian	In preparation
Czech	Final
Danish	Final
Dutch	Final
English	Final
Finnish	Final
French	Final
German	Final
Greek	Final
Hebrew	Final
Hungarian	Final
Italian	Final
Japanese	Final
Korean	Pending
Lithuanian	In preparation
Malaysian	Pending
Norwegian	Final
Polish	Final
Portuguese	Final
Brazilian Portuguese	Final
Romanian	In preparation
Russian	Final
Serbian	Final
Slovak	Final
Slovenian	Final
Sotho	In preparation
Spanish	Final
American Spanish	Final
Argentinian Spanish	Final
Swedish	Final
Turkish	Final

Modules

The core questionnaire, EORTC QLQ-C30, has been developed for use in all types of cancer populations in order to allow comparisons of data between studies and diagnosis. A disadvantage of such a 'generic cancer measure' may be its inability to measure disease and/or study specific aspects of QOL. Therefore a modular approach was chosen. Disease-specific modules have been rigorously developed in accordance with standardized guidelines.[37] The modules can provide more detailed information relevant to QOL in specific patient populations, such as disease symptoms related to specific tumour site (head and neck, prostate, etc.), side-effects associated with given treatment (radiation and/or mucosites), or specific domains associated with disease and/or treatment (sexuality, body image, spirituality, family support, etc.).

Four modules have been cross-culturally developed and validated. These are the Lung Cancer Module (QLQ-LC13),[38] the Breast Cancer Module (QLQ-BR23),[39] the Head and Neck Cancer Module (QLQ-H&N37)[40] and the Oesophageal Cancer Module (QLQ-OES24).[41] Furthermore, a series of other modules are in the process of being finalized, such as a palliative-care module, a body image module, a sexuality module, a gynaecological cancer module, a colorectal cancer module, a bladder cancer module and a prostate cancer module.

The EORTC QLQ-C30 and modules are copyrighted, and may not be used without prior consent from the Quality of Life Unit at the EORTC Data Centre.†

Functional assessment of cancer therapy (FACT-G)

FACT-G was developed in the English language (in the USA) as an approach to measure self-reported HRQOL in cancer clinical trials. It has been tested and revised, and the third ver-

sion (FACT Version 3)[42] is now available. It consists of five domains: physical well-being (seven items), social well-being (seven items), emotional well-being (six items), relationship with doctor (two items) and functional well-being (seven items). Five additional experimental items collecting information about how much each domain affects QOL is added. There are currently twelve disease-specific subscales, which are intended to use only in conjunction with FACT-G (Table 12.3).[42] FACT has been translated into a number of languages, including Dutch, French, German, Italian, Norwegian, Swedish, Spanish and Canadian French.

HRQOL CANCER-SPECIFIC SCALES: COMMENTS

No gold standard can be recommended to measure HRQOL in malignant disease. Two of the most recent developed measures, the EORTC QLQ-C30 and FACT-G, are similar in some ways. Both are multidimensional, and consist of scales measuring domains of physical, social and psychological nature. Both generate subscales for specific domains, in contrast to the FLIC (which was developed much earlier), where all QOL domains are scored as an overall measure. Using the scoring system in the FLIC, information may be lost, and the instrument's ability to detect differences between groups may be reduced. Both the EORTC QLQ-C30 and FACT-G have developed modules or subscales to be used in conjunction with a core (general) instrument. Very few, if any, direct head-to-head comparison between the QLQ-C30 and FACT-G have been well performed. Therefore it is difficult to determine on the basis of empirical evidence which of the two instruments should be used in a given situation. The same also goes for other cancer-specific instruments, such as the FLIC, RSCL and CARES. It is therefore recommended that a careful review be undertaken of all available instruments with regard to content, layout and quality of translation. Furthermore, in order to make comparisons, existing data in similar cancer groups may also be taken into consideration when

†EORTC Data Centre, Avenue E Meunier 83, 1200 Brussels, Belgium (Fax +32 2 772 35 45; Tel +32 2 774 16 61).

Table 12.3 FACT-G

Cancer subscales	Cancer treatment subscales
Bladder cancer	Biological response modifier and/or retinoid therapy
Brain cancer	Bone marrow transplantation
Breast cancer	Chemotherapy neurotoxity
Central nervous system	
Cervical cancer	**Cancer/HIV subscales**
Colorectal cancer	Anorexia/cachexia
Head and neck cancer	Faecal incontinence
Lung cancer	Fatigue/anemia
Oesophageal cancer	
Ovarian cancer	**Additional subscales**
Pancreatic cancer	Benign urinary incontinence (FAIT)
Prostate cancer	HIV infection (FAHI)
	Multiple sclerosis (FAMS)
	Non-life-threatening conditions (FANLT)
	Spirituality

decisions are made about which instrument to use.

NORM DATA: EORTC QLQ-C30

Values representing the normal population are often absent for HRQOL measures. Such norms may be used as a guideline when interpreting scores obtained in different patient populations and as a standard when HRQOL measures are used in resource allocation. Studies have been published presenting normal values for generic instruments such as SF-36,[43] GHQ[44] and NHP.[45]

In order to obtain norms, a Norwegian population-based sample was chosen randomly from the Norwegian Population Registry.[46] A total of 3000 was approached, receiving a survey package consisting of the EORTC QLQ-C30 and a form asking about sociodemographic data, and past or present illness and health.

A response rate of 68% was obtained. The internal consistency measured by the Cronbach alpha coefficients was satisfactory for most scales. The mean scales for the entire population and male and female genders are given in Table 12.4 and Figure 12.1. Men reported better function on all scales. Function was reduced and symptoms were increased with increasing age (for more details see original publication[46]). Factors such as education and employment, living situation (including marital status) also seemed to have influence in some of the scales within the QLQ-C30.

The trends regarding the distribution of scores related to sociodemographic variables were comparable to those seen in data from other population surveys exploring general instruments. Age seemed to influence the scores in the cohort, with a gradual decline in mean scores for all functioning scales except 'emotional'. This may be a natural process, and, together with others (i.e. education and living situation), should be taken into consideration when interpretation and comparison of QOL data between studies is performed. The data may serve as guidelines when comparing results from cancer patients. Cancer popula-

Table 12.4 EORTC QLQ-C30: mean scores on scales and items for all respondents by gender

	Male (n = 1016)	Female (n = 949)	Total (n = 1965)
Functioning scales[a]			
Cognitive	87.7	86.8	86.5
Emotional	85.4	80.8	82.8
Physical	93.2	88.2	90.0
Role	93.4	93.9	92.8
Role, new	85.7	80.6	83.3
Social	87.7	84.8	85.8
Global QOL[a]	75.4	70.3	73.7
Global health QOL[a]	77.3	71.8	15.3
Symptom scales[b]			
Fatigue	25.0	31.7	28.8
Nausea/vomiting	2.9	4.2	4.0
Pain	16.9	23.4	20.5
Single items[b]			
Appetite loss	5.7	8.3	7.5
Constipation	7.1	13.4	10.7
Diarrhoea	9.3	8.0	9.4
Dyspnoea	13.4	14.0	14.3
Financial impact	7.3	9.6	9.0
Sleep disturbance	15.5	24.6	20.4

[a] Higher score indicates better function.
[b] Higher score indicates more symptoms.

tions have substantially lower scores on functioning scales, and report more symptoms, depending upon stage of disease, treatment received and tumour progression. For example, in comparing the norm data with a cohort of patients with malignant myeloma,[47] the difference exceeded 10 for 8 of the 15 scales/items, with the largest difference being for role functioning and overall QOL.

It has been debated what to consider as a clinical significant difference in the various scales within the EORTC QLQ-C30. Some investigators have argued that a difference of

10–15 may be of substantial value. The norm data may give a similar indication. However, more empirical data are necessary before any final recommendation can be given.

In a normal population emesis is an infrequent symptom compared for example with pain and fatigue. Data from the normal Norwegian cohort on the emesis scale are shown in Tables 12.5(A) and (B). The mean score on the emesis scale is very low, 4.0 (SD 12.1), which corresponds to only 4% of the population giving a rating of 'quite a bit' or 'very much' for the nausea item. As expected with

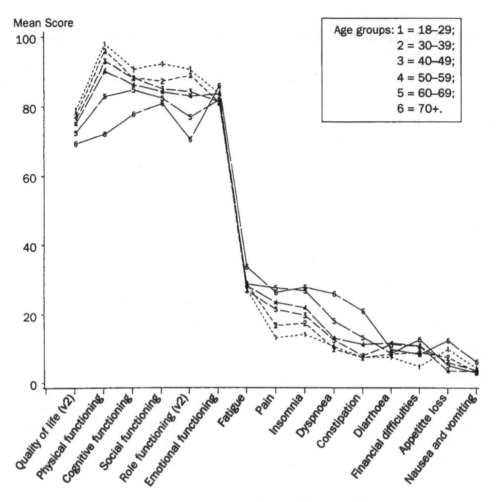

Figure 12.1 Mean age profiles for scale and item scores of the EORTC QLQ-C30 (+3)

such a low prevalence, emesis has a low correlation with overall QOL ($r = 0.3$), while pain and fatigue have correlations of 0.6 and 0.7 respectively.

While nausea and vomiting are of less importance in a normal population, patients with cancer frequently report these very distressing symptoms. In the National Hospice Study,[48] 62% of terminal patients reported nausea and vomiting at some time during their last six weeks of life. The prevalence has been estimated to be at least 40%. In advanced cancer these symptoms develop independently of chemotherapy, and are probably due directly or indirectly to the

tumour. In contrast to chemotherapy-induced emesis, the impact of 5-HT$_3$ antagonists on emesis in this patient population is questionable. The pathophysiological basis of the symptoms is not well understood; therefore optimal treatment strategies are difficult to design.

QOL AND EMESIS

In all cancer-specific HRQOL measures, emesis is incorporated as one of several questions. For example, in QLQ-C30, two questions make up the so-called nausea and vomiting scale, asking

Table 12.5(A) Mean and median scores of the EORTC QLQ-C30 in a normal Norwegian population

	Mean	SD
Pain	20.5	(27.3)
Nausea, vomiting	4.0	(12.1)
Fatigue	28.8	(24.4)
Quality of life	75.3	(23.4)

Table 12.5(B) Normal Norwegian population: percentage of population in the various cells of the four-point Likert scale

	Not at all	A little	Quite a bit	Very much
Pain	55	26	14	5
Nausea	88	10	3	1
Tired	33	45	15	7

about the experience of these two symptoms during the last week on a four-point Likert scale.

There is no doubt that emesis is an important symptom of cancer and its treatment. It may be hypothesized that the cause of emesis may have major impact on patients' interpretation of the symptom and that it has a major influence on QOL. Detailed prospective analyses of the impact of nausea and vomiting on overall QOL are rare. In a cohort of 294 patients with breast cancer treated at the Royal Marsden Hospital, UK between 1986 and 1987, the influence of emesis on overall QOL was assessed.[49] Emesis was measured using a linear analogue scale, and overall QOL using the Uniscale. By using a multiple-regression model, relationships between various QOL dimensions, namely activity of daily living, symptoms, emotional well-being, nausea/vomiting, appearance/ attractiveness and overall QOL, were assessed. The only variable not to explain significant Uniscale variance was nausea/vomiting. Only a minority of these patients (62/294) were currently

receiving chemotherapy. Later in the questionnaire, it was asked specifically how these symptoms were experienced over the last 24 hours. The finding may be a reflection of the importance of emesis in a general cancer population, not reflecting the acute phase of the chemotherapy.

In another report the consequences of chemotherapy-induced emesis were studied in 122 patients from an outpatient oncological unit. The FLIC was used to measure HRQOL while the functional living index emesis (FLIE),[50] which was specifically developed to evaluate chemotherapy-induced nausea and vomiting, was assessed to measure these symptoms. Data from this study indicated that symptoms of post-chemotherapy nausea and vomiting impact upon patients' normal function. A significant reduction in HRQOL (FLIC scores) was seen in patients who experienced emesis. In the group of patients who did not experience emesis, HRQOL was not significantly reduced between baseline and three days post-chemotherapy.

The effect of chemotherapy-induced emesis may be influenced by factors such as pre-chemotherapy HRQOL,[51] coping mechanism and treatment intention.[52] It has been hypothesized that disease prognosis may be an important factor influencing how patients perceive their treatment. When the treatment is given with a palliative intention, it seems of major importance to keep the unpleasant symptoms at a minimum. However, even in patients with locally advanced lung cancer, low correlations were found between treatment-related factors and overall QOL.[53] In contrast much higher correlations were found between treatment-related symptoms and overall QOL. These unexpected findings may indicate that the individual patient's perception of symptoms may differ from that of the health-care professions.

Studies evaluating the relationship between emesis and overall QOL may shed light on the understanding of distress related to cancer treatment and the disease itself. With the availability of improved control of chemotherapy-related emesis using 5-HT$_3$ receptor antagonists in combination with other drugs, emesis may have a lower impact on overall QOL. However, before any final conclusions can be drawn, prospective large studies assessing the relationship between emesis and HRQOL should be undertaken.

HRQOL as a predictor of emesis

As mentioned previously, the possible association between HRQOL and emesis has been assessed in several studies.[49,50,54] In order to improve the treatment of emesis during cancer treatment, the ability to predict patients at higher risk may improve emetic control. In a Canadian study, Osoba et al[8] used data from a large cohort consisting of 832 chemotherapy naive patients. HRQOL was measured using the EORTC QLQ-C30 within seven days prior to chemotherapy. In the univariate analysis ten of the HRQOL measures were associated with post-chemotherapy emesis. In order to develop a model of predictive characteristics to explore post-chemotherapy emesis, HRQOL measures plus patient and treatment characteristics were considered in a multivariate regression model. Low social function, pre-existing nausea, emetogenecity of chemotherapy, the use of maintenance antiemetics and female gender were associated with both nausea and vomiting post chemotherapy. In a risk-factor analysis, the incidents of post-chemotherapy nausea increased from 20% in those having no risk factors to 76% of those having any four of the actual risk factors. These data show the importance of measuring HRQOL in cancer chemotherapy. A suggestion would be to use HRQOL indicators in future studies to replicate these findings and shed further light on the association between HRQOL and emesis.

ACKNOWLEDGEMENTS

I should like to thank Marianne Jensen Hjermstad for support with data from the EORTC QLQ-C30 Norwegian Norm Study and Helene Flottorp for work with the manuscript.

REFERENCES

1. Bradburn NM, Caplovitz D, *Reports on Happiness. A Pilot Study of Behavior Related to Mental Health.* Chicago: Aldine, 1965.
2. Andrews FM, Whitey SB, *Social indicators of Well-Being: Americans' Perception of Life Quality.* New York: Plenum, 1976.
3. Priestman TJ, Baum M, Evaluation of quality of life in patients receiving treatment for advanced breast cancer. *Lancet* 1976; ii: 899–901.
4. Karnofsky DA, Abelmann WH, Craver LF, Burchenal JH, The use of nitrogen mustards in the palliative treatment of carcinoma. With particular reference to bronchogenic carcinoma. *Cancer* 1948; 1: 634–56.
5. Coates A, Abrahams S, Kaye S et al, On the receiving end – patient perception of the side effects of cancer chemotherapy. *Eur J Cancer Oncol* 1983; 19: 203–8.

6. Earl HM, Rudd RM, Spiro SG et al, A randomised trial of planned versus as required chemotherapy in small cell lung cancer: a Cancer Research Campaign trial. *Br J Cancer* 1991; **64**: 566–72.

7. Coates AS, Gebski V, Signorini D et al, for the Australian New Zealand Breast Cancer Trials Group, Prognostic value of quality of life scores during chemotherapy for advanced breast cancer. *J Clin Oncol* 1992; **10**: 1833–8.

8. Osoba D, Zee B, Pater J et al, for the Quality of Life and Symptom Control Committees of the National Cancer Institute of Canada Clinical Trials Group, Determinants of postchemotherapy nausea and vomiting on patients with cancer. *J Clin Oncol* 1997; **15**: 116–23.

9. Kaasa S, Mastekaasa A, Lund E, Prognostic factors for patients with inoperable non-small cell lung cancer, limited disease. The importance of patients' subjective experience of disease and psychosocial wellbeing. *Radiother Oncol* 1989; **15**: 235–42.

10. Ganz PA, Lee JJ, Siau J, Quality of life assessment. An independent prognostic variable for survival in lung cancer. *Cancer* 1991; **67**: 3131–5.

11. Lindley CM, Hirsch JD, O'Neill CV et al, Quality of life consequences of chemotherapy-induced emesis. *Qual Life Res* 1992; **1**: 331–40.

12. O'Brien BJ, Rusthoven J, Rochi A et al, Impact of chemotherapy-associated nausea and vomiting on patient's functional status and costs: survey of five Canadian centres. *Can Med Assoc J* 1993; **149**: 296–302.

13. Spilker B (ed.), *Quality of Life and Pharmacoeconomics in Clinical Trials.* Philadelphia: Lippincott–Raven, 1996.

14. Osoba D, *Effect of Cancer on Quality of Life.* Boston: CRC Press, 1991.

15. The Constitution of the World Health Organization. *WHO Chronicle* 1947; 29.

16. Bergner M, Bobbit RA, Carter WB, Gilson BS. The Sickness Impact Profile; development and final revision of a health status measure. *Med Care* 1981; **19**: 787–805.

17. Ware JE, Sherbourne CD, The MOS 36-item Short-Form Health Status Survey (SF-36): 1. Conceptual framework and item selection. *Med Care* 1992; **30**: 473–83.

18. Hunt SM, McKanna SP, McEwen J et al, The Nottingham Health Profile: subjective health status and medical consultations. *Soc Sci Med* 1981; **15A**: 221–9.

19. Kaplan RM, Feeny D, Revicki DA, Methods for assessing relative importance in preference based outcome measures. *Qual Life Res* 1993; **2**: 467–75.

20. Ware JE, Keller SD, Gandek B et al, for the IQOLA Project Group. Evaluating transplantations of health status questionnaires. Methods from the IQOLA Project. *Int J Techn Assessm Health Care* 1995; **11**: 525–51.

21. Schipper H, Clinch J, McMurray A et al, Measuring the quality of life of cancer patients: The Functional Living Index – Cancer: development and validation. *J Clin Oncol* 1984; **2**: 472–83.

22. de Haes JC, van Knippenberg FJ, Neijt JP, Measuring psychological and physical distress in cancer patients: structure and application of the Rotterdam Symptom Check List. *Br J Cancer* 1990; **62**: 1034–8.

23. Schag CAC, Ganz PA, Heinrich RL, Cancer Rehabilitation Evaluation System – Short Form (CARES-SF): a cancer specific rehabilitation and quality of life instrument. *Cancer* 1991; **68**: 1406–13.

24. Aaronson NK, Ahmedzai S, Bergman B et al, The European Organization for Research and Treatment of Cancer QLQ-C30: a quality of life instrument for use in international clinical trials in oncology. *J Natl Cancer Inst* 1993; **85**: 365–76.

25. Cella DF, Tulsky DS, Gray F et al, The Functional Assessment of Cancer Therapy scale: development and validation of the general measure. *J Clin Oncol* 1993; **11**: 570–9.

26. Aaronson NK, Cull AM, Kaasa S, Sprangers MAG, The European Organization for Research and Treatment of Cancer (EORTC). Modular approach to quality of life assessment in oncology: an update. In: *Quality of Life and Pharmacoeconomics in Clinical Trials*, 2nd edn (Spilker B, ed.). Philadelphia: Lippincott–Raven, 1996: 179–89.

27. Kaasa S, Bjordal K, Aaronson N et al, The EORTC Core Quality of Life Questionnaire QLQ-C30: validity and reliability when analysed with patients treated with palliative radiotherapy. *Eur J Cancer* 1995; **31A**: 2260–3.

28. Bjordal K, Kaasa S, Psychometric validation of the EORTC Core Quality of Life Questionnaire, 30-iem version and a diagnosis-specific module for head and neck cancer patients. *Acta Oncol* 1992; **31**: 311–21.

29. Bjordal K, Kaasa S, Mastekaasa A, Quality of life in patients treated for head and neck cancer: a follow-up study 7 to 11 years after radiotherapy. *Int J Radiat Oncol Biol Phys* 1994; **28**: 847–56.

30. de Boer JB, Sprangers MAG, Aarondon NK et al,

The feasibility, reliability and validity of the EORTC QLQ-C30 in assessing the quality of life in patients with a symptomatic HHIV infection or AIDS (CVC IV). *Psychol Health* 1994; **9**: 65–77.

31. Fosså S, Quality of life assessment in unselected oncologic out-patients: a pilot study. *Int J Oncol* 1994; **4**: 1393–7.

32. Osoba D, Zee B, Warr D et al, Psychometric properties and responsiveness of the EORTC Quality of Life Questionnaire (QLQ-C30) in patients with breast, ovarian and lung cancer. *Qual Life Res* 1994; **3**: 353–64.

33. Ringdal GI, Ringdal K, Testing the EORTC Quality of Life Questionnaire on cancer patients with heterogeneous diagnoses. *Qual Life Res* 1993; **2**: 129–40.

34. Hjermstad MJ, Fosså SD, Bjordal K et al, Test/retest study for the European Organization for Research and Treatment of Cancer Core Quality of Life Questionnaire. *J Clin Oncol* 1995; **13**: 1249–54.

35. Niezgode HE, Pater JL, A validation study of the domains of the Core EORTC Quality of Life Questionnaire. *Qual Life Res* 1993; **2**: 319–25.

36. Fayers P, Aaronson N, Bjordal K et al, *EORTC QLQ-C30 Scoring Manual*. Brussels: The EORTC Study Group on Quality of Life, EORTC Data Center, 1995.

37. Sprangers MAG, Cull A, Bjordal K et al, The European Organization for Research and Treatment of Cancer approach to quality of life assessment: guidelines for developing questionnaire modules. *Qual Life Res* 1993; **2**: 287–95.

38. Bergman B, Aaronson NK, Adhmedzai et al, The EORTC QLQ-LC13: a modular supplement to the EORTC Core Quality of Life Questionnaire (QLQ-C30) for use in lung cancer clinical trials. *Eur J Cancer* 1994; **30**: 635–42.

39. Sprangers MAG, Groenvold M, Arraras JI et al, for The European Organization for Research and Treatment of Cancer, Breast Cancer–Specific Quality of Life Questionnaire Module: first results from a three-country field study. *J Clin Oncol* 1996; **10**: 2756–68.

40. Bjordal K, Ahlner-Elmqvist M, Tollesson E et al, Development of a European Organization for Research and Treatment of Cancer (EORTC) questionnaire module to be used in quality of life assessment in head and neck cancer patients. *Acta Oncol* 1992; **31**: 311–21.

41. Blazeby JM, Alderson D, Winstone K et al, on behalf of the EORTC Quality of Life Study Group, Development of an EORTC Questionnaire Module to be used in quality of life assessment for patients with oesophageal cancer. *Eur J Cancer* 1996; **11**: 1912–17.

42. Bonomi AE, Cella DF, Hahn EA et al, Multilingual translation for the Functional Assessment of Cancer Therapy (FACT) quality of life measurement system. *Qual Life Res* 1996; **5**: 302–20.

43. Jenkinson C, Coulter A, Wright L, Short form 36 (SF-36) health survey questionnaire: normative data for adults of working age. *Br Med J* 1992; **306**: 1437–40.

44. Goldberg D, Williams P, *A Users Guide to the General Health Questionnaire*. Berkshire: NFER–Nelson, 1988.

45. Hunt SM, McKenna SP, McEven J et al, The Nottingham Health Profile: subjective health status and medical consultations. *Soc Sci Med* 1981; **15A**: 221–9.

46. Hjermstad MJ, Fayers PM, Bjordal K, Kaasa S, Health related quality of life in the general population assessed by the EORTC Core Quality of Life Questionnaire – the EORTC QLQ-C30 (+3). Submitted for publication.

47. Wisloff F, Eika S, Hippe E et al, Measurement of health-related quality of life in multiple myeloma. *Br J Haematol* 1996; **92**: 604–13.

48. Reuben DB, Mor V, Nausea and vomiting in terminal cancer patients, National Hospice Study. *Arch Intern Med* 1986; **146**: 2021–3.

49. Bliss JM, Robertson B, Selby PJ, The impact of nausea and vomiting upon quality of life measures. *Br J Cancer* 1992; **66**(Suppl XIX): S14–23.

50. Lindley CM, Hirsch JD, O'Neill SV et al, Quality of life consequences of chemotherapy-induced emesis. *Qual Life Res* 1992; **1**: 331–40.

51. Osoba D, Zee B, Warr D et al, Quality of life studies in chemotherapy-induced emesis. *Oncology* 1996; **53**(Suppl 1): 92–5.

52. Schmoll H-J, Quality of life measurement in antiemetic trials: a discussion of Professor Selby's paper. *Br J Cancer* 1992; **66**(Suppl XIX): S24–5.

53. Kaasa S, Mastekaasa A, Psychosocial well-being of patients with inoperable non-small cell lung cancer. *Acta Oncol* 1988; **27**: 829–35.

54. Soukop M, Management of cyclophosphamide-induced emesis over repeat courses. *Oncology* 1996; **53**(Suppl 1): 39–45.

13

Patients' point of view

Anne L Swinbourne, Martin HN Tattersall

CONTENTS • Introduction • Post-treatment nausea and vomiting • Role of non-pharmacological factors • Anticipatory nausea and vomiting • Implications for clinical practice

INTRODUCTION

The public perception is that nausea and vomiting are two of the inevitable and significant side-effects of cancer chemotherapy. Nausea and vomiting are indeed experienced by many patients after chemotherapy infusion to differing degrees of severity. While some drugs are more likely than others to cause nausea and vomiting, the factors that influence the variation in patient reports of these side-effects are not clear. This chapter will attempt to outline how patients perceive nausea and vomiting, as well as some of the factors that may contribute to the variation in patient reports. This will be done by examining the severity, frequency and duration of post-treatment nausea and vomiting and anticipatory side-effects of treatment.

POST-TREATMENT NAUSEA AND VOMITING

In an oft-cited study, Coates et al[1] surveyed 99 chemotherapy patients and asked them to rank the relative severity of 73 commonly experienced treatment side-effects. Patients overwhelmingly reported post-treatment vomiting and then nausea as the side-effects that both-

ered them the most. These side-effects occupied the top two positions on a rank list of severity regardless of the patient's diagnosis, treatment protocol, and objective or subjective response to treatment. When responses were broken down by patient characteristics, regardless of sex, age, marital status and domestic situation, nausea and vomiting were always rated among the top three side-effects in terms of severity.

A decade later, the survey was repeated in a similar population.[2] While nausea was reported by over 70% of patients and was ranked overall as the most severe side-effect, vomiting was experienced by 50% of the sample and had dropped in rank to 5th in severity. Tiredness, loss of hair and the effect of treatment on family were now ranked as being of more concern than vomiting. This drop was evident in all patient subgroups, but was most marked in the over-60 age group, who ranked vomiting as 15th in severity and reported significantly less nausea than younger patients. Not surprisingly, patients receiving cisplatin rated both post-chemotherapy nausea and post-chemotherapy vomiting as significantly more severe when compared with patients on all other regimens. Over the entire sample in the first 24 hours post treatment, 51% of patients experienced nausea and 24% vomiting that was rated as causing a significant level of discomfort.

One other major change in the ranking was patients' increased concern about the effect of their treatment on family members. This was rated 10th in 1983, and rose in rank to 4th in 1993. Poor control of delayed emesis after some drug treatments[3,4] combined with a shift towards treating patients on an outpatient basis[5] means that more families now have to care for patients at home post therapy, and are exposed to the occurrence of side-effects such as nausea and vomiting. Cancer-chemotherapy patients typically experience a decrease in their ability to function at pretreatment levels for a period after treatment due to side-effects such as nausea and vomiting. If the family member being cared for is normally a parent, the reversal in roles may add to the distress of a family already coping with a cancer diagnosis. That this distress is evident to the patient is reflected in the ranking of this concern.

It is notable that nausea maintained its importance at the top of the ranking, whilst the ranking of vomiting dropped. These findings are consistent with those of other authors. Morrow[6] has presented a summary of data collected over the period 1978–1990, which indicates that patient self-report of the frequency of post-treatment nausea has remained constant, with prevalence rates ranging between 62% and 72%. This pattern of results may indicate that while the introduction of new antiemetic drugs has resulted in better control over vomiting, there has been less corresponding improvement in control over nausea.[7,8] The studies presented by Morrow[6] all use the same standardized self-report instrument, which facilitates comparison across surveys not only of frequency but also of severity of nausea. It appears from these data that the severity of nausea has also remained remarkably consistent over this time period, with roughly one-third of the patients rating nausea as 'moderate' and another third describing it as 'severe' to 'intolerable'. These data confirm the frequency and severity of chemotherapy-induced nausea as a significant problem for many cancer patients.

There are several aspects of patients' percep-

tion of post-treatment nausea and vomiting that are not clear from a review of the literature. Although many data are available on patients' perception of the frequency and severity of post-treatment nausea and vomiting, the perception of duration has been less explored,[9,10] even though it may be just as important to the patient. It is feasible that long-duration, low-grade nausea may be perceived by the patient as being more aversive and disruptive than a short-duration intense bout of nausea and vomiting. At least the latter is over and done with and the patient can go back to their day-to-day routine. Some support for this view comes from Love et al,[11] who reported that post-treatment nausea and vomiting showed a significant positive correlation with overall treatment distress and that this correlation rose significantly for those patients whose nausea lasted more than 24 hours post-treatment.

The issue of duration comes to the fore when trying to assess the impact of delayed side-effects of treatment. Delayed nausea and vomiting is by definition that which is experienced more than 24 hours after chemotherapy administration. Patients report two main patterns of delayed side-effects.

Firstly, there is nausea and vomiting that starts within the 24 hours post-chemotherapy and *persists* into the days beyond. Secondly, there is nausea and vomiting that is reported as *first* occurring beyond 24 hours post-treatment. Love et al[11] report that of the patients who experienced nausea in their sample at any time over the first six cycles, 70% reported at least one episode that persisted beyond 24 hours. In the Griffin et al[2] study, delayed nausea severe enough to cause significant discomfort was reported by 57% of the sample. Vomiting over the same period was reported by 29% of patients. This represents an increase of 6% and 5% over reported rates for acute nausea and vomiting respectively. Owing to the design of the study, what this increase actually represents cannot be determined. For example, it may represent an escalation in severity in pre-existing acute nausea and vomiting, or it may represent 'new' cases of distress.

Morrow et al[3] followed 327 patients from

three major North American centres over several chemotherapy cycles. These authors attempted to separate persistent nausea from nausea that first occurs more than 24 hours post-treatment. Their results indicate that for approximately one-third of patients their first experience of nausea occurred more than 24 hours post-treatment. Delayed vomiting first developed 24 hours post-treatment in 26% of the same sample. Vomiting that first occurred beyond 24 hours post-treatment was rated as less severe than acute vomiting, and a steady decrease in the percentage of patients reporting delayed vomiting episodes over the second and third days post-treatment was observed. By contrast, the pattern for delayed nausea was remarkably steady. The severity ratings of delayed and acute nausea were comparable within the sample, and the frequency of reported delayed episodes remained steady at 10–15% over days 2 and 3 post-treatment. The overwhelming majority of delayed nausea and vomiting episodes started in the morning, and persisted throughout the 24 hour period on 56% of the occasions that it was reported.

Given that the treatment regimens of all patients in this study included antiemetic drugs standard for the alleviation of post-treatment nausea and vomiting, these data indicate that delayed nausea and vomiting constitutes a significant clinical problem. Evidence suggests that the presently available antiemetic drugs control acute substantially better than delayed nausea and vomiting.[6,8]

There is evidence that patients who experience delayed nausea rate treatment as significantly more distressing overall than patients not reporting delayed symptoms.[11] This may be due to the more pronounced disruption of normal function experienced by these individuals. While most patients expect some period of nausea and/or vomiting to occur post-treatment,[11] to wake up still feeling sick if not sicker the day after treatment may invoke feelings of disappointment, which in turn may compound feelings of distress. Patients need to be informed if their treatment is likely to have a delayed pattern of nausea and emesis. They need to know that this may happen, since this allows them to

modify their expectations and prepare for possible eventualities. If they are outpatients, they need to be provided with appropriate antiemetics, detailed instructions on how and when to take these drugs, and told who to contact in the event of intolerable distress. They need to be reassured that something can be done.

ROLE OF NON-PHARMACOLOGICAL FACTORS

Although patients consistently rate nausea and vomiting as two of the most frequent and distressing side-effects of chemotherapy, the objective degree of drug toxicity may not be proportional to the level of distress that treatment causes the individual. The psychological literature indicates that a person's appraisal and perception of an event depends on a multiplicity of factors, of which the nature of the objective event is only one of many possible influences.[12,13] The goal of treatment and the stage of the patient's disease may influence a patient's perceptions and tolerance of side-effects. For example, patients may be willing to tolerate higher levels of nausea and vomiting if they perceive that the treatment is being effective. There is little comparative survey data on this issue. Coates et al[1] reported that there was little difference in the ranking of severity of side-effects between patients who thought that they were improving and those who felt that chemotherapy was not successful, which seems to indicate that treatment response may not influence perceptions of side-effects. It is also likely that any assessment of the role of treatment success in influencing patients' perceptions would be hopelessly confounded by factors such as differences in the emetogenic potential of protocols, disease status and treatment goal.

Additionally, the number of cycles of chemotherapy patients have had may enter in as a confounder. Patients who have had several cycles of chemotherapy have probably formed a firmer opinion about the success/failure of their treatment than patients who have had fewer cycles, even though the former are also more likely to experience post-treatment nausea and vomiting.[7] Although one of the best predictors of post-treatment distress is the amount of distress experienced on the previous cycle, the overall picture seems to be that the more treatment cycles the patient has had, the higher the risk of post-treatment nausea and vomiting.[7,8,14] It seems that even patients who experience complete protection from nausea and vomiting in the early cycles are still at risk as treatment continues.[8]

One way to investigate perceptions of treatment and associated toxicity is to assess the cost/benefit ratio involved. To investigate the relationship between toxicity, tumour response and patients' perceptions of the morbidity of treatment, Slevin et al[15] presented subjects with two hypothetical treatment regimens: one with severe side-effects, including high levels of nausea and vomiting, the other with mild side-effects including little or no nausea and vomiting. Subjects were asked to indicate the level of benefit in three areas (chance of cure, prolonging of life, and relief of symptoms) that would make a course of each chemotherapy regimen acceptable to them. The investigators compared cancer patients who were about to commence cytotoxic therapy with matched non-patient controls and a variety of medical professionals. They found that while the matched non-patient controls wanted greater benefit for any risk of side-effects, patients were willing to take significantly greater risks for less potential benefit, while medical professionals fell between the two groups. Patients were also more likely to accept the intensive treatment than the matched control group. In fact, no patient indicated that they would refuse either treatment. Experience with chemotherapy did not seem to effect patients' willingness to undergo the hypothetical treatment regimens. A subsample of patients were reassessed 3 months after starting their chemotherapy, and their responses remained stable.

It has been argued that since the Slevin et al[15] study used patients who had decided to have chemotherapy, they were not representative of the wider population of cancer patients. In a replication study, Bremnes et al[16] widened the subject pool to include all patients with a diagnosis of cancer on a first referral to an oncology unit. No treatment recommendation had yet been made, and the questionnaire was administered at the time of their first physical examination. These researchers found that, in contrast to the earlier study, cancer patients wanted significantly more chance of cure for any risk than the non-patient control group. This result was qualified by age effects. Patients older than 60 years wanted significantly more chance of cure, prolonging of life, and relief of symptoms for risk of toxicity than patients less than 50 years old. In the less than 50 years age group, patients were significantly more willing to accept high toxicity for small benefit than were controls. In contrast to the Slevin et al[15] study, it was reported that 9% of patients indicated that they would categorically refuse treatment, and refusal was positively correlated with age.

Reasons for the differences between these two studies more than likely lie in the patient populations. The finding that patients found any treatment, including one with high toxicity, more acceptable in the Slevin et al[15] study may reflect the fact that these individuals were actually about to commence chemotherapy, while the decision about treatment was still in the future for those patients in the Bremnes et al[16] study. It thus seems that perceptions of treatment and likely associated toxicity are influenced by where patients are in the treatment decision-making process. The closer the real possibility of chemotherapy, the more likely it is that individuals perceive the treatment and associated toxicity as acceptable. This may reflect mechanisms of cognitive dissonance coming into play as patients reconcile the reality of their situation with their dislike of treatment. Patients who have a lot to live for, for example those with dependent young children, are more likely to accept increased toxicity for minimal increases in survival.[15-17]

The patients' perceptions contrast with that of the cancer doctors surveyed in these studies. The responses of cancer doctors tended, on the whole, to lie between the conservatism of the controls and the willingness of the patient groups. Contrary to popular belief, it may be that while cancer doctors perceive chemotherapy as a more acceptable treatment than does the non-patient population, the doctors are not more enthusiastic than their patients when it comes to participation in potentially toxic chemotherapy regimens. This view is supported by doctor surrogate studies and investigations of patient information preferences.[18-20]

Patients' perceptions of chemotherapy differ not only across but also within particular patient subgroups. The wide variation in objective and subjective experience of side-effects between patients – even those with comparable disease and drug regimen – has resulted in a large body of investigation into the effects of non-pharmacological factors on patient experience. The results are conflicting. Past designs have confounded ratings of treatment side-effects with the emetogenic potential of the chemotherapy, number of treatment cycles and stage of disease, as well as patient variables such as age and sex. To avoid confounding and to examine the role of non-pharmacological factors on post-treatment side-effects, Jacobsen et al[21] used a prospective design and recruited only female patients all having the same adjuvant chemotherapy for breast cancer. On the basis of past research into individual differences in perception and reaction to stressful events, as well as reports from the field of oncology,[22-24] they decided to examine the contribution of patients' expectations, anxiety levels, and previous experience with non-treatment related nausea and vomiting. It was hypothesized that high levels of each of these factors would be associated with the occurrence of self-reported post-treatment nausea and vomiting. The results bore out these hypotheses. Patients who expected to be sick after chemotherapy tended to report post-treatment nausea more frequently than patients with no such expectations. They also reported nausea of greater severity and longer duration. High levels of pretreatment anxiety tended to be associated with a higher frequency and intensity of post-treatment nausea. Additionally, patients who reported more episodes of post-treatment nausea were significantly more likely to have experienced nausea when anxious in the past. A past history of motion sickness was associated with nausea of longer duration.

No significant relationship was found between reported past history of nausea and vomiting and patients' expectations of the occurrence of post-treatment nausea. Individual differences in distress may be based in part upon the extent and manner in which patients expect, monitor and interpret their physical symptoms. Patients who expect to be sick may perhaps keep a 'closer eye' on physiological reactions, thus detecting and reporting any aversive sensations.

Subsequent research examined the effect that patients' awareness of physiological changes has on their interpretation and perception of an event. In several studies, Miller[25-28] has identified two patterns of behaviour that have discriminated between levels of reported distress in a variety of stressful medical settings. Patients who are classed as 'monitors' tend to attend closely to threat-relevant stimuli, to be more attentive to the negative aspects of an event, and to engage in more intrusive ideation. 'Blunters', on the other hand, tend to avoid attending to those aspects of an event that may be distressing, using distraction techniques to turn their attention and thoughts away from the situation. Both these attentional styles can be very effective forms of coping in particular situations. However, a growing body of evidence indicates that a monitoring style increases perceived distress in situations where the stressor is mostly out of the individual's control.[29,30] Such stressors may be chronic illness and aversive medical procedures.

Monitors are reported to experience greater treatment side-effects and report more distress during procedures than blunters. For example, Miller and Mangen[31] reported that, when undergoing colposcopy after an abnormal PAP smear, monitors tended to display significantly more agitation than blunters as rated by observers. Monitors also reported significantly more pain and discomfort over the 5-day period following the procedure. Blunters reported a steadily declining pattern of discomfort over this period, whilst 'monitors' did not report a significant decrease in discomfort until the third day. If the distinction between coping styles can be extended to the chemotherapy context then monitors should be more likely to report post-treatment nausea and vomiting and rate it as more severe and of longer duration than patients who use a blunting coping style.

Some evidence for this conceptualisation has been reported. Gard et al[32] found that patients who utilized a monitoring coping style reported significantly more post-treatment nausea than blunters. While there were no differences in rated severity of the nausea between the two coping style groups, 'monitors' reported nausea of significantly longer duration. This was despite the fact that significantly more of the 'monitors' were taking some sort of antiemetic medication. One conclusion may be that patients with a monitoring attentional style may be over-reporting symptoms by interpreting any plausible sensation as nausea, for example, mis-labelling gastrointestinal sensations due to anxiety as nausea caused by treatment. While there is some evidence that patients who employ a monitoring attentional style are accurate in their detection and reporting of bodily sensations,[33] data on the accuracy of their interpretation of these sensations is limited.

ANTICIPATORY NAUSEA AND VOMITING

In the context of cancer treatment, anticipatory nausea and/or vomiting (ANV) refers to the occurrence of nausea and vomiting before a chemotherapy session in the absence of any pharmacological agent. The best supported theory of the development of ANV contends that it develops via a classical (Pavlovian) conditioning process. A full discussion of the evidence for this view is presented in Chapter 10. Briefly, the chemotherapy is postulated to be the initial unconditioned stimulus that elicits the unconditioned response of nausea and vomiting. Chemotherapy drug administration takes place in the presence of many other stimuli, such as the clinic environs and the staff who work there, as well as internal stimuli such as cognitions and emotional states. Over repeated treatment administrations, these contextual stimuli become associated with post-treatment distress to the extent that exposure to these cues comes to elicit nausea and vomiting. In other words, stimuli associated with the treatment administration eventually come to act as conditioned stimuli eliciting the now-conditioned response of nausea and vomiting.

Prevalence rates varying between 14% and 63% have been reported.[34] A recent review of prospective studies indicated that before the second cycle of chemotherapy around 10% of patients across studies reported ANV. This figure increased to between 22% and 40% of patients by the sixth cycle.[6] Part of this variance may come from the differing definitions of ANV that investigators employ. Some investigators assess nausea and vomiting independently, while others combine the two. Overall, patients report anticipatory nausea more often than anticipatory vomiting,[35,36] and there is some indication that females tend to report anticipatory vomiting more often than males.[36] ANV tends to develop within the first six treatment cycles,[37] and appears to become more severe over the course of treatment.[38] However, the pattern of occurrence is not one of regular episodes systematically increasing in severity. While most patients who experience ANV report repeated episodes, they tend to experience it intermittently.[37,39]

Typically, patients report that ANV tends to be less severe than post-treatment nausea and vomiting,[35,36] and there are some indications that although prevalence rates have remained steady, reported severity has declined.[35,40] This may be due in part to the increased efficacy of antiemetic treatment. As mentioned earlier, while there has been mixed success with the control of post-treatment nausea, there has been significant improvement in the control of post-treatment vomiting. It is possible that this has resulted in the experience of post-treatment distress as a whole being perceived by patients as just as frequent but less severe than in the past. If ANV has its genesis in a conditioning process then any decrease in post-treatment distress will affect the extent of anticipatory distress. The evidence appears to support this interpretation.

Despite these changes, around 17% of patients report anticipatory nausea and 5% report anticipatory vomiting of an intensity sufficient to cause them significant discomfort.[2] This is of concern for several reasons. The experience of ANV is significantly positively correlated with patient ratings of overall treatment difficulty, emotional distress caused by chemotherapy, and disruption of social life and employment.[11] Patients who develop ANV tend to be those suffering the more intense post-treatment side-effects, experiencing anxiety, and general distress about treatment. These are patients who are most at risk of discontinuing or interrupting treatment.[39,41] To develop ANV might be the straw that breaks the camel's back.

These feelings may be compounded by an inability to communicate their distress to relevant others. Patients seem to be aware that ANV is a predominantly psychological phenomenon, unlike post-treatment nausea and vomiting. When asked what they think is causing their ANV, the majority of patients give a psychological rationale postulating nervousness, anxiety or the more general 'it's in my head' as a cause.[6,42] This explanation brings little comfort, since some patients feel that this is a sign they are losing their minds or that they should be able to cope with this by themselves. Whatever the reason, patients may avoid reporting ANV to the medical staff or others for fear of ridicule or on the basis that they do not perceive it to be a 'medical' problem.[6,42] As a result, these patients do not have access to interventions that can help relieve anticipatory side-effects.

IMPLICATIONS FOR CLINICAL PRACTICE

There is broad acceptance in the developed world that patients are participants in medical decisions about their care. An informed patient is also one who can anticipate and prepare for events that may occur. An informed patient is one who has the best chance of coping and benefiting from treatment. Forewarned is forearmed.

The experience of cancer chemotherapy and of its side-effects varies greatly not only between individuals but also for the same individual over time. This variability makes the prediction of morbidity very difficult. Even two patients receiving the same chemotherapy protocol may report very different patterns of and reactions to nausea and vomiting. The degree of distress experienced appears to result from a complex interaction of pharmacological and non-pharmacological factors.

This review has identified some patient variables that influence the extent of nausea and vomiting associated with cancer chemotherapy. Age, anxiety levels, past history of nausea and vomiting, and patient expectations are factors that may need to be considered when designing an antiemetic policy. Physicians also need to be aware of the high prevalence of ANV and know that patients may not spontaneously bring its occurrence to their attention. Including questions about any anticipatory distress in routine assessments of treatment toxicity is one way to elicit this information. Behavioural techniques that are effective in reducing the incidence and severity of ANV need to be brought to the patient's attention.

The control of post-treatment nausea and vomiting has important implications for the overall experience of treatment. Patients' perceptions of post-treatment nausea and vomiting are significantly correlated with overall ratings of the level of distress and disruption caused by treatment.[11] Any reduction in the extent of these side-effects should result in the treatment experience becoming easier for the majority of patients. It is plausible that improved control of treatment-related nausea and vomiting could have a flow-on effect to levels of compliance and completion of treatment.

REFERENCES

1. Coates A, Abraham S, Kaye SB et al, On the receiving end – patient perception of the side-effects of chemotherapy. *Eur J Cancer Clin Oncol* 1983; **19**: 203–8.
2. Griffin AM, Butow PN, Coates AS et al, On the receiving end. V: Patient perception of the side effects of cancer chemotherapy in 1993. *Ann Oncol* 1996; **7**: 189–95.
3. Morrow GR, Hickok JT, Burish TG, Rosenthal SN, Frequency and clinical implications of delayed nausea and delayed emesis. *Am J Clin Oncol* 1996; **19**: 199–203.
4. Rhodes VA, Watson PM, Johnson MH, Patterns of nausea and vomiting in chemotherapy patients: a preliminary study. *Oncol Nurs Forum* 1985; **12**(3): 42–8.
5. Cooper S, Georgiou V, The impact of cytotoxic chemotherapy-perspectives from patients, specialists and nurses. *Eur J Cancer* 1992; **28A** (Suppl 1): S36–8.
6. Morrow GR, Behavioural factors influencing the development and expression of chemotherapy induced side effects. *Br J Cancer* 1992; **66**(Suppl XIX): S54–61.
7. Morrow GR, Hickok JT, Rosenthal SN, Progress in reducing nausea and emesis. *Cancer* 1995; **76**: 343–57.
8. Martin M, Myths and realities of antiemetic treatment. *Br J Cancer* 1992; **66**(Suppl XIX): S46–51.
9. Morrow GR, The assessment of nausea and vomiting. *Cancer* 1984; **53**: 2267–78.
10. Kaye SB, How should nausea be assessed in patients receiving chemotherapy? *Cancer Treat Rev* 1991; **18**: 85–93.
11. Love RR, Leventhal H, Easterling DV, Nerenz DR, Side effects and emotional distress during cancer chemotherapy. *Cancer* 1989; **63**: 604–12.
12. Lazarus RS, Coping theory and research: past, present, and future. *Psychosom Med* 1993; **55**: 234–47.
13. Folkman S, Lazarus RS, Dunkel-Schetter C et al, Dynamics of a stressful encounter: cognitive appraisal coping and encounter outcomes. *J Pers Soc Psychol* 1986; **50**: 992–1003.
14. Jacobsen PB, Andrykowski MA, Redd WH et al, Nonpharmacologic factors in the development of posttreatment nausea with adjuvant chemotherapy for breast cancer. *Cancer* 1988; **61**: 379–85.
15. Slevin ML, Stubbs L, Plant HJ et al, Attitudes to chemotherapy: comparing views of patients with cancer with those of their doctors, nurses, and general public. *Br Med J* 1990; **300**: 1458–60.
16. Bremnes RM, Anderson K, Wist EA, Cancer patients, doctors and nurses vary in their willingness to undertake cancer chemotherapy. *Eur J Cancer* 1995; **31A**: 1955–9.
17. Coates AS, Simes RJ, Patient assessment of adjuvant treatment in operable breast cancer. In: *Introducing New Treatments for Cancer: Practical, Ethical and Legal Problems* (Williams CJ, ed.). Chichester: Wiley, 1992: 447–58.
18. Turner S, Maher EJ, Young T et al, What are the information priorities for cancer patients involved in treatment decisions? An experienced surrogate study in Hodgkin's disease. *Br J Cancer* 1996; **73**: 222–7.
19. Mackillop WJ, Ward GK, O'Sullivan B, The use of expert surrogates to evaluate clinical trials in non-small cell lung cancer. *Br J Cancer* 1986; **54**: 661–7.
20. Penman DT, Holland JC, Bahna GF et al, Informed consent for investigational chemotherapy: patients' and physicians' perceptions. *J Clin Oncol* 1984; **2**: 849–55.
21. Jacobsen PB, Andrykowski MA, Redd WH et al, Nonpharmacologic factors in the development of posttreatment nausea with adjuvant chemotherapy for breast cancer. *Cancer* 1988; **61**: 379–85.
22. Cassileth BR, Lusk EJ, Bodenheimer BJ et al, Chemotherapeutic toxicity – the relationship between patients' pretreatment expectations and posttreatment results. *Am J Clin Oncol* 1985; **8**: 419–25.
23. Cohen RE, Blanchard EB, Ruckdeschel JC, Smolen RC, Prevalence and correlates of posttreatment and anticipatory nausea and vomiting in cancer chemotherapy. *J Psychosom Res* 1986; **30**: 643–54.
24. Morrow GR, Susceptibility to motion sickness and the development of anticipatory nausea and vomiting in cancer patients undergoing chemotherapy. *Cancer Treat Rep* 1984; **68**: 1177–8.
25. Miller SM, Brody DS, Summerton J, Styles of coping with threat: implications for health. *J Pers Soc Psychol* 1988; **54**(1): 142–8.
26. Miller SM, Roussi P, Altman D et al, Effects of coping style on psychological reactions of low-income, minority women to colposcopy. *J Rep Med* 1994; **39**: 711–8.
27. Miller SM, Monitoring and blunting: validation of a questionnaire to assess styles of information

seeking under threat. *J Pers Soc Psychol* 1987; **52:** 345–53.

28. Miller SM, Monitoring versus blunting styles of coping with cancer influence the information patients want and need about their disease. Implications for cancer screening and management. *Cancer* 1995; **76:** 167–77.

29. Miller SM, Rodoletz M, Mangan CE et al, Applications of the monitoring process model to coping with severe long-term medical threats. *Health Psychol* 1996; **15:** 216–25.

30. Davey GC, Tallis F, Hodgson S, The relationship between information-seeking and information-avoiding coping styles and the reporting of psychological and physical symptoms. *J Psychosom Res* 1993; **37:** 333–44.

31. Miller SM, Mangan CE, Interacting effects of information and coping style in adapting to gynecologic stress: should the doctor tell all? *J Pers Soc Psychol* 1983; **45:** 223–36.

32. Gard D, Edwards PW, Harris J, McCormack G, Sensitizing effects of pretreatment measures on cancer chemotherapy nausea and vomiting. *J Con Clin Psychol* 1988; **56:** 80–4.

33. Steptoe A, Vogele C, Individual differences in the perception of bodily sensations: the role of treait anxiety and coping style. *Behav Res Ther* 1992; **30:** 597–607.

34. Morrow GR, Dobkin PL, Anticipatory nausea and vomiting in cancer patients undergoing chemotherapy treatment: prevalence, etiology, and behavioral interventions. *Clin Psychol Rev* 1988; **8:** 517–56.

35. Stefanek ME, Sheidler RN, Fetting JH, Anticipatory nausea and vomiting: Does it still remain a significant clinical problem. *Cancer* 1988; **62:** 2654–7.

36. Boakes RA, Tarrier N, Barnes BW, Tattersall MHN, Prevalence of anticiptaory nausea and other side-effects in cancer patients receiving chemotherapy. *Eur J Cancer* 1993; **29A:** 866–70.

37. Nerenz D, Leventhal H, Easterling DV, Love RR, Anxiety and drug taste as predictors of anticipatory nausea in cancer chemotherapy. *J Clin Psychol* 1986; **4:** 224–33.

38. van Kommen R, Redd WH, Personality factors associated with anticipatory nausea/vomiting in patients receiving cancer chemotherapy. *Health Psychol* 1985; **4:** 189–204.

39. Andrykowski MA, Jacobsen PB, Marks E et al, Prevalence, predictors, and course of anticipatory nausea in women receiving adjuvant chemotherapy for breast cancer. *Cancer* 1988; **62:** 2607–13.

40. Carey MP, Burish TG, Etiology and treatment of the psychological side effect associated with cancer chemotherapy: A critical review and discussion. *Psychol Bull* 1988; **104:** 307–25.

41. Fallowfield L, Behavioural interventions and psychological aspects of care during chemotherapy. *Eur J Cancer* 1992; **28A**(Suppl 1): S39–41.

42. Redd WH, Jacobsen PB, Andrykowski MA, Behavioral side effects of adjuvant chemotherapy. *Recent Results Cancer Res* 1989; **115:** 272–8.

14

Emesis: A challenge for nurses

Helen Gall

INTRODUCTION

The patient with cancer, whether newly diagnosed or one who has been on treatment for some time, will have to attempt to cope with the distress and anguish associated with the knowledge of having a life-threatening disease. This is not only true for the patient, but also extends to family, friends and those involved in the treatment. Cancer treatment, especially chemotherapy, is well known for its unpleasant side-effects. Many consider that the side-effects are part of the treatment, and therefore need to be accepted as something that is 'normal' considering the often poor prognosis of the patient. Patients experience nausea and vomiting as the most distressful side-effect.[1] This is often the reason why some patients may refuse further treatment or may not complete the treatment course in progress.[2,3] If this is the case, and the patient with a potentially curable disease does refuse further treatment, the side-effects of nausea and vomiting could be considered a potentially fatal toxicity.[3-5]

In 1988 a survey was carried out among nurses who were attending the Fifth International Conference on Cancer Care held in London: 260 completed questionnaires were returned. Nurses were asked to identify the three most distressing side-effects of cancer therapy. Nearly 85% of the responders mentioned nausea and vomiting, followed by alopecia (60%), fatigue (30%), diarrhoea (10%) and pain (9%).[6]

Uncontrolled nausea and vomiting lead to decreased nutritional intake and serious metabolic derangements, and decreases in patients' sense of well-being, both mentally and physically, and their ability for self-care.[3,7]

As chemotherapeutic drugs become more aggressive and the regimes more complex and intense, the severity of the potential side-effects increases. This is also true regarding nausea and vomiting. As nurses have become more active in carrying out their own research projects, the subject of emesis has received more attention during the last 10 years. The development and subsequent use of $5-HT_3$ receptor antagonists has given many patients complete or improved relief from these unpleasant side-effects.

THE ROLE

Coping with emesis presents a challenge to nurses. Nurses spend more time every day with the patient than any other member of the healthcare team, and are therefore in an ideal position to encourage, support and assist the patient. Patients who are experiencing nausea and vomiting for the first time have new (personal) demands for self-care actions. Patients' ability to respond appropriately is dependent on the knowledge of how to cope, and the capacity to do so.[7]

Emesis may be complicated by other factors, either a side-effect or a symptom of the disease, for example pain. Patients may be very distressed by the vomiting; this distress may be equal to if not greater than the actual discomfort from the vomiting. This is particularly true with the unexpectedness of anticipatory vomiting, which may result in extreme embarrassment. Reassuring the patient and establishing a balance between being honest and realistic about the severity and duration of the emesis is a sensitive issue, and requires the input of a skilled nurse.

The role of the nurse may be divided into different categories, namely assessing the (potential) problem, educating the patient and family, carrying out basic nursing care, counselling the patient (and family), administration of anti-emetic drugs and offering alternative approaches to managing the symptoms.

In each category it is essential to assess the severity of the problem, then, together with the patient, to define realistic goals to solve or alleviate the problems, plan nursing care interventions that will achieve these goals, implement the chosen interventions, and afterwards evaluate the effect of the care given. Where necessary, the plan may be adjusted according to the needs of the patient and the evaluation of the interventions. Each phase of the nursing process needs to be carefully worked out to ensure that the patient receives a personal nursing care programme that is tailored to his or her requirements.

ASSESSMENT

For the nurse to assess the potential problems accurately he or she requires detailed knowledge of the chemotherapy regime and the potential side-effects that may be expected. The initial contact with the patient and family sets the scene for an open relationship of trust and confidence. During the initial assessment, the nurse acquires knowledge regarding predisposing factors for nausea and vomiting. These include[4]

- gender (women are more prone to vomiting than men);
- alcohol use (patients accustomed to a high intake vomit less than low to moderate drinkers);
- previous experiences (the number of emetic incidences tends to increase with each additional course of chemotherapy);
- anxiety levels (more anxious patients experience more nausea and vomiting).

Past experiences with nausea and vomiting not related to chemotherapy, for example during pregnancy, influenza or due to 'nerves', increases the risk of emesis.[8] Strategies that were helpful with previous incidences may be useful with the current treatment.

As nausea and vomiting are two completely different side-effects, they should be assessed separately. Nausea may occur in the absence of vomiting and may be equally distressing; and if poorly controlled, it may cause additional anxiety and distress to the patient, family or carers, including friends and nursing staff.[9] Nausea is subjective and patient-dependent. Measurement of nausea is most frequently obtained using a Likert-scale self-report ranging from 0 to 10 (0 is no nausea and 10 is the most severe degree one can imagine) or a report of nausea expressed in number of hours.[10,11]

While the patient is being treated, the nurse will continue the assessment process by observing and documenting the duration, frequency, amount and appearance of the vomitus.[8] The experience of (or lack of) nausea and vomiting will strongly influence each following treatment cycle.

EDUCATION

Prior to the first treatment, patients and families need to receive information regarding the treatment plan and the possible side-effects. Often it is the physician who will inform the patient initially. After consent to be treated has been obtained, the nurse may continue the education process by reinforcing the available information and supplying additional practical information. This should emphasize the minimal symptom experience pattern, namely that patients be told to expect little or no nausea and vomiting during or post treatment.[7] With the currently used antiemetic schedules, the response has been greatly improved.

Information includes how the treatment is to be given, how long it will take and which drugs are to be administered. Explanations include possible side-effects that the chemotherapy and antiemetic drugs may have, the cause of the nausea and vomiting, how to care and cope with being nauseated and vomiting, what sort of measures are likely to give relief, and what precautions are required when handling vomitus containing cytostatic drugs. The nurse may also need to dispel any preconceived ideas regarding the incidence and severity of the emetic episodes.[4,12] All verbal information should be supported with written information.

COUNSELLING

The nurse spends more time with the patient than any other member of the healthcare team,[2,12] and is in an excellent position to gain trust and confidence. In his or her role as counsellor, the nurse should establish a good relationship with the patient and family. It is this initial contact that will establish the basis for supporting the patient during the entire treatment plan.[13,14] This is especially important when the same nurse is responsible for the patient's care through the whole treatment period.

Prior to the first treatment, the patient is likely to be anxious and nervous, as it is an unknown experience.[2] As the nurse prepares the patient, the setting needs to be relaxed and comfortable, with the impression that there is no need to rush. The nurse should be calm, and create an atmosphere of trust, ensuring that he or she is a continuous resource for supplying reassurance, support and empathy, always ready to repeat information already given. Points that the patient has not fully understood should be explained. The patient needs to know that his or her best interests are the motivating reason for treatment, in spite of possible side-effects.

Having assessed the patient's vulnerability to stress, it is essential to ensure that there is adequate support for both patient and family. Psychological well-being is important to the patient, as it will help him or her to cope with the treatment burden and the potential side-effects, to preserve family and social relationships and to continue to lead a normal life.[13]

BASIC NURSING CARE

This may include being there for the patient when an emetic episode occurs, having a receptacle for the vomitus within easy reach of the patient, providing a mouthwash and a cool, refreshing face-cloth, and removing unpleasant sights and odours quickly. The patient's fluid balance is regulated, attention is given to the electrolyte balance based on laboratory results, and fluid and dietary requirements are attended to.

In the past many believed that patients would tolerate treatment better, with less nausea and vomiting, if they did not eat or drink prior to, during or after the chemotherapy administration. The benefit of nil per os or only clear fluids versus light meals has been explored. Eating less or not at all has not been shown to decrease the amount of nausea and vomiting.[15] Many patients prefer to have something in their stomachs, and they may be encouraged to eat light food and to assess what they tolerate best. By allowing patients to choose their dietary requirements, they are able to exert more control over the situation and improve self-care abilities.

ADMINISTRATION OF ANTIEMETIC DRUGS

At present there are a number of drugs used in the treatment of nausea and vomiting. No single antiemetic prevents nausea and vomiting in all patients or with every course of chemotherapy. Even with very effective antiemetic drugs or combinations of drugs, complete response, defined as no vomiting and no nausea, is not achieved in all patients.

The antiemetic plan should include the drugs that work best for the patient, including the dosage, route and frequency. It is the nurse who observes the intensity, duration, frequency and the amount of stress experienced with each emetic attack and who should communicate this to the treating physician. The latter will then be able to adjust the prescribed drugs by increasing the dose, or adopting a more frequent regime, or a change in drugs or administration route.[8,9,12]

From the first course of chemotherapy, the patient should receive adequate antiemetic treatment. Nausea and vomiting should not be considered a necessary side-effect of chemotherapy, but must be avoided at all costs. The old rule that prevention is better than cure still holds true today. Patients who experience nausea and vomiting with the first course are more likely to have problems with following courses of chemotherapy, and are at a greater risk of developing anticipatory nausea and vomiting.

All antiemetic drugs should be given on a regular basis. Needless to say, all medications, interventions and incidents must be documented in the patient's records. This is valuable information when discussing dose adjustments or changes in antiemetic drugs.[8,10]

NON-MEDICAL INTERVENTIONS

A number of non-medical interventions have been described in the nursing literature, with varying results. These interventions vary from aerobic exercises, to distraction, to music therapy, to guided imagery or to relaxation techniques. The effectiveness seems to be more prominent in reducing nausea.[8,11]

Winningham and MacVicar[16] reported the use of aerobic exercise in a group of patients being treated for breast cancer. Patients were randomized into three groups, namely experimental exercise ($n = 16$), placebo ($n = 14$) and control ($n = 12$) groups. The results of this study indicate that moderate aerobic exercise may be beneficial as an adjunctive self-care measure to antiemetic therapy in controlling chemotherapy-induced nausea and in promoting physical well-being.

Music therapy has been used to help patients with the coping process. Most people can relate to and enjoy music. It helps to relax the person and provide a restful atmosphere. Orchestral music is most effective, and may be classical, folk, popular, rock, mood or jazz, depending on the taste of the patient.[2,17] The effect will depend on the degree to which the patient relates to the music used. When music is to be used in an open area, for instance a waiting room, a general type of music should be used so that most people can relate to it.

Relaxation and visualization therapy have been used in a number of clinics with good effect.[2,18-21] Patients are taught, prior to the commencement of chemotherapy, progressive muscle relaxation, and this may be followed by guided imagery. They are encouraged to use the learned techniques at regular intervals during and after the chemotherapy.

BREATHING EXERCISES AND DIVERSIONAL THERAPY

Patients who are sceptical about using relaxation techniques combined with guided imagery or visualization may be happy to use deep breathing exercises as described by Cobb.[18] Diversion or distraction can be very varied, and may take the form of reading, handwork, puzzles, television, videos, etc.[2] This is often used intuitively by many nurses, and focuses on allowing the patient to concentrate on something other than the symptoms and distress experienced.[22]

CONCLUSIONS

Nausea and vomiting are two unpleasant side-effects of chemotherapy that cause patients and carers great distress. Management of these side-effects is a challenge for all nurses, and requires effective nursing skills and a thorough knowledge of the problem and the possible interventions. When nausea and vomiting have been well controlled, the patient will experience a sense of well-being and improved quality of life. The time saved in the caring of the patient will then be available for support and teaching.

The nurse will also benefit, since his or her own personal feeling of being powerless decreases, job satisfaction increases and there is an increase in personal well-being.

REFERENCES

1. Coates A, Abraham S, Kaye SB et al, On the receiving end – patient perception of the side effects of cancer chemotherapy. *Eur J Cancer Clin Oncol* 1983; **19**: 203–8.
2. Pervan V, Practical aspects of dealing with cancer therapy-induced nausea and vomiting. *Semin Oncol Nurs* 1990; **6**(Suppl 1): 3–5.
3. Cotanch PH, Measuring nausea and vomiting in clinical nursing research. *Oncology Nursing Forum* 1984; **11**: 92–4.
4. Hawthorn J, The emetic potential of cancer treatments. In: *The Management of Nausea and Vomiting Induced by Chemotherapy and Radiotherapy* (International Training Package for Nurses). Glaxo Holdings, 1991.
5. Cotanch PH, Measuring nausea and vomiting. In: *Instruments for Clinical Nursing Research* (Frank-Stromborg M, ed.). Norwalk, CT: Appleton & Lange, 1988: 313–21.
6. Pritchard PA, Speechly VD, What do nurses know about emesis? *International Cancer Nursing News* 1989; **1**: 6–8.
7. Rhodes VA, Watson PM, Johnson MH et al, Patterns of nausea, vomiting, and distress in patients receiving antineoplastic drug protocols. *Oncology Nursing Forum* 1987; **14**: 35–44.
8. Wickham R, Managing chemotherapy-related nausea and vomiting: the state of the art. *Oncology Nursing Forum* 1989; **16**: 563–74.
9. Jenns K, Importance of nausea. *Cancer Nursing* 1994; **17**(6): 488–93.
10. Bachmann-Mettler I, Assessing nausea and vomiting. In: *Cancer Nursing: The Balance. Proceedings of the Sixth International Conference on Cancer Nursing* (Pritchard AP, ed.). Harrow, Middlesex: Scutari Press, 1990: 130–2.
11. Devine EC, Westlake SK, The effects of psycho-educational care provided to adults with cancer: meta-analysis of 116 studies. *Oncology Nursing Forum* 1995; **22**: 1369–81.
12. Dulfer S, Nurses and cancer therapy – emesis. *International Cancer Nursing News* 1990; **2**(1/2): 12–14.
13. Ouwerkerk J, Keizer HJ, Psychologic aspects of the treatment of emesis in cancer nursing. *Semin Oncology Nursing* 1990; **6**(Suppl 1): 6–9.
14. Maher M, The conduct of clinical trials in the area of emesis control. *Semin Oncology Nursing* 1990; **6**(Suppl 1): 10–13.
15. Peters CAH, Myths of antiemetic administration. *Cancer Nursing* 1989; **12**: 102–106.
16. Winningham ML, MacVicar MG, The effect of aerobic exercise on patient reports of nausea. *Oncology Nursing Forum* 1988; **15**: 447–50.
17. Cook JD, Music as an intervention in the oncology setting. *Cancer Nursing* 1986; **9**: 23–8.
18. Cobb SC, Teaching relaxation techniques to cancer patients. *Cancer Nursing* 1984; **7**: 157–61.
19. Troesch LM, Blust Rodehaver C, Delaney EA, Yanes B, The influence of guided imagery on chemotherapy-related nausea and vomiting. *Oncology Nursing Forum* 1993; **20**: 1179–85.
20. Scott DW, Donahue DC, Mastrovito RC, Hakes TB, Comparative trial of clinical relaxation and an antiemetic drug regime in reducing chemotherapy-related nausea and vomiting. *Cancer Nursing* 1986; **9**: 178–87.
21. Arakawa S, Use of relaxation to reduce side effects of chemotherapy in Japanese patients. *Cancer Nursing* 1995; **18**: 60–6.
22. Grant M, Nausea, vomiting and anorexia. *Semin Oncology Nursing* 1987; **3**: 277–86.

15

Nausea and vomiting in children

Richard F Stevens

INTRODUCTION

Paediatric malignancy is uncommon, and accounts for less than 2% of cancer occurring in all age groups.[1] Nevertheless, there has been a dramatic improvement in the cure rate for children with malignant disease over the last three decades. This improvement has been the result of, in the main, more intensive chemotherapeutic and radiotherapeutic regimens. The fundamental aim of treatment for childhood malignancy remains the goal of cure, and disease palliation is usually not considered as the first option. This increasingly aggressive approach to treatment has, however, resulted in increased toxicity, and in particular the acute side-effects associated with myelosuppression, alopecia, and nausea and vomiting.

IMPLICATIONS OF CHEMOTHERAPY-RELATED NAUSEA AND VOMITING IN CHILDREN

For many years, the association of intense nausea and vomiting with intensive chemotherapy was accepted almost as an unavoidable side-effect. However, it has become increasingly evi-

dent that nausea and vomiting rank very highly as some of the most distressing side-effects of anti-cancer (Table 15.1).

Nausea and vomiting associated with chemotherapy can be severe, and can continue for some time after the therapy has stopped.[3] This may result in dehydration and electrolyte imbalance, which has the potential for increasing the nephrotoxicity of chemotherapy.[4]

Table 15.1 Rank order of the side-effects of chemotherapy[2]

Vomiting
Nausea
Alopecia
Thought of impending treatment
Timetable for treatment in clinic
Need for a needle
Breathlessness
Feeling tired
Difficulty with sleeping

In cancer patients, nausea (the sensation of the imminent need to vomit) and vomiting itself (the forceful expulsion of gastric contents) are not the mild, transient symptoms associated with other disease states. Rather, they may be severe and prolonged. These symptoms may become debilitating, and children may become physically incapable of receiving further cancer chemotherapy or become so distressed physically or emotionally that they or their parents may actually refuse further treatment.

It has been estimated that nausea and vomiting can result in 25–50% of adult patients delaying one or more scheduled courses of chemotherapy or even refusing further treatment.[5]

FACTORS AFFECTING CHEMOTHERAPY-INDUCED EMESIS

Not every child receiving cancer chemotherapy will experience nausea and vomiting. However, it has been estimated that these symptoms will occur in up to 70% of patients.[6] It is also well recognized that children are more prone to vomiting than adults. The nature and pharmacology of the chemotherapy prescribed is by far the most important factor contributing to drug-induced emesis. Table 15.2 gives an indication of the emetogenic potential of chemotherapeutic drugs. These range from the relatively weak emetogens such as the vinca alkaloids to the platinum drugs, which cause emesis in the vast majority of children. It is only to be expected that the dose, schedule and route of administration of these cytotoxics can also influence their emetogenic potential. Combination chemotherapy given over a prolonged period of time tends to have the most dramatic effect.

Other factors can make a significant contribution towards the development of emesis in children. Whether patients are new to chemotherapy or have received treatment before can effect their susceptibility to nausea and vomiting.[7] Poor control of emesis during previous therapy increase the chances of nausea and vomiting during subsequent chemotherapy.[8] Anxiety,[9] motion sickness[10] and previous

bad experiences of emesis[11] also contribute in no little fashion to nausea and vomiting. Anticipatory vomiting may be a problem; it is often the result of conditioning, and may occur before the administration of further courses of chemotherapy.[12]

The pattern of emesis is not the same for all cytotoxic agents or modes of radiotherapy. Acute post-chemotherapy emesis has been most extensively studied, and usually occurs during the first 24 hours after administration of the cytotoxic agent. It is usually associated with the most severe emesis, and may well be associated with nausea and vomiting that starts the day after treatment and continues for several days (delayed emesis).[13] The pattern of acute emesis can depend on the type of chemotherapy. Cisplatin tends to cause a peak of emesis 4–8 hours after therapy, whereas high-dose cyclophosphamide and carboplatin have the most severe effect 10–12 hours after therapy.[14]

Emesis associated with radiotherapy is usually the result of treatment to the epigastric region or upper abdomen or of total body irradiation (TBI). The level of emesis tends to be dose-related, and adults tend to be more susceptible than children.[15]

CLINICAL PRESENTATION

Childhood emesis associated with cytotoxic chemotherapy and radiotherapy can be variable both in the symptoms that present and in their intensity. These variations are the result of differences in patients' responses to identical treatment regimens as well as the wide variety of treatment protocols involved. It is therefore important to evaluate the emetogenic potential of the treatment before initiating antiemetic therapy (see Table 15.2).

Symptoms range from nausea to retching and vomiting, and frequently occur in a cyclic fashion if not treated early and effectively. Retching is the result of the same physiological mechanisms as vomiting, but there is no expulsion of gastric contents. Children often find retching more distressing because of the strain on abdominal muscles and no apparent relief of

Table 15.2 The emetogenic potential of commonly used chemotherapy and radiotherapy in children

HIGH EMETOGENIC POTENTIAL A	Cisplatin Carboplatin High-dose cyclophosphamide (>1 g/m²) High-dose cytosine arabinoside (>0.5 g/m²) Ifosfamide Total body irradiation
B	Actinomycin D Adriamycin Busulphan Cyclophosphamide (0.5–1 g/m²) Cytosine arabinoside (100–500 mg/m²) Daunorubicin Epirubicin M-amsa High-dose methotrexate (>3 g/m²) Mitoxantrone Procarbazine
C	Low-dose cyclophosphamide (<0.5 g/m²) Low-dose cytosine arabinoside (<100 mg/m²) Methotrexate (<3 g/m²) Intrathecal triple chemotherapy Chest, abdominal and spinal radiotherapy
D LOW EMETOGENIC POTENTIAL	L-Asparaginase Bleomycin Vinblastine Vincristine VP 16 (etoposide)

symptoms. Anticipatory emesis may occur at any time before treatment starts, and is usually the result of a conditioned response. It is therefore important to try and control emesis during the early courses of therapy.

PRINCIPLES OF TREATMENT

There are three main aspects to the treatment of nausea and vomiting in children undergoing cytotoxic chemotherapy: prophylaxis, duration of therapy, and individualization of treatment.

Prophylaxis

The aim of prophylactic treatment is to block the vomiting receptor sites (either central or peripheral) before stimulation by the emetogenic agent. Treatment must therefore be started prior to the commencement of chemotherapy or radiotherapy. All antiemetics are more effective when used prophylactically; the exact timing of therapy depends on several factors including the nature of the chemotherapy, the child's previous pattern of emesis, and the route of administration of the antiemetic. More reliable and rapid control can be achieved when antiemetics are given parenterally, and the intravenous route is most commonly used because patients are frequently thrombocytopenic and invariably require some form of venous access for the subsequent chemotherapy. Oral therapy has obvious advantages for children and staff alike, but may not be as effective in achieving emesis control. Nevertheless, it is frequently possible to commence therapy via the intravenous route and then maintain emesis control with oral medication.

Duration of therapy

Having achieved emesis control, it is important to maintain control by adopting a regular rather than an 'on-demand' approach. 'Breakthrough' emesis can be particularly difficult to treat. When parental therapy is indicated (as it is in the majority of situations), a loading dose followed by regular therapy is the most appropriate, regardless of the patient's symptoms. The transfer from intravenous to oral therapy can be contemplated once emetic control has been achieved.

Individualization of treatment

Not all antiemetic regimens are equally effective in all children.

Table 15.2 illustrates some of the cytotoxic drugs used in the treatment of childhood malignancy in a roughly decreasing order of emetogenic potential. The chemotherapeutic agents at the lower end of the scale may induce moderate nausea with little or no associated vomiting, whereas those at the opposite end may produce debilitating nausea accompanied by severe vomiting.

The severity of vomiting also differs between children, with some patients experiencing few emetic episodes over a period of days whereas others may show severe nausea and vomiting over only a few hours. Symptoms may appear almost instantaneously after the start of chemotherapy or may be delayed for hours. Combination chemotherapy naturally increases the risk of more severe and prolonged emesis.

The psychological status of the child also has an important role in formulating antiemetic therapy. Positive suggestion (e.g. close proximity of another vomiting child) and the placebo effect of therapy are well recognized.[16] Children who suffer from motion sickness are more prone to the side-effects of cancer chemotherapy.[17] Hypnosis or desensitization may be helpful additions in the control of emesis.[18] Conditioned patient responses, such as vomiting soon after arrival in the outpatient clinic, are difficult to control. But a friendly atmosphere that offers calm, privacy and reassurance to the child without obvious stimuli such as the sight or smell of food help considerably.

THE PHARMACOLOGICAL APPROACH TO THE CONTROL OF EMESIS IN CHILDREN

Until recently, there has been a relatively poor understanding of the basis of chemotherapy-induced emesis, and therapy was frequently prescribed empirically. Which drug to use was based mainly on overt symptoms rather than an accurate understanding on the underlying physiology. For example, sedation and a reduced level of anxiety were found to reduce symptoms of nausea and vomiting, and therefore benzodiazepines became a popular choice of therapy. Dopamine antagonists, which stimulate gastric motility, have been shown to be effective in relieving nausea associated with gastric stasis. Corticosteroids are known to produce a slight feeling of 'well-being', and may help in the control of emesis.

Table 15.3 illustrates some of the diverse range of compounds that have been used in the control of nausea and vomiting in children. The table is not comprehensive, and is influenced by availability and marketing in different parts of

Table 15.3 Medications used in the management of childhood emesis associated with chemo-radiotherapy

Class	Examples	Mode of action	Side-effects
Phenothiazines	Chlorpromazine, prochlorperazine	Dopamine blockage at chemoreceptor trigger zone (CTZ), plus variable cholinergic and adrenergic receptor blockade	Extrapyramidal reactions, sedation, dry mouth
Antihistamines	Promethazine, cyclizine	Exact mode of action unknown; block labyrinthine impulses; sedative effect	Drowsiness
Dopamine antagonists	Metoclopramide, domperidone	Dopamine receptor blockade at CTZ; increase in gastric emptying	Extrapyramidal reactions, diarrhoea
Butyrophenones	Haloperidol, droperidol	Dopamine receptor blockade at CTZ	Extrapyramidal reactions, sedation
Cannabinoids	Nabilone	Central antiemetic action – site unknown	Hypotension, dizziness, CNS disturbance
Corticosteroids	Methylprednisolone, dexamethasone	Uncertain; reduced prostaglandin synthesis	Dyspepsia, fluid retention, hyperglycaemia
Benzodiazepines	Lorazepam	Central antiemetic action – site unknown	Sedation, respiratory depression
5-HT$_3$ receptor antagonists	Ondansetron, granisetron	Blocking of selective 5-HT$_3$ receptor sites both centrally and in the GI tract	Few and mild; some constipation and headaches

the world. Some of the drugs listed also go under different non-generic names.

Phenothiazines

The phenothiazines were the most commonly used antiemetics historically. They influence dopamine blockade at the chemoreceptor trigger zone (CTZ), and may also directly depress the vomiting centre. They also have variable cholinergic and adrenergic receptor blockage. Chlorpromazine has limited antiemetic activity and a relatively high incidence of side-effects, including hypotension, sedation, abnormal liver function, blood dyscrasias and unwanted potentiation of the sedative effects of narcotics and barbiturates. The piperazine class includes prochlorperazine, perphenazine, trifluoperazine and thiethylperazine. These agents have greater antiemetic action and produce less sedation. However, side-effects are relatively common in children; they result mainly from dopamine antagonism, and are manifested clinically by a variety of extrapyramidal reactions, including restlessness, akathisia (involuntary limb shaking), torticollis and occulogyric crises.[19] Although these reactions may be controlled to some effect by drugs such as diphenhydramine or lorazepam, this is obviously undesirable in children, and the effects can be very distressing to patient, parent and professional alike.

Antihistamines

Although many antihistamines have antiemetic potential, there is no real correlation between antiemetic activity and individual antihistamines. Promethazine and cyclizine may be useful in the control of mild to moderate emesis, particularly in the younger child, where a sedative effect may be useful.

Metoclopramide

Metoclopramide is a derivative of procainamide. It has a central action by blocking dopamine receptors at the CTZ and also by stimulating gastric emptying. It has a spectrum of activity resembling that of the phenothiazines, but its additional effect on the gastrointestinal tract offers additional advantages. There has been a tendency in adults undergoing chemo-radiotherapy to increase the dose of metoclopramide with the aim of achieving better emesis control. This has resulted, however, in an increased incidence of side-effects, particularly extrapyramidal reactions,[20] and therefore has not proved popular in children, where the incidence of neurological side-effects may exceed 10%.

Domperidone

Domperidone also acts at the CTZ. It has no effect on gastric emptying, but has the advantage over metoclopramide and the phenothiazines of being less likely to cause central effects such as sedation or dystonic reactions because it does not readily cross the blood–brain barrier.

Benzodiazepines

Lorazepam has little or no direct antiemetic effect in children. Nevertheless, it is sometimes useful when used in combination, since it produces amnesia and can reduce anticipatory nausea and vomiting by reducing unwanted previous experiences of chemotherapy.[21]

Cannabinoids

The cannabinoids, the active ingredients of marijuana, have proven antiemetic activity in older children and adolescents. Although the exact mechanism of action is unknown, it is thought that they exert their effect via central nervous system depression. Nabilone is a synthetic cannabinoid, and may be particularly useful in adolescents, but side-effects including drowsiness, dizziness and the development of a 'high', are not uncommon.[22]

Butyrophenones

Droperidol is a potent blocker of dopamine receptors at the CTZ. Experience of its use in children is limited. When used in higher doses, it does have some antiemetic activity, but side-effects, including tachycardia, agitation, somnolence and in particular extrapyramidal reactions, are not uncommon. Haloperidol is also sometimes used as an antiemetic, but it is not recommended for children.

Corticosteroids

The exact mode of action of corticosteroids is unknown, although it is suggested that the effect may be prostaglandin-modulated. Dexamethasone has been most widely studied, and appears to be most effective when used in combination.[23,24] It appears to be a safe, effective adjunct to antiemetic regimens.

5-HT₃ antagonists

The mode of action of these agents has already been discussed in Chapter 3. In summary, they probably prevent emesis by blocking 5-HT₃ receptors at two sites:

- the vagal nerves that innervate the gastrointestinal tract;
- the same vagal nerves in the chemoreceptor trigger zone (CTZ) and hindbrain vomiting system.

Not all the 5-HT₃ receptor antagonists are available in all parts of the world, and they may not be available in both oral and intravenous forms. Granisetron (SmithKline Beecham) does not have a product licence for oral use in children in the UK, and tropisetron (Sandoz) does not have a product licence for use in children at all. As a result, most of the clinical data relate to the use of ondansetron in children.

Ondansetron has been used in comparative and non-comparative studies.[25,26] Analysis of its efficacy is complicated by the variety and complexity of chemotherapy, but overall at least two-thirds of patients experience fewer than three emetic episodes on their worst day of chemotherapy (which can last for up to 10 days) with highly emetogenic chemotherapy such as cisplatin, ifosfamide and cyclophosphamide, and with total body irradiation. At least 80% of children experienced better control than previously with alternative antiemetics.

In many children, good antiemetic control can be established with intravenous therapy, and continuing control can be maintained with oral medication.[27] There is also the potential for dose modification and other combinations, for example 5-HT₃ antagonists and dexamethasone, in particularly difficult patient groups.[28]

The 5-HT₃ antagonists appear to be very well tolerated in children, with few major side-effects.[29] Mild headaches, constipation and transient alterations in liver-function tests have been reported, but extrapyramidal reactions appear to be absent.

These agents have significant cost implications, but there are suggestions that when the overall cost of using cheaper but less effective medication is taken into consideration, the differences are relatively small.[30] Nevertheless, they have helped significantly in the control of emesis, and have influenced the overall quality of life for children undergoing intensive cancer chemotherapy.[31]

APPROACH TO THERAPY

It makes sense for each paediatric oncology unit to formulate its own policy for the control of emesis. Differences will naturally exist between centres, based on ward environment, nursing and psychological support, patient diagnostic profile, etc.

Table 15.4 outlines a possible approach to the management of chemotherapy-induced emesis in children, with the drugs being graded from high to low emetogenicity. This table should only be considered as a basic outline, but it does offer a structure that can be suitably modified on the basis of local circumstances and developments.

THE FUTURE

Despite recent significant advances, problems in the control of chemotherapy-induced emesis in children and adolescents remain. Different drug dosings and combinations are required for particular clinical situations. The place of alternative and complementary therapies such as hypnosis, relaxation therapy and acupuncture need to be evaluated. Some of these therapies could be provided by parents, relatives and even siblings with the aim of achieving a more

Table 15.4 An outline of emesis control in children

Emetogenic potential (on scale A to D, see Table 15.2 for details)		Younger children	Older children
High	A	*Before therapy* 5-HT$_3$ antagonist i.v., with or without i.v. dexamethasone	*Before therapy* 5-HT$_3$ antagonist, i.v., with or without i.v. dexamethasone
		After therapy 5-HT$_3$ antagonist i.v. or oral ± dexamethasone ± metoclopramide	*After therapy* 5-HT$_3$ antagonist i.v. or oral ± dexamethasone ± prochlorperazine
	B	*Before therapy* 5-HT$_3$ antagonist i.v.	*Before therapy* 5-HT$_3$ antagonist i.v.
		After therapy 5-HT$_3$ antagonist i.v. or oral ± metoclopramide	*After therapy* 5-HT$_3$ antagonist i.v. or oral ± metoclopramide
	C	Metoclopramide oral or i.v.	Prochlorperazine oral or i.v. or promethazine i.v.
	D	No medication	No medication

relaxed patient environment. Unfortunately, these alternative and complementary approaches are time-consuming, and also have financial implications.

It is hoped that the recent progress in the understanding of the physiology of emesis will provide a more scientific and rational background to the development of further antiemetic agents.

CONCLUSIONS

To date, there is no antiemetic agent or regimen that will totally prevent chemotherapy-induced emesis in all paediatric patients. However, careful attention to the individual needs of the child and a knowledge of the previous pattern of nausea and vomiting followed by the implementation of prophylactic and continuous therapy will increase the effectiveness of any antiemetic regimen.

For many years, emesis has been one of the Cinderellas of medical oncology, and has been judged with a higher priority by patients than their healthcare professionals. A better understanding of the underlying physiology of emesis has allowed a more rational approach, and has resulted in considerable improvement in the quality of life for many patients.

REFERENCES

1. Stiller CA, Centralisation of treatment and survival rates for cancer. *Arch Dis Child* 1988; 63: 23–30.
2. Coates A, Abraham S, Kaye SB et al, On the receiving end – patient perception of the side-effects of cancer chemotherapy. *Eur J Cancer Oncol* 1983; 19: 203–8.
3. Kris MG, Gralla RJ, Clark RA et al, Incidence, course and severity of delayed nausea and vomiting following the administration of high dose cisplatin. *J Clin Oncol* 1985; 3: 1379–84.
4. Madias NE, Harrington JT, Platinum nephrotoxicity. *Am J Med* 1978; 65: 307–14.
5. Laszlo J, Nausea and vomiting as major complications of cancer chemotherapy. *Drugs* 1983; 25: 1–7.
6. Morrow GR, Chemotherapy related nausea and vomiting: etiology and management. *CAA Cancer Treat J* 1989; 39: 89–104.
7. Roila F, Tonato M, Basurto C, Antiemetic activity of high doses of metoclopramide in cisplatin treated patients: a randomised double blind trial of the Italian Oncology Group for Clinical Research. *J Clin Oncol* 1988; 5: 141–9.
8. Marty M, Ondansetron and chemotherapy induced emesis. In: *Proceedings of 3rd National Congress on Neo-Adjuvant Chemotherapy*, 35–41. Paris, 1991.
9. Nesse RM, Carli T, Curtis GC et al, Pre-treatment nausea in cancer chemotherapy: a conditioned response? *Psychosom Med* 1990; 42: 43–6.
10. Morrow GR, The assessment of nausea and vomiting. *Cancer* 1984; 53: 2267–80.
11. Andrykowsky MA, Redd WH, Hatfield AK, Development of anticipatory nausea: A prospective analysis. *J Consult Clin Psychol* 1985; 53: 447–54.
12. Morrow GR, Morrell CM, Behavioural treatment of the anticipatory nausea and vomiting induced by cancer chemotherapy. *N Engl J Med* 1982; 307: 1476–80.
13. Kris MG, Gralla RJ, Clark RA et al, Incidence, course and severity of delayed nausea and vomiting following the administration of high-dose cisplatin. *J Clin Oncol* 1985; 3: 1379–84.
14. Martin M, Diaz-Rubio E, Sanches A et al, The natural course of emesis after carboplatin treatment. *Acta Oncol* 1990; 29: 593–5.
15. Priestman T, Radiation induced emesis. *Clinician* 1988; 6: 40–3.
16. Parson JA, Webster JH, Dowd J, Evaluation of the placebo effect in the treatment of radiation sickness. *Acta Radiol* 1961; 56: 129–40.
17. Morrow GR, The effect of a susceptibility to motion sickness on the side effects of cancer chemotherapy. *Cancer* 1988; 55: 2766–70.
18. Zelter L, Le Baron S, Zelter PM, The effectiveness of behavioural intervention for reduction of nausea and vomiting in children and adolescents receiving chemotherapy. *J Clin Oncol* 1984; 2: 683–90.
19. Silva KL, Muller PJ, Pearce J, Acute drug induced extrapyramidal syndromes. *Practitioner* 1973; 211: 316–20.
20. Gralla RJ, Itri LM, Pisko SE et al, Anti-emetic efficacy of high dose metoclopramide: randomised trials with placebo and prochlorperazine in patients with chemotherapy induced nausea and vomiting. *N Eng J Med* 1981; 305: 905–9.
21. Laszlo J, Clark RA, Hanson DC, Lorazepam in cancer patients treated with cisplatin: A drug having antiemetic, amnesic and anxiolytic effects. *J Clin Oncol* 1985; 3: 864–9.
22. Sallan SE, Cronin CM, Zelen M et al, Antiemetics in patients receiving chemotherapy for cancer. *N Engl J Med* 1979; 302: 134–8.
23. Bruera ED, Roca E, Cedara L et al, Improved control of chemotherapy induced emesis by addition of dexamethasone to metolopramide in patients resistant to metoclopramide. *Cancer Treat Rep* 1983; 67: 381.
24. DrapKin RL, Sokol GH, Paladine WJ et al, The antiemetic effect and dose–response of dexamethasone in patients receiving cisplatinum. *Proc Am Soc Clin Oncol* 1982; 199: 61.
25. Stevens RF, A review of ondansetron as prophylaxis for chemotherapy and radiotherapy induced emesis in children. In: *Ondansetron – Clinical Experience in Adults and Children*. Hannover, 1992: 26–32.
26. Hewitt M, McQuade B, Stevens RF, The efficacy and safety of ondansetron in the prophylaxis of cancer-chemotherapy induced nausea and vomiting in children. *Clin Oncol* 1993; 5: 11–14.
27. Pinkerton CR, Williams D, Wooton C et al, 5HT$_3$ antagonist ondansetron – an effective outpatient anti-emetic in cancer treatment. *Arch Dis Child* 1990; 65: 822–5.
28. Alvarez O, Freeman A, Bedros A et al, Randomised double-blind crossover ondansetron–dexamethasone versus ondansetron–placebo study for the treatment of chemotherapy-

induced nausea and vomiting in paediatric patients with malignancies. *J Ped Haem Oncol* 1995; **17**: 145–50.

29. Yarker YE, McTavish D, Granisetron: an update of its therapeutic use in nausea and vomiting induced by antineoplastic therapy. *Drugs* 1994; **48**: 761–93.

30. Cunningham D, Gore M, Davidson N et al, The real cost of emesis – an economic analysis of ondansetron vs metoclopramide in controlling emesis in patients receiving chemotherapy for cancer. *Eur J Cancer* 1993; **29**: 303–6.

31. Laupert A, The role of nurses in the nutrition and management of emesis in children with cancer. In: *Ondansetron – Management of Emesis in Children with Cancer.* Hannover, 1992: 40–3.

16

Side-effects of antiemetics

Caroline Duhem, Fernand Ries, Mario Dicato

CONTENTS • Introduction • Side-effects of non-5-HT$_3$ RA antiemetics • Side-effects of 5-HT$_3$ RA-containing regimens • Conclusions

INTRODUCTION

The introduction of 5-hydroxytryptamine type 3 (5-HT$_3$) receptor antagonists (5HT$_3$ RA) in the current pharmacopeia has dramatically improved the management of chemotherapy- and radiotherapy-induced emesis. The wide experience acquired with these drugs in daily practice since the early 1990s has confirmed the remarkable safety profile reported in preliminary clinical trials.

Moreover, ondansetron, the pioneer compound in this class of drugs, showed great efficacy and appeared not to have any limiting side-effects. No significant improvements in either efficacy or toxicity have been brought by more recent 5-HT$_3$ RA compounds.

This chapter summarizes the more frequent side-effects encountered with former and current antiemetic drugs, with special attention to 5-HT$_3$ RAs.

SIDE-EFFECTS OF NON-5-HT$_3$ RA ANTIEMETICS

Before the '5-HT$_3$ RAs era', several drugs were available for the oncologist, allowing in most instances an acceptable control of nausea and vomiting but at the price of frequent, sometimes distressing side-effects.

Common doses and administration schedules of these agents are given in Table 16.1.

Substituted benzamides

Metoclopramide was the first drug in this class to be used as an antiemetic, and has been subsequently the most common-prescribed agent for chemotherapy-induced emesis. In most trials, the frequency of occurrence and the severity of side-effects associated with metoclopramide were largely dependent on the dose, the route of administration and the age of the treated patients.

With high-dose metoclopramide, side-effects like fatigue, sedation, lethargy and drowsiness are commonly experienced (15–40% of cases), but the more distressing ones are related to the dopamine-antagonist activity of metoclopramide, and consist of extrapyramidal reactions, anxiety, restlessness, hyperactivity and tremors.[1-5] Acute dystonic reactions are more common in younger patients (20–30% in those less than 30 years old, 2–3% in older patients)[6]

Table 16.1 Non-5-HT₃ RA antiemetics: dose and administration schedules

Antiemetic agent	Route	Dose range	Frequency of administration
Substituted benzamides			
• Metoclopramide	i.v.	1–3 mg/kg	Every 2 h
	Oral	1–3 mg/kg	Every 2–4 h
• Alizapride	i.v./i.m.	1–3 mg/kg	Every 2 h
	Oral	1–3 mg/kg	Every 2–4 h
Butyrophenones			
• Haloperidol	i.v./i.m.	1–3 mg/kg	} Every 2–4 h
	Oral	1–3 mg/kg	
• Droperidol	i.v.	0.5–2 mg	Every 4 h
Corticosteroids			
• Dexamethasone	i.v.	4–20 mg	} Once a day or every 4–6 h
	Oral		
• Methylprednisolone	i.v.	250–500 mg	
Phenothiazines			
• Prochlorperazine	Oral	5–10 mg	Every 2–4 h
	Rectal	25 mg	Every 4–6 h
	i.m./i.v.	10–20 mg	Every 3–6 h
• Chlorpromazine	Oral	25–50 mg	} Every 3–6 h
	i.m./i.v.	25 mg	
Benzodiazepine			
• Lorazepam	i.v.	1–2 mg/m²	Every 4 h
Cannabinoid			
• THC	Oral	5–10 mg/m²	Every 3–4 h

and when the drug is given orally on consecutive days, making the control of cisplatin-induced emesis really problematic in multiple-day chemotherapy for germ cell tumors, for instance, before availability of 5-HT₃ RAs.[4]

Generally, combined antiemetic regimens were, of course, designed to improve their efficacy, but also to alleviate some of these side-effects (such as the use of a benzodiazepine to control restlessness or a benzodiazepine, benztropine or diphenhydramine to limit dystonia).

Another benzamide derivative, alizapride, was later developed in an attempt to improve antiemetic efficacy and reduce dystonic reactions. However, the results obtained with this compound have been conflicting, and alizapride did not offer any obvious advantage over metoclopramide in terms of efficacy or reduced side-effects.

Butyrophenones

Haloperidol and droperidol are both effective antiemetics, although less active than metoclopramide in cisplatin-induced nausea and vomiting. Their toxicity profile is similar to that of benzamides, including sedation, dystonic reactions and restlessness (attributed to their common dopamine-blocking effect). Moreover, a mild degree of hypotension is occasionally observed.[5]

Phenothiazines

This class of compounds, including prochlorperazine and chlorpromazine, did not bring any advantage in terms of efficacy (comparable in these compounds to butyrophenones). In addition, a significant degree of orthostatic hypotension, especially after i.v. administration, was observed, limiting its use as outpatient therapy.[5,7]

Corticosteroids

A short course of corticosteroids produces only mild side-effects, except sometimes a certain degradation of pre-existing conditions like diabetes or psychosis. Steroids do not decrease the efficacy of chemotherapy. Their low degree of toxicity and their different mechanism of action make them ideal candidates for use in combination with other antiemetics. However, dosage and routes of administration have not been studied adequately.

Benzodiazepines

Benzodiazepines such as lorazepam are not suitable for use as single antiemetic agents, but can be useful in combination in a multidrug antiemetic regimen.

Lorazepam can alleviate metoclopramide-induced restlessness and decrease anxiety, and may have a light antiemetic activity. However, lorazepam-induced sedation may become a problem if patients have to travel home alone after chemotherapy.[8] Marginally, a certain degree of memory loss has caused difficulties when lorazepam has been evaluated in clinical studies.

Cannabinoids

Trials with cannabinoids were encouraged by anecdotal reports of decreased emesis in younger patients who used marijuana while receiving chemotherapy. Delta-9-tetrahydrocannabinol (THC) and subsequently the synthetic cannabinoids nabilone and levonantradol exhibit significant antiemetic activity, but side-effects are frequent, though generally manageable.[5] They include sedation, dry mouth, orthostatic hypotension, ataxia, dizziness, and euphoria or dysphoria. These drugs are not used frequently in current antiemetic regimens.

SIDE-EFFECTS OF 5-HT$_3$ RA-CONTAINING REGIMENS

Side effects of 5-HT$_3$ RAs are generally mild, and almost never limit their clinical use. The most frequent problems involve the gastrointestinal tract and the central nervous system, probably resulting from the interaction at the two main target sites of these drugs, namely the vagal afferent nerves in the gastrointestinal mucosa and the same vagal nerves in the brainstem vomiting system.[9]

Headache and constipation are commonly reported by patients in the hours or days following 5-HT$_3$ RA administration, while other (rare) possible side-effects are occasionally noted with uncertain cause–effect relation with the prescribed antiemetics.

The most common side-effects, with their frequencies of occurrence, are given in Table 16.2.

Neurological side-effects

In the published studies, headache is reported as the most common adverse event, at an

Table 16.2 Major side-effects occurring in 5-HT₃ RA-pretreated patients receiving cisplatin-containing regimens

Side-effect	Average percentage
• Headache	15–25%
• Constipation	10–20%
• Diarrhea	10–15%
• Abdominal discomfort	5–10%
• Flushing	1–5%
• Sedation	1–5%

incidence varying between 5 and 50% with all 5-HT₃ RAs.[2-4,10-12] This large range is probably related to the variability in the appreciation of the symptom and in the studied population, but a frequency of 15–25% is generally recognized. Headache is generally unimportant and easily controlled by acetaminophen (paracetamol) when any treatment is needed. A previous history of recurrent, severe headache or migraine does not seem to be predictive of occurrence of those induced by 5-HT₃ RAs.[13] The incidence of headache is apparently not affected by the adjunction of dexamethasone in the antiemetic protocol.[14]

No extrapyramidal reactions have been described, except in two case reports, and in one of these the relationship between the antiemetic and the reported dystonic reaction is questionable.[15]

A mild degree of drowsiness is described by a small minority of patients (<5%), but the low incidence and low severity of this short-lasting sedation mean that it is not essential to prevent patients systematically from driving after treatment.

Gastrointestinal side-effects

Constipation is frequently experienced in adults (10–20%), especially older patients;[2-4,11,12] children may be less likely to report constipation than adults.[16,17] Moreover, in most trials when vincristine is part of the chemotherapy, constipation may have been attributed to the vinca alkaloid and not reported. Again, this adverse event is generally mild to moderate in severity, and easily prevented by soft laxative drugs in subsequent administration of 5-HT₃ RAs. In rare instances, mostly in patients also receiving opioids and/or presenting concurrent gastrointestinal symptoms, hospitalization has been required for fecal impaction resulting in obstruction.[2] However, this extreme condition has always been reversible with conservative treatment.

Paradoxically, diarrhea is reported in almost the same proportion of patients (10–15%), followed occasionally by adverse events, such as hiccups, abdominal discomfort and heartburn. All of these are probably diverse, mild counterparts to the major, highly beneficial way of action of 5-HT₃ RAs on upper gastrointestinal tract motility in control of chemotherapy-induced emesis.[9]

Cardiac side-effects

Some concern was raised about potential arrhythmogenic effects of 5-HT₃ RAs after several clinical studies had reported some treatment-emergent ECG variations characterized by small increases in PR, QRs duration and QTc intervals, especially at higher dose levels of antiemetics.[18-21] This observation could be due to the presence of 5-HT receptors in human atrial tissue.[22] However, the magnitude of these ECG changes from baseline, culminating 1–2 hours after 5-HT₃ RA treatment, never exceeded 10–18%. They were all transient, asymptomatic and not clinically significant. None of these compounds has been associated with heart block (>grade 1), heart failure or any symptomatic arrhythmia, even in studies assessing the safety of 5-HT₃ RA compounds in association with chemotherapy presenting potential acute arryhthmogenic effects (anthracyclines ± paclitaxel).

At present, there are no contraindications in cardiac conditions or with any concomitant antiarryhthmic medication or chemotherapy to the use of 5-HT$_3$ RAs in any antiemetic study protocol or in the clinical use.

Vascular side-effects

In 1992, Coates et al[23] reported on eight cases of chemotherapy-treated patients developing severe clinical features suggestive of extensive microangiopathy (thrombocytopenia, renal insufficiency and thrombotic events). These seemed to occur with an unusually high incidence after ondansetron administration. Although no clear causal link could be established between both events, and other alternative explanations could be hypothetized in these heavily treated patients, this clustering of adverse events (fatal in two cases) in the early 5-HT$_3$ RA clinical era led to some concern. However, even after the attention of clinical oncologists had been drawn to these potentially severe consequences, no such observations were subsequently reproduced for ondansetron or any other 5-HT$_3$ RAs, making the Coates case reports probably circumstantial.

Short-lasting flushing is occasionally experienced by a minority of patients (1–5%) receiving 5-HT$_3$ RAs without any notable vital-sign modification or significant discomfort.

Laboratory findings

Transitory increases (up to 150% of baseline value) of transaminase levels have been reported in 5–15% of patients treated with 5-HT$_3$ RAs and cisplatin-containing regimens in pilot studies. However, they have not been observed in patients receiving 5-HT$_3$ RAs in moderately emetogenic chemotherapies or in normal-volunteer studies, suggesting the probable role of cisplatin itself. Likewise, ondansetron was suspected to enhance the

nephrotoxicity of the third-generation platinum compound, Zeniplatin, in phase II trials because of the higher proportion and severity of nephrotoxic events in the ondansetron-treated group of patients (44%) when compared with other antiemetic protocols (3%).[24] However, the wide experience now acquired with 5-HT$_3$ RAs in high-dose cisplatin-treated patients has proved their lack of inherent nephrotoxicity, making the former observation rather circumstantial; the role of 5-HT$_3$ RAs in the development of platinum-induced nephrotoxicity is merely neutral.

Finally, it is notable that 5-HT$_3$ RAs do not interact significantly with any important drug metabolism, particularly with chemotherapeutic agents, and cannot be suspected of decreasing their efficacy or enhancing their toxicity when used in combination.

Comments

Importance of 5-HT$_3$ RA subtype and dose
In general, adverse events are reported by 25–75% of patients in preclinical studies, depending on the examined populations, and the definitions and grading of the side-effects by the investigator: most of them are often not objective, and vary greatly with patient sensitivity.

Concerning the 5-HT$_3$ RAs themselves, there are no significant differences in the incidence or severity of side-effects,[11,25,26] according to their subtype in randomized studies where they have been compared for their efficacity and their safety profile.[26]

There does not seem to be any dose-dependent increase in the incidence of side-effects or their severity in studies where this parameter has been evaluated,[27–29] except for ECG changes (increases in PR, QRs and QTc periods) for ondansetron[27] and dolasetron.[19] Conflicting data are reported concerning the dose-dependent incidence of ondansetron-induced headache (8 mg versus 32 mg).

Finally, there is no increase if any adverse event following repeated exposure to 5-HT$_3$ RA compounds, and their safety profile in repeated courses was comparable to that seen following acute treatment in chemotherapy-naive patients.[29-31]

Importance of emesis inducer

The underlying disease, the concurrent medical condition of the patient and the toxic effects of the antineoplastic drugs or of radiotherapy complicate the evaluation of the side-effects of antiemetic drugs in the clinic. These may therefore be optimally appreciated when compared with other antiemetics rather than in normal volunteers.

Antiemetic studies were first performed for highly emetogenetic chemotherapy (mainly containing high-dose cisplatin) and then in moderately emetogenic chemotherapy[32,33] or radiotherapy. Overall, the proportion of patients experiencing adverse events is higher in cisplatin-containing regimens (around 50%) than in moderately emetogenic chemotherapy (15–25%) or radiotherapy (15–25%).

In the small series where these parameters have been assessed, adverse events with $5\text{-}HT_3$ RAs occur in about 60% of patients receiving high-dose chemotherapy, followed by marrow or peripheral blood stem cell support preceded or not by total-body irradiation.[34-36] However, the reported values are probably not very reli-able, because of the multifactorial origin of symptoms like diarrhea or headache in such situations and the lack of comparison with non-$5\text{-}HT_3$ RA-containing regimens.

CONCLUSIONS

Drugs like $5\text{-}HT_3$ RA antiemetics, just like most hematopoietic growth factors currently available, have their full significance as part of 'supportive care'. They represent a significant advance in the management of nausea and vomiting, which are among the most distressing adverse experiences encountered after anticancer treatments, at the price of trivial side-effects. Their relative innocuity is due to their specific, targeted mechanism of action, the counterpart of this being their poor efficacy in emesis patterns (like delayed emesis) that probably develop through different pathways than $5\text{-}HT_3$ receptor stimulation.

Among $5\text{-}HT_3$ RAs that are currently available or under development, the choice should be made on the basis of the route of administration, the pharmacokinetics and the local cost. No demonstrated advantages can be reasonably anticipated on the basis of efficacy or safety profile in these agents.

REFERENCES

1. Gralla RJ, Itri M, Pisko SE et al, Antiemetic efficacy of high-dose metoclopramide: randomized trials with placebo and prochlorperazine in patients with chemotherapy-induced nausea and vomiting. *N Engl J Med* 1981; 305: 905–9.
2. De Mulder P, Seynaeve C, Vermorken J et al, Ondansetron compared with high-dose metoclopramide in prophylaxis of acute and delayed cisplatin-induced nausea and vomiting. *Ann Int Med* 1990; 113: 834–40.
3. Marty M, Pouillart P, Scholl S et al, Comparison of the 5-hydroxytryptamine₃ (serotonin) antagonist ondansetron (GR 38032F) with high-dose metoclopramide in the control of cisplatin-induced emesis. *N Engl J Med* 1990; 322: 816–21.
4. Sledge GN, Einhorn LH, Nagy C, House K,

Phase III double-blind comparison of intravenous ondansetron and metoclopramide as antiemetic therapy for patients receiving multiple-day cisplatin-based chemotherapy. *Cancer* 1992; 70: 2524–8.
5. Gralla RJ, Tyson LB, Borden LB et al, Antiemetic therapy: a review of recent studies and a report of a random assignment trial comparing metoclopramide with delta-9-tetrahydrocannabinol. *Cancer Treat Rep* 1984; 68: 163–72.
6. Kris MG, Tyson LB, Gralla RJ et al, Extrapyramidal reactions with high-dose metoclopramide. *N Engl J Med* 1983; 309: 433–4.
7. Carr BI, Bertrand M, Browning S et al, A comparison of the antiemetic efficacy of prochlorperazine and metoclopramide for the treatment of cisplatin-induced emesis: a prospective random-

ized double-blind study. *J Clin Oncol* 1985; **3**: 1127–32.

8. Kris MG, Gralla RJ, Clark RA et al, Antiemetic control and prevention of side effects of anti-cancer therapy with lorazepam or diphenhydramine when used in combination with metoclopramide plus dexamethasone. A double-blind, randomized trial. *Cancer* 1987; **60**: 2816–22.

9. Freeman AJ, Cunningham KT, Tyers MB, Selectivity of 5-HT3 receptor antagonists and antiemetic mechanisms of action. *Anti Cancer Drugs* 1993; **3**: 79–85.

10. Einhorn LH, Nagy C, Werner K, Finn AL, Ondansetron: a new antiemetic for patients receiving cisplatin chemotherapy. *J Clin Oncol* 1990; **8**: 731–5.

11. Andrews PA, Bhandari P, Davey PT et al, Are all 5-HT$_3$ receptor antagonists the same? *Eur J Cancer* 1992; **28A** (Suppl 1): 2–6.

12. De Bruijn KM, Tropisetron: a review of the clinical experience. *Drugs* 1992; **43**(Suppl 3): 11–22.

13. Veniziano M, Framarino Dei Malatesta M, Bandiera AF et al, Ondansetron-induced headache; our experience in gynecological cancer. *Eur J Gynaecol Oncol* 1995; **16**: 203–7.

14. Smith DB, Newlands ES, Rustin GJS et al, Comparison of ondansetron plus dexamethasone as a antiemetic prophylaxis during cisplatin-containing chemotherapy. *Lancet* 1991; **338**: 487–90.

15. Kanarek BB, Curnow R, Palmer J, Cook SF, Ondansetron: confusing documentation surrounding an extrapyramidal reaction. *J Clin Oncol* 1992; **10**: 506–7.

16. Billett AL, Sallan SE, Antiemetics in children receiving cancer chemotherapy. *Support Care Cancer* 1994; **2**: 279–85.

17. Jurgens H, MacQuade B, Ondansetron as prophylaxis for chemotherapy and radiotherapy-induced emesis in children. *Oncology* 1992; **49**: 279–85.

18. Watanabe H, Kasegawa A, Shinopaki T et al, Possible cardiac side effects of granisetron, an antiemetic agent, in patients with bone and soft tissue sarcoma receiving cytotoxic chemotherapy. *Cancer Chemother Pharmacol* 1995; **35**: 278–82.

19. Hesketh PJ, Gandara DR, Hesketh A et al, Dose-ranging evaluation of the anti-emetic efficacy of intravenous dolasetron in patients receiving chemotherapy with doxorubicin or cyclophosphamide. *Support Care Cancer* 1996; **4**: 141–6.

20. Kris MG, Grunberg S, Gralla RJ et al, Dose-ranging evaluation of the serotonin antagonist dolasetron mesylate in patients receiving high-dose cisplatin. *Clin Oncol* 1994; **12**: 1045–9.

21. Lifsey DS, Gralla RJ, Clark RA et al, Electrocardiographic changes with serotonin antagonist antiemetics: rate of occurrence and clinical relevance. *Proc Am Soc Clin Oncol* 1993; **12**: 1611.

22. Kaumann AJ, Sanders L, Brown AM et al, A 5-hydroxytryptamine receptor in human ratrium. *Br J Pharmacol* 1990; **100**: 879–85.

23. Coates AS, Childs A, Cox K et al, Seven vascular adverse effects with thrombocytopenia and renal failure following emetogenic chemotherapy and ondansetron. *Ann Oncol* 1992; **3**: 719–22.

24. Aamdal S, Can ondansetron hydrochloride (Zofran®) enhance the nephrotic potential of other drugs? *Ann Oncol* 1992; **3**: 774.

25. Stewart A, MacQuade B, Cronje JD et al, Ondansetron compared with granisetron in the prophylaxis of cyclophosphamide-induced emesis in out-patients: a multicenter, double-blind, double-dummy, randomized, parallel-group study. *Oncology* 1995; (Suppl 2): 202–10.

26. Aapro MS, Always more 'setrons': how many do we need? *Support Care Cancer* 1997; **5**: 1–2.

27. Fraschini G, Ciociola A, Esparza L et al, Evaluation of three oral dosages of ondansetron in the prevention of nausea and emesis associated with cyclophosphamide–doxorubicin chemotherapy. *J Clin Oncol* 1991; **9**: 1268–74.

28. Beck TM, Hesketh PJ, Madajewicz S et al, Stratified, randomized, double-blind comparison of intravenous ondansetron administered as a multiple-dose regimen versus two single-dose regimens in the prevention of cisplatin-induced nausea and vomiting. *Clin Oncol* 1992; **10**: 1969–75.

29. Perez E, Navari R, Kaplan H et al, Efficacy and safety of different doses of granisetron for the prophylaxis of cisplatin-induced emesis. *Support Care Cancer* 1997; **5**: 31–7.

30. Cunningham D, Dicato M, Verweij J et al, Optimum anti-emetic therapy for cisplatin induced emesis over repeat courses: ondansetron plus dexamethasone plus lorazepam compared with metoclopramide, dexamethasone plus lorazepam. *Ann Oncol* 1996; **7**: 277–82.

31. Roila F, Control of acute cisplatin induced emesis over repeat courses of chemotherapy. *Oncology* 1996; **53**(Suppl 1): 65–72.

32. Levitt M, Warr D, Yelle L et al, Ondansetron compared with dexamethasone and metoclopramide as antiemetics in the chemotherapy of

breast cancer with cyclophosphamide methotrexate and fluorouracil. *N Engl J Med* 1993; 328: 1081–4.

33. Schmoll HJ, Casper J, Management of other non-cisplatin-induced emesis. *Oncology* 1996; 53 (Suppl 1): 51–5.

34. Prentice HG, Efficacy and safety of granisetron in the treatment of emesis induced by total body irradiation, a comparison with standard antiemetic therapy. *Proc Am Soc Clin Oncol* 1993; 12: 1574.

35. Barbounis V, Koumalgis G, Vassilomanolakis M et al, A phase II study of ondansetron as antiemetic prophylaxis in patients receiving high-dose polychemotherapy and stem cell transplantation. *Support Care Cancer* 1995; 3: 301–6.

36. Or R, Drakas P, Nagler A et al, The anti-emetic efficacy and tolerability of tropisetron in patients conditioned with high-dose chemotherapy (with and without total body irradiation) prior to bone marrow transplantation. *Support Care Cancer* 1994; 2: 245–8.

Index

T - #0329 - 101024 - C0 - 246/189/13 [15] - CB - 9781853172670 - Gloss Lamination